SECOND EDITION

MEDICAL CARE IN THE NURSING HOME

NOTICE

SECOND EDITION

Medical Care in the Nursing Home

Joseph G. Ouslander, M.D.
Professor of Medicine
Director, Division of Geriatric Medicine and Gerontology and Chief of Medicine, Wesley Woods Geriatric Center at Emory University, Atlanta, Georgia
Director, Atlanta Veterans Administration Rehabilitation Research and Development Center

Dan Osterweil, M.D.
Medical Director, Jewish Homes for the Aging of Greater Los Angeles
Associate Professor, Multicampus Division of Geriatric Medicine and Gerontology
UCLA School of Medicine, Los Angeles, California

John Morley, M.D.
Dammert Professor of Gerontology
Division of Geriatric Medicine
St. Louis University Medical Center
Director of GRECC
Veterans Administration Medical Center
St. Louis, Missouri

Foreword by Robert L. Kane, M.D.

McGraw-Hill
HEALTH PROFESSIONS DIVISION

New York St. Louis San Francisco Bogotá Caracas
Lisbon London Madrid Mexico City Milan Montreal
New Delhi San Juan Singapore Sydney Tokyo Toronto

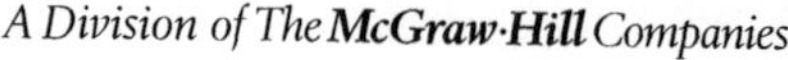

McGraw-Hill
A Division of The McGraw-Hill Companies

MEDICAL CARE IN THE NURSING HOME
Second Edition

1 2 3 4 5 6 7 8 9 0 DOC DOC 9 8 7 6

ISBN 0-07-048209-8

This book was set in Times Roman by Keyword Publishing Services.
The editors were Martin J. Wonsiewicz and Peter McCurdy;
the production supervisor was Richard Ruzycka.
The cover was designed by Matthew Dvorozniak.
Project supervision was done by Keyword Publishing Services.
R. R. Donnelley & Sons, Inc., was printer and binder.

This book is printed on acid-free paper.

Library of Congress Cataloging-in-Publication Data

Ouslander, Joseph G.
Medical care in the nursing home/Joseph Ouslander, Dan Osterweil, John Morley.—2nd ed.
p. cm.
Includes bibliographical references and index.
ISBN 0-07-048209-8
1. Nursing home care. I. Osterweil, Dan. II. Morley, John E. III. Title.
[DNLM: 1. Long-Term Care—in old age. 2. Homes for the Aged. 3. Nursing Homes. 4. Physician's Role. WT 31 0933m 1997]
RC954.3.087 1997
362.1′6—dc20
DNLM/DLC
for Library of Congress 96-43576

CONTENTS

FOREWORD

The American nursing home has come a long way even since the first edition of this book was written. Trends that were beginning then have become more established. Managed care has emerged as a major force and promises to play a dominant role in shaping health care. The role of the nursing home is changing as a result of these converging forces. To a limited degree the nursing home is playing an active role in shaping its own destiny, but primarily it is responding to external forces.

Diversification is a major theme for nursing home care. The multiple roles played by the nursing home in serving a heterogeneous constituency have reached a stage where it is time to question again whether one institution can adequately respond. Pressures to specialize are taking several forms. Special care units are developing to handle defined populations, such as those with dementia.

Accountability has assumed center stage. In the past several years we have witnessed the universal requirement for comparable data collection in all nursing homes across the country. Although the potential for using this information has not yet been realized, it is not hard to envision looking at outcomes of care for individual residents over time and making (case-mix corrected) comparisons across institutions. It is only a short step to comparing the outcomes of care for those treated in nursing homes to comparable clients cared for in other settings.

Managed care presents both a threat and an opportunity. In the short term, nursing homes are pursuing new managed care business as alternatives to hospital care. As managed care moves from an emphasis on acute care to including long-term care, the effects on nursing homes could be dramatic. In a search for the most cost-effective means of providing care, managed care could become the catalyst for long-term care reform, providing a more competitive environment for community-based care. Traditional institutional models will no longer suffice. Managed care will inevitably press for closer linkages between the medical and nursing aspects of long-term care. With growing recognition that primary care can affect the use of expensive hospital care, the nursing home will be viewed as a joint production unit, whose productivity will be measured in terms of overall success, not separate analyses of various aspects of care.

Just as the nursing home seems doomed to repeat the history of the hospital, nursing homes are now caring for patients who would have been in the hospital decades ago. The dramatic shortening of hospital lengths of stay has created a demand for what is now being called "subacute care." In effect, an earlier model of what was then "progressive patient care" in the hospital has been reinvented as a new form of care in a new setting. It remains to be seen whether care delivered to recently discharged hospital patients will be better in nursing homes than in other post-hospital settings such as home care. Informal feedback from those providing such care suggests that it requires a different mind set from traditional nursing home care, one more akin to hospital care.

At the other end of the continuum, nursing homes have been challenged as the best way to meet the needs and wishes of the cognitively intact physically disabled (and even of many mentally disabled). More individualized care in settings where residents can have private space that they can control seems to be favored. Various versions of assisted living models are springing up. These seem to offer less expensive, more individualized care with more emphasis on personal preferences and less on technology.

All these changes promise that the nursing home medical director will face a series of challenges in the ensuing years. Under the pressures for single points of accountability, medical direction will have to become actively involved in management decisions and planning. Expectations for performance will increase under the pressure of higher standards and greater competition. Although we may not be able to forecast accurately just what changes will occur, it is safe to predict that future nursing home medical directors will have to be better trained and better informed. Books like this one will play an important role in helping to make that transition.

Robert L. Kane, M.D.
Minnesota Chair in Long-Term Care and Aging
University of Minnesota School of Public Health

PREFACE

Two concerns motivated us to write the first edition of *Medical Care in the Nursing Home*. First, the need and demand for nursing home care will continue to grow over the next several decades as our older population continues to live into extreme old age in increasing numbers. While noninstitutional long-term services are becoming more accessible, they will not be practical or appropriate for a substantial proportion of the frail and dependent geriatric population. Second, we believe that substantial improvements in the medical care provided in nursing homes are necessary and feasible, and that these improvements will also have positive effects on the quality of life of nursing home residents, their loved ones, and the staff that cares for them.

We embarked on the second edition because several important developments have impacted medical care in the nursing home setting over the last several years. Federal rules and regulations contained in OBRA 1987 were fully implemented just as the first edition was being published. The Resident Assessment Instrument, which includes the Minimum Data Set (MDS) and the Resident Assessment Protocols (RAPs), now serve as clinical practice guidelines for nursing home professionals. While the impacts of the MDS and RAPs on the outcomes of nursing home residents remain largely unknown, we believe they serve as a useful common approach and we have incorporated relevant elements of these assessment tools throughout the text. The nursing home population continues to grow more dependent and medically ill. The latter is the result of the continued trend to discharge patients from acute hospitals sicker and quicker, as well as the growth of capitated managed care systems in which there is a strong financial incentive to treat acutely ill patients in less expensive settings than the acute hospital. "Subacute care" has emerged as an important aspect of nursing home care, and the medical instability of many patients now being admitted to nursing homes has created a myriad of clinical, administrative, and financial challenges for nursing home providers. Understanding of the most appropriate diagnostic assessment and therapeutic strategies for common conditions in the nursing home population continues to increase, and we have attempted to incorporate new findings throughout the text. The role of the nursing home medical director has, through the work of the American Medical Directors Association (AMDA) and several other organizations, become more clearly defined, more sophisticated, and held in higher professional respect. We have included numerous examples of administrative policies and procedures which we hope will be helpful to medical directors as their jobs become more complex and challenging.

We thank the numerous individuals who reviewed and provided input to the first edition, as well as Dr. Rick L. Smith, who thoroughly reviewed and provided thoughtful suggestions for several of the chapters in this edition. We also thank Ms. Laura Hodson, whose expert secretarial assistance made this book possible. Most importantly, we thank the nursing home residents and health professionals who have taught us so much about nursing home care, and our families, who again tolerated numerous days and nights without our presence so that we could produce this second edition.

PART ONE

GENERAL AND ADMINISTRATIVE ASPECTS OF MEDICAL CARE IN THE NURSING HOME

IS ANYBODY LISTENING?

I am an 84-year-old woman, and the only crime which I have committed is that I have an illness which is called chronic. I have severe arthritis and about five years ago I broke my hip. While I was recuperating in the hospital, I realized that I would need extra help at home. But there was no one.... So I wound up at a convalescent hospital in the middle of Los Angeles. All kinds of people are thrown together here. I sit and watch, day after day. As I look around this room, I see the pathetic ones (maybe the lucky ones—who knows?) who have lost their minds, and the poor souls who should be out but nobody comes to get them, and the sick ones who are in pain. We are all locked up together....

For the last few years I have been reading about the changes in Medicare regulations. All I can see from these improvements is that nurses spend more time writing. For, after all, how do you regulate caring? Most of the nurses' aides who work here are from other countries. Even those who can speak English don't have much in common with us. So they hurry to get their work done as quickly as possible. There are a few caring people who work here, but there are so many of us who are needy for that kind of honest attention.

A doctor comes to see me once a month. He spends approximately three to five seconds with me and then a few more minutes writing in the chart or joking with the nurses. (My own doctor doesn't come to convalescent hospitals, so I had to take this one.)....

I noticed that most of the physicians who come here don't even pay attention to things like whether their patients' fingernails are trimmed or whether their bodies are foul-smelling. Last week when the doctor came to see me, I hadn't had a bath in 10 days because the nurse's aide took too long on her coffee break. She wrote in the chart that she gave me a shower—anyway, who would check or care? I would be labeled as a complainer or losing my memory, and that would be worse....

I remember how I used to bake pies and cakes and cookies for friends and neighbors and their children. In the five years I have been here, I have had no choice—no choice of when I want to eat or what I want to eat....

As I write this, I keep wishing I were exaggerating....

I am writing this because many of you may live to be old like me, and by then it will be too late. You, too, will be stuck here and wonder why nothing is being done, and you, too, will wonder if there is any justice in life. Right now, I pray every night that I may die in my sleep and get this nightmare of what someone has called life over with, if it means living in this prison day after day.

(Abstracted from an anonymous letter published in the Los Angeles Times, September 23, 1979.)

CHAPTER
ONE

DEMOGRAPHICS AND ECONOMICS OF NURSING HOME CARE

INTRODUCTION

Nursing home care continues to be a growing industry. Currently there are close to 16,000 licensed nursing homes (NHs) and between 1.5 million and 2 million NH beds. This is almost triple the number of acute care hospitals and double the number of acute care hospital beds. Expenditures for NH care now exceed $50 billion, of which close to half comprises public monies.

Several sociodemographic factors are going to dramatically increase the demand for and cost of NH care over the next several decades.

The purpose of this chapter is to review, briefly and graphically, demographic and economic factors that are relevant to current and future NH care. An awareness of these factors is important for all physicians and health professionals who care for NH residents.

DEMOGRAPHICS AND THE DEMAND FOR NURSING HOME CARE

Three basic factors contribute to the need for NH care: (1) the number of frail people with such severe functional disabilities that they cannot live independently or with mental, behavioral, or physical conditions that make management by a community caregiver difficult; (2) the social support system available for individuals who cannot live independently; and (3) the availability, accessibility, and financing of community long-term-care resources. **Table 1-1** summarizes these factors.

The frail geriatric population is the most rapidly growing segment of our society. **Figure 1-1** depicts this growth over the next several decades. By the year 2030, the number of Americans older than 65 will double, to over 60 million. Average life expectancy at age 65 now approaches 10 years; even at age 85, it is still close to 5 years (**Fig. 1-2**). This will result in more than doubling the number of those age 85 and older by the year 2030—a group currently numbering close to 3 million. With the dramatic growth of the "old old" population will come an increased number of people with the conditions listed in **Table 1-1**, which contribute to NH admission.

Table 1-1 Factors affecting the need for nursing home admission

Factors
Characteristics of the individual
Age, sex, race
Marital status
Living arrangements
Degree of mobility
Ability to perform basic and instrumental activities of daily living
Urinary incontinence
Behavior problems
Mental status
Memory impairment
Mood disturbance
Tendency for falls
Clinical prognosis
Income
Payment eligibility
Need for special services
Characteristics of the support system
Family capability
Health and function of spouse (if married)
Presence of responsible relative (usually adult child)
Family structure of responsible relative
Employment status of responsible relative
Physician availability
Amount of care currently received from family and others
Community resources
Formal community resources (See Table 1-2)
Informal support systems
Presence of long-term care institutions
Characteristics of long-term care institutions

Source: After Kane RL, Ouslander JG and Abrass IB: *Essentials of Clinical Geriatrics*, 3d ed. McGraw-Hill, New York, 1994.

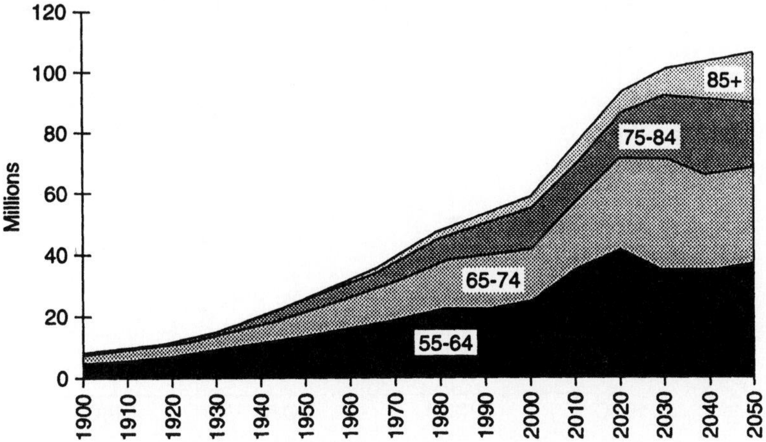

Figure 1-1 Actual and projected growth of the U.S. geriatric population. (After Kane RL, Ouslander JG, and Abrass IB: *Essentials of Clinical Geriatrics*, 3d ed. New York, McGraw-Hill, 1994.)

Recent data suggest that close to 40 percent of community-dwelling individuals aged 85 and older have some degree of dementia. Thus, as depicted in **Fig. 1-3**, the number of people with dementia and associated disorders will also rise dramatically. At the same time, the social support system is unlikely to improve and may worsen. Among those of age 75 and above, about

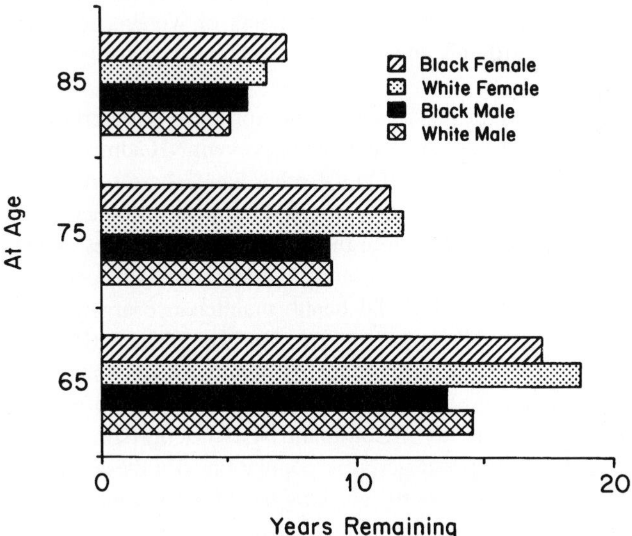

Figure 1-2 Life expectancy in the geriatric population. (After Kane RL, Ouslander JG, and Abrass IB: *Essentials of Clinical Geriatrics*, 2d ed. New York, McGraw-Hill, 1989.)

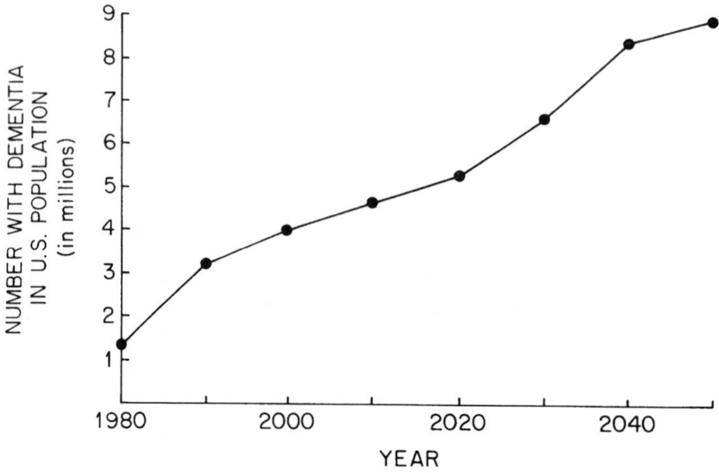

Figure 1-3 Projected number of persons with dementia in the U.S. population. (Based on prevalence estimates and projections from the National Institute on Aging and U.S. Bureau of Census.)

20 percent of men and 50 percent of women live alone. Of the elderly who live alone, close to one-third have no children, and between 40 percent and 50 percent see their children once a week or more often (**Fig. 1-4**). Most formal and informal long-term care services are currently arranged for or provided by daughters. The cohort of people who are growing old at the present time have had fewer children and tend to be geographically separate from the children they do have. In addition, increasing numbers of women are working, which will make it more difficult and stressful for them to care for a frail parent or grandparent.

There is a variety of services available for the frail elderly outside of NHs (**Table 1-2**). These services clearly delay or prevent NH admission in a subgroup of the frail geriatric population. On the other hand, these services are generally not well coordinated and are not reimbursed by most insurance and government programs (see below). Better coordination of these services is being fostered through case managers, hospital and community-based geriatric programs, innovated programs such as social health maintenance organizations (SHMO) and the Program for All-Inclusive Care for the Elderly (PACE), and other strategies. The increasing number of such programs and the increasing number of elderly who, either themselves or through their children, can afford these services will improve the accessibility of community-based long-term care services for a subgroup of the growing frail geriatric population. But these factors will not be enough to dramatically reduce the growing need for NH care. Even among those who are able to live in the community despite severe functional impairments, many eventually come to a time when it is in their and their caregivers' best interests to consider entry into a NH.

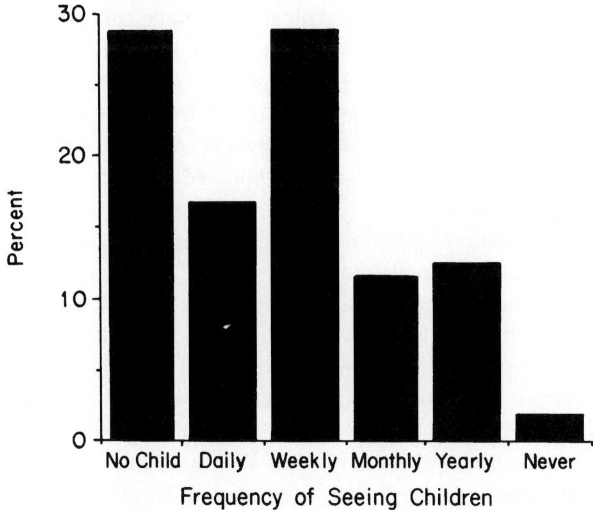

Figure 1-4 Frequency of seeing children among community-dwelling elderly who live alone. (After Kane RL, Ouslander JG, and Abrass IB: *Essentials of Clinical Geriatrics*, 2d ed. New York, McGraw-Hill, 1989.)

Table 1-2 Examples of formal community services available outside of nursing homes

Housing
- Senior apartments
- Residential care facilities
- Assisted living
- Foster care
- Life care community

Health promotion activities
- Wellness programs
- Exercise classes
- Family and patient education
- Nutrition consultation
- Meal programs
- Volunteer programs

Outreach
- Screening clinics
- Mobile vans
- Discharge planning
- Case management
- Information and referral
- Meals-On-Wheels
- Transportation
- Emergency response system
- Respite care

Outpatient centers
- Geriatric clinics
- Psychosocial counseling
- Rehabilitation
- Adult day care
- Day hospital

Home health
- Home health agencies
  - Medicare-certified
  - Private
  - Visiting nurse association
- Hospice
- Homemaker
- Chore
- Home infusion therapies
- Durable medical equipment

Acute inpatient units
- Geriatric
- Rehabilitation
- Psychiatric
- Alcohol/substance abuse

Current rates of NH usage vary with age, sex, race, and NH bed availability. As can be seen in **Fig. 1-5**, the percentage of blacks in NHs is generally lower than that of whites; a greater proportion of white women than white men in each age group are in an NH; and the proportion in NHs increases dramatically with age to close to 25 percent among white women aged 85 and older. **Table 1-3** lists the number of NHs, and NH beds per 1000 people aged 65 and older; they vary substantially from state to state.

Even these statistics are, however, deceiving, because point prevalence rates underestimate the actual number of people who spend time in an NH. This number is much higher, because a subgroup of NH residents turns over rapidly. Data on length of NH stay are somewhat difficult to interpret because they will vary depending on whether they are calculated in a cohort of admissions, current NH residents, or discharges. **Figure 1-6** depicts the median length of stay based on discharge status (alive versus dead). As can be seen, in either case median length of stay is less than 6 months. In fact, close to half of all NH admissions stay less than 6 months, although many are readmitted after a stay in an acute care hospital. The trend towards shorter lengths of stay is growing with the growth of subacute care. The number of hospital-based skilled nursing facilities grew from 652 in 1986 to almost 2000 in 1994. Overall 34 percent of long-term care facilities were providing subacute care in 1994. Thus the prevalence of NH use depicted in **Fig. 1-5** and **Table 1-3** underestimates the lifetime risk of NH admission. Current estimates suggest that the risk of NH admission now approaches 43 percent for those who turned 65 in 1990 (52 percent in women and 33 percent in men). Of those who enter a NH, 55 percent will have a total lifetime use of one year or more, and 21 percent five years or more.

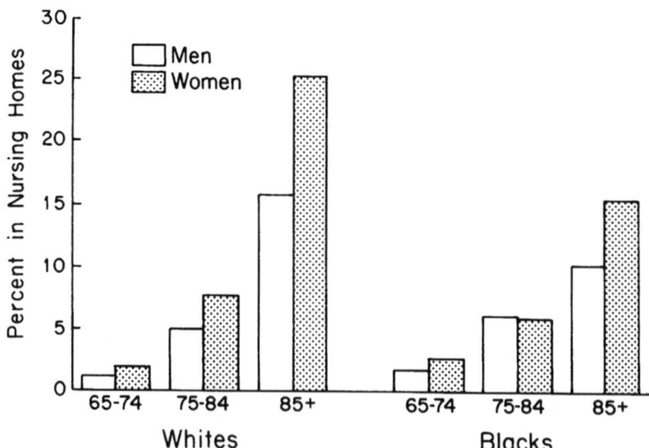

Figure 1-5 Percent of population age 65 and older in nursing homes by age, sex, and race. (Based on 1985 data from the National Center for Health Statistics.)

Table 1-3 Number of nursing homes and licensed beds in each state by bed size

State	≤100 beds		101–200 beds		200 + beds		Total NHS	Total Beds	Beds per 1000 age 65 +
	NHS	Beds	NHS	Beds	NHS	Beds			
Alabama	96	6,492	100	13,580	8	2,039	204	22,111	41.1
Alaska	13	584	1	101	1	224	15	909	36.4
Arizona	40	2,798	73	10,180	11	2,640	124	15,618	30.4
Arkansas	121	9,173	108	13,324	7	1,752	236	24,249	67.7
California	808	58,639	300	42,708	53	13,186	1,161	114,533	35.3
Colorado	104	6,767	81	10,929	9	1,621	192	19,317	55.4
Connecticut	120	8,179	127	17,857	20	5,220	267	31,256	68.4
Delaware	27	1,702	20	2,575	—	—	47	4,277	50.3
District of Columbia	7	318	5	832	6	2,008	18	3,158	41.0
Florida	184	11,913	385	50,625	34	8,710	603	71,248	28.7
Georgia	165	13,100	136	17,783	24	6,003	325	36,886	54.0
Hawaii	14	887	7	923	2	540	23	2,350	17.7
Idaho	33	2,103	22	2,840	1	216	56	5,159	40.6
Illinois	355	25,812	294	40,338	122	31,766	771	97,916	66.9

Table 1-3 (*Continued*)

State	≤100 beds		101–200 beds		200 + beds		Total NHS	Total Beds	Beds per 1000 age 65 +
	NHS	Beds	NHS	Beds	NHS	Beds			
Indiana	299	19,319	203	28,269	37	10,227	539	57,815	80.5
Iowa	326	20,830	90	11,391	7	2,131	423	34,352	79.3
Kansas	300	19,529	64	8,152	5	1,135	369	28,816	82.3
Kentucky	157	10,937	87	11,415	5	1,427	249	23,779	49.9
Louisiana	89	6,879	181	24,846	22	5,025	292	36,750	76.4
Maine	107	6,506	21	2,607	3	718	131	9,831	58.5
Maryland	74	4,805	115	16,785	24	6,812	213	28,402	52.7
Massachusetts	288	16,710	236	31,436	20	4,747	544	52,893	63.4
Michigan	176	11,966	208	28,156	37	9,051	421	49,173	42.7
Minnesota	208	14,366	138	19,060	28	7,839	374	41,265	73.4
Mississippi	72	4,605	70	8,936	5	1,340	147	14,881	45.7
Missouri	300	19,196	224	29,326	26	6,965	550	55,487	75.6
Montana	46	2,875	16	2,133	2	501	64	5,509	49.6
Nebraska	153	9,769	45	5,993	4	1,157	202	16,919	74.5

Nevada	11	889	16	2,298	2	468	29	3,655	25.0
New Hampshire	44	2,722	24	3,034	6	1,622	74	7,378	56.3
New Jersey	105	5,330	170	24,255	54	15,722	329	45,307	42.9
New Mexico	37	2,284	29	3,507	2	797	68	6,588	38.1
New York	157	11,186	259	39,693	157	51,629	573	102,508	43.2
North Carolina	164	11,551	166	22,021	8	2,139	338	35,711	42.2
North Dakota	48	3,084	20	2,719	1	223	69	6,026	64.8
Ohio	649	43,551	246	33,462	59	14,310	954	91,323	62.7
Oklahoma	268	17,903	125	15,764	9	2,124	402	35,791	82.3
Oregon	109	7,110	56	7,017	2	412	167	14,539	35.5
Pennsylvania	225	13,385	345	47,646	86	27,766	656	88,797	47.2
Rhode Island	58	3,225	39	5,450	6	1,492	103	10,167	66.5
South Carolina	98	6,858	60	8,383	3	767	161	16,008	38.4
South Dakota	86	5,389	15	1,971	1	222	102	7,582	72.2
Tennessee	115	8,113	154	21,685	16	4,966	285	34,764	54.3
Texas	516	37,100	551	72,304	46	11,410	1,113	120,814	67.2
Utah	59	3,557	25	3,213	—	—	84	6,770	42.3

Table 1-3 *(Continued)*

State	≤100 beds		101–200 beds		200 + beds		Total	Total	Beds per 1000
	NHS	Beds	NHS	Beds	NHS	Beds	NHS	Beds	age 65 +
Vermont	31	1,523	13	1,792	—	—	44	3,315	48.8
Virginia	111	6,609	124	17,927	18	4,854	253	29,390	42.2
Washington	139	9,721	115	15,440	15	3,369	269	28,530	47.6
West Virginia	58	3,768	45	5,782	1	205	104	9,755	35.5
Wisconsin	188	12,677	141	19,072	51	14,523	380	46,272	69.3
Wyoming	14	950	10	1,300	1	211	25	2,461	49.2
TOTAL	**7,972**	**535,244**	**6,105**	**828,835**	**1,065**	**294,231**	**15,142**	**1,658,310**	**53.2**

Source: After Marion Merrell Dow Managed Care Digest Series, Institutional Digest, 1995.

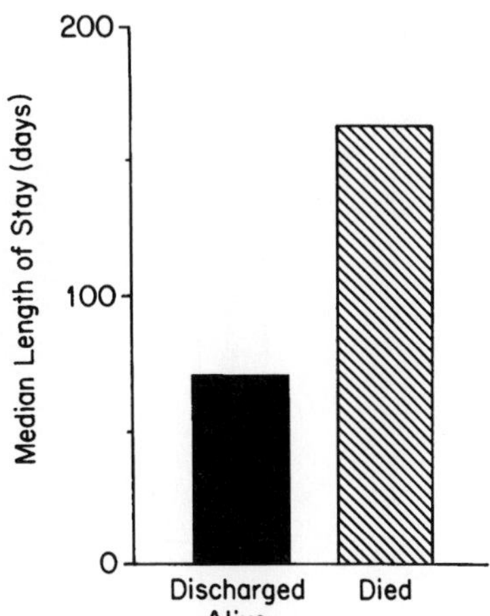

Figure 1-6 Median length of stay in nursing homes among residents who were discharged alive versus residents who died in the nursing home. (After Kane RL, Ouslander JG, and Abrass IB: *Essentials of Clinical Geriatrics*, 2d ed. New York, McGraw-Hill 1989.)

All these factors will contribute to a growing demand for NH care over the next several decades. The number of NH residents is expected to more than double over the next 30 years and to exceed 5 million by the year 2040 (**Fig. 1-7**). This increased number of NH residents will be accompanied by dramatic—and, to many, frightening—increases in the cost of caring for this population.

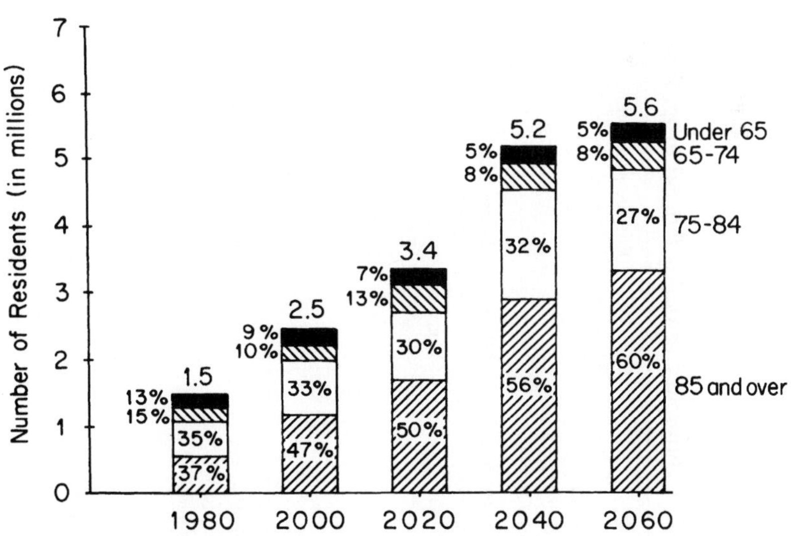

Figure 1-7 Projected growth in the nursing home population. (Based on estimates from the National Center for Health Statistics, 1977.)

Table 1-4 Summary of major federal programs for the elderly

Program	Eligible population	Services covered	Deductibles and copayments
Medicare (Title XVIII of the Social Security Act)			
Part A: Hospital insurance	All persons eligible for Social Security and others with chronic disabilities such as end-stage renal disease plus voluntary enrollees 65 +	Per benefit period, "reasonable cost" for 90 days of hospital care plus 60 lifetime reservation days; 100 days of skilled nursing facility (SNF) per benefit period; home health visits including 80 hours/year of respite care; hospice care (if terminal)	Full coverage for hospital care after a deductible of about 1 day for days 2–60 For SNF care, for each benefit period (up to 100 days) the first 20 are fully covered; for days 21–100 a copayment (~ $90/day applies)
Part B: Supplemental medical insurance	All those covered under Part A who elect coverage; participants pay a monthly premium	80 percent of "reasonable cost" for physicians' services; supplies and services related to physician services; outpatient, physical and speech therapy; diagnostic tests and radiographs; mammogram; surgical dressings; prosthetics; ambulance	Deductible and 20 percent copayment (No copay after a limit reached)
Medicaid (Title XIX of the Social Security Act)	Eligibility criteria vary from state to state. Persons receiving Supplemental Security Income (SSI) or receiving SSI and state supplement or meeting lower eligibility	Mandatory services for categorically needy: Inpatient hospital services; SNF; limited home health care; laboratory tests and radiographs; family planning; early	None, once patient spends down to eligibility level Spend-down based on income and assets

	standards used for medical assistance criteria in 1972 or eligible for SSI or were in institutions and eligible for Medicaid in 1973; medically needy who do not qualify for SSI but have high medical expenses are eligible for Medicaid in some states	and periodic screening; diagnosis and treatment for children through age 20 Optional services vary from state to state: Dental care; therapies; drugs; intermediate care facilities; extended home health care; private duty nurse; eyeglasses; prostheses; personal care services; medical transportation and home health care services (states can limit the amount and duration of services)	
Social Services Block Grant (Title XX of the Social Security Act)	All recipients of Aid to Families with Dependent Children (AFDC) and SSI; optionally, those earning up to 115 percent of state median income and residents of specific geographic areas	Day care; protective services; family counseling; home-based services; employment, education and training; health-related services; information and referral; transportation; day service family planning; legal services; home-delivered and congregate meals	Fees are charged to those with incomes greater than 80 percent of state's median income
Title III of the Older Americans Act	All persons 60 years and older; low-income, minority, and isolated older persons are special targets	Homemaker; home-delivered meals; home health aides; transportation; legal services; counseling; information and referral plus 19 others. (50 percent of funds must go to those listed)	Some payment may be requested

This information applies as of July 1993.

Source: After Kane RL, Ouslander JG and Abrass IB: *Essentials of Clinical Geriatrics*, 3d ed. McGraw-Hill, New York, 1994.

ECONOMIC CONSIDERATIONS

Overview

NH care is expensive. Currently the United States spends close to $50 billion for NH care, and the expenditures are escalating rapidly. Medicare spending on NH care increased 150 percent between 1990 and 1993, to almost $0.5 billion. From the NH resident's perspective, care in a decent facility can cost anywhere from $30,000 to $45,000 per year.

Who pays for NH care? A recent survey of older people found that the majority thought the answer was Medicare. **Table 1-4** summarizes major federal programs that support health and other types of care for the elderly. As shown, Medicare does provide for 150 days of skilled care in a nursing facility (after a 3-day acute care hospitalization) but through various mechanisms sharply restricts its expenditures on this type of care. Thus, while Medicare funds about half the per capita health expenditures of the elderly, and its expenditures for subacute SNF care are increasing, it contributes very little to the cost of NH care (**Fig. 1-8**). Overall, Medicare supports less than 3 percent of this cost. As shown in **Fig. 1-9**, only 1 percent of Medicare dollars went to NH care in 1984, in contrast to 68 percent of Medicaid expenditures and 42 percent of out-of-pocket expenditures for health care by the elderly. While the absolute number of dollars is increasing, the relative proportions of expenditures is remaining about the same.

Medicare limits its expenditures for NH care by narrowly defining skilled (as opposed to custodial) care and by limiting the duration of the "skilled" benefit. Decisions about skilled care are generally determined by the interdisciplinary care team and are reviewed periodically by local intermediaries, who sometimes do not precisely define their guidelines. Thus, decisions about what constitutes skilled care may vary across the country. Medicare also limits its reimbursement for physician services in NHs (see below). This creates several potentially negative incentives, which are discussed further in Chapter 5.

The fact that over 90 percent of NH care is paid for by either out-of-pocket expenditures or by Medicaid (**Figs. 1-8 and 1-9**) has led to a phenomenon known as "spend down." Individuals who need NH care and do not qualify for the Medicare skilled benefit, or whose Medicare coverage has been terminated through the facility-based utilization review process, must spend down their assets until they are impoverished and can pass the means test for Medicaid. Because of the high cost of NH care, the virtual lack of private insurance coverage for it and the prevalence of near poverty among the elderly (about 12 percent are below the poverty line and close to one-third are between the poverty line and double it), most elderly who require NH care for longer than a few weeks end up spending down to qualify for Medicaid. Given the daily private-pay cost of a NH bed (approximate range $80–120), it does not take long for most older individuals to become impoverished and qualify for Medicaid.

Many government officials, providers, and consumers recognize the need to change the system of reimbursement for NH care. But change will not occur

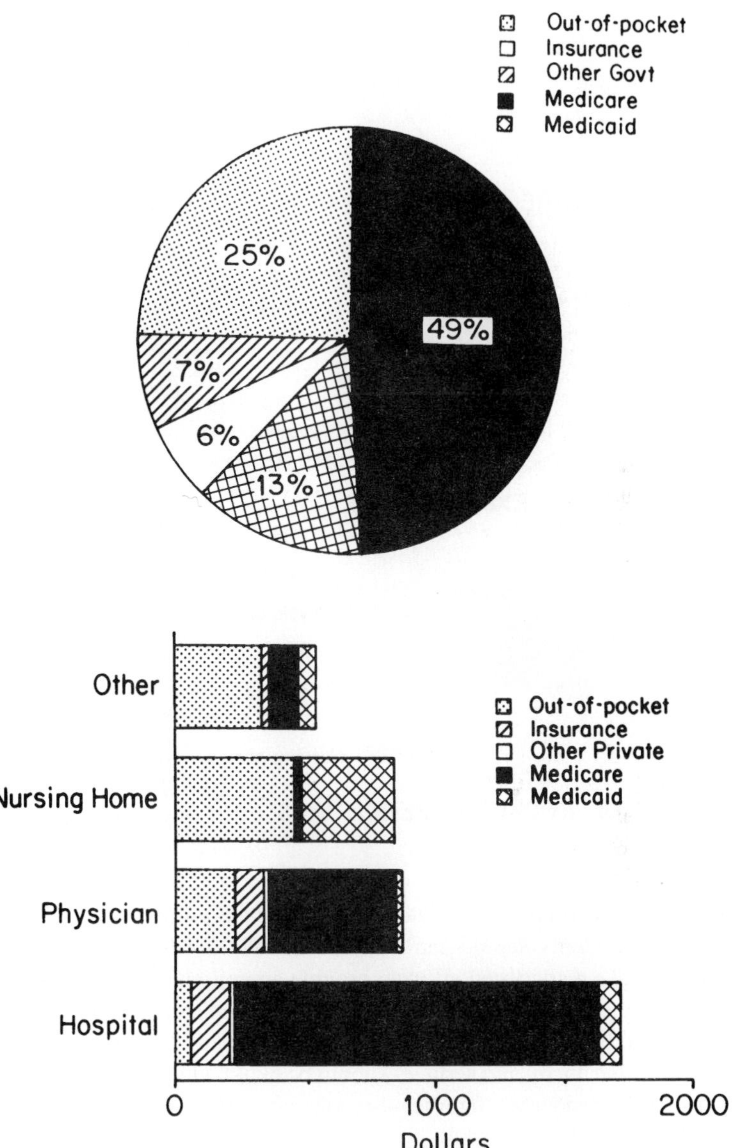

Figure 1-8 Top: Sources of overall health care expenditures for the geriatric population. Bottom: Per capita health care expenditures by type of care and source for the geriatric population. Based on 1984 data. (After Kane RL, Ouslander JG, and Abrass IB: *Essentials of Clinical Geriatrics*, 2d ed. New York, McGraw-Hill, 1989.)

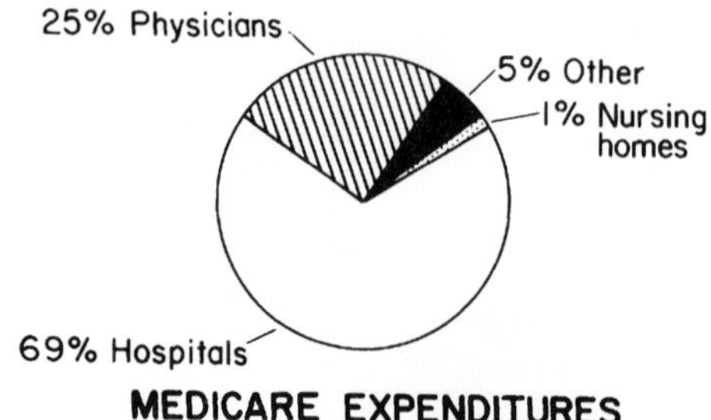

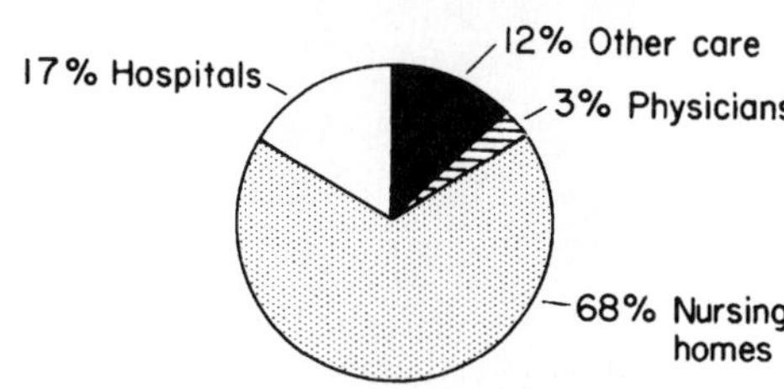

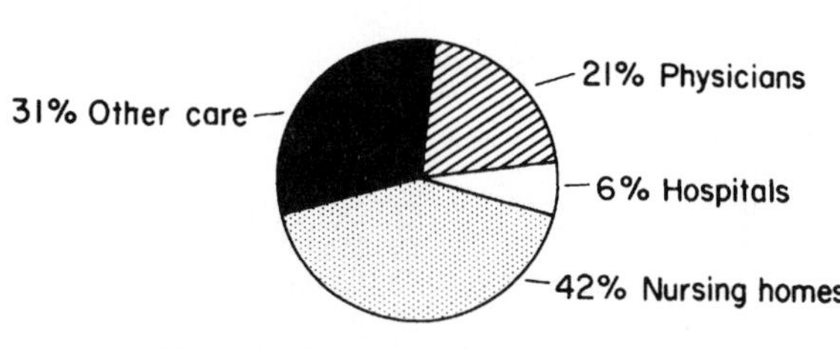

Figure 1-9 Proportions of Medicare, Medicaid, and out-of-pocket expenditures used for different types of care by the geriatric population. Based on data from the United States Special Committee on Aging, 1986. (After Kane RA and Kane RL: *Long Term Care: Principles, Programs, and Policies.* New York, Springer, 1987.)

rapidly. In the meantime, physicians and other health professionals who provide care to NH residents should familiarize themselves with the reimbursement system and make a concerted effort to provide appropriate care in the most cost-effective manner possible. Whenever feasible, Medicare coverage of skilled nursing should be considered, even if for only brief periods of time. Strategies to provide desirable uncovered services should be explored with NH administrators, residents, and residents' families—recognizing that there will always be limitations.

Nursing Home Reimbursement

Nursing home care at present consists of two payment levels: routine (or custodial) and skilled nursing care. The latter is significantly higher. In California, for example, the per diem Medicare rates for routine care are 1.6

Table 1-5 Examples of average per diem rates for nursing home care[a]

	Routine	Ancillary	Total
Medicare	$125	$292	$417
HMO	117	118	235
Private	92	8	100
MediCal	77	1	78

[a]Based on daily rates for skilled nursing beds in California, 1995.

times the MediCal rate, and, including the ancillary cost, it is five-fold the MediCal rate. This discrepancy has provided a strong incentive for the nursing home industry to shift its focus from routine, chronic care ("custodial") to the more complex skilled nursing or subacute level of care (See Chapter 6). The mechanism that establishes Medicare rates is rather complex, and includes direct costs as well as a proportion of indirect costs (administrative, space). **Table 1-5** provides examples of average per diem rates for skilled nursing care.

Medical Provider Reimbursement

One of the most sweeping changes in reimbursement for nursing home care came about with the physician payment reform. The reform by the Health Care Financing Administration (HCFA) included the relative value units (RVUs) basing physician payments on time and effort, overhead costs including malpractice premiums, and geographic practice costs (GPCS) that vary from locale to locale and for surgical, medical and other specialties. These changes have affected physicians' reimbursement for NH evaluation and management (E/M) services quite favorably. This method recognized the additional cognitive effort required to comply with all the regulatory demand posed by the Omnibus Budget Reconciliation Act (OBRA 87). The law allowed for a period of transition and adjustments of the fee schedule, which was scheduled to be fully implemented by January of 1996. The reform has recognized special issues that are unique to NH physician services. These include the frequency of comprehensive assessment hospital discharge and NH admission procedures. Coverage for required visits and use of physician extenders for NH care are also included.

The reform also introduced clear requirements for the use of specific E/M codes. This provision was intended to upgrade the services rendered, stating that payment is directly related to work performed and that failing to document work done may lead to payment denial should the NH records be audited as the regulations have mandated. **Table 1-6** lists key elements for scoring the complexity of the history and physical exam. **Table 1-7** lists the documentation required for the most common CPT codes used for NH care.

Table 1-6 Key components for determining the complexity of the history and physician exam

History of Present Illness (HPI)	Review of Systems (ROS)	Past History, Family or Social (PFSH)	Exam	Type of History and Exam
1–3 HPI findings	N/A	N/A	One affected body area or organ system and other related organ systems	Problem-focused
1 to 3 HPI findings	1 or more systems reviewed	N/A	One affected body area of organ system	Expanded, problem-focused
4 or more HPI findings	2 to 9 systems reviewed	One-plus related family or social history	Affected body area(s) or organ system plus symptomatic organ(s)	Detailed
4 or more HPI findings	10 to 14 systems reviewed	3 (1 each related HPI, ROS, PFSH)	General, multi-system (8–12 organs) or complete single organ	Comprehensive

After the initial required visit performed by the physician, other required visits may alternate between personal visits by the physician and visits by a physician assistant (PA), nurse practitioner (NP), or a clinical nurse specialist (CNS) who are employed by the physician. At least one of every three visits must be performed by the physician (See Chapter 9). The appropriate E/M codes performed by team members should be identified with a modifier to indicate which practitioner performed the team visit:

AM Physician team member
AU Physician assistant team member
AL Nurse practitioner team member
AY Clinical nurse specialist team member

THE FUTURE

Given the growing demand for NH care, the present reimbursement system, and the staggering federal deficit, what does the future hold? It is beyond the scope

Table 1-7 Nursing home CPT evaluation and management codes

Code	History and Exam Key Components	Medical decision Key components	Time Minutes
99301 3 of 3 key components Annual Assessment	Detailed history Comprehensive exam	Straightforward, low complexity	30
99302 3 of 3 key components Creation of a new plan of care is required	Detailed history Comprehensive exam	Moderate to high complexity	40
99303 3 of 3 key components Admission or readmission Creation of a new plan of care is required	Comprehensive history and exam	Moderate to high complexity	50
99311 2 of 3 key components	Problem-focused history and exam	Straightforward, low complexity	15
99312 2 of 3 key components	Expanded, focused history and exam	Moderate complexity	25
99313 2 of 3 key components	Detailed history and exam	Moderate to high complexity	35

of this book to discuss health policy in any detail. Just a few issues relevant to the future of NH care will be covered briefly. First, it is clear that more reimbursement for long-term care, whether it be community-based or in a NH, will be necessary. This will require public and private input. From the government standpoint, some shifting of the focus from acute, expensive, high-technology care toward the care of frail functionally impaired elderly will be necessary. Current demonstration programs involving case management and SHMOs are efforts in this direction. Other capitated programs, such as PACE, are evolving, and many states are considering or implementing capitated Medicaid programs. The fostering of tax incentives for families caring for this population, for tax-deferred savings for long-term-care needs, and the use of reverse mortgages for paying for NH care are being considered. From the private perspective, the development of continuing care (life care) retirement communities that include NHs and the development of long-term-care insurance policies are examples of evolving strategies to deal with the costs of long-term care

Whatever changes in the reimbursement system do occur over the next several years, one thing seems certain: some type of case-mix reimbursement will become national. Several states already do reimburse on the basis of their own measures of case mix. The Health Care Financing Administration is in the process of testing case-mix reimbursement based translating data derived from the minimum data set (MDS) into resource utilization groups (RUGs).

Figure 1-10 illustrates an example of a RUG classification system. Each RUG category is reimbursed at a different level. The potential problem with the

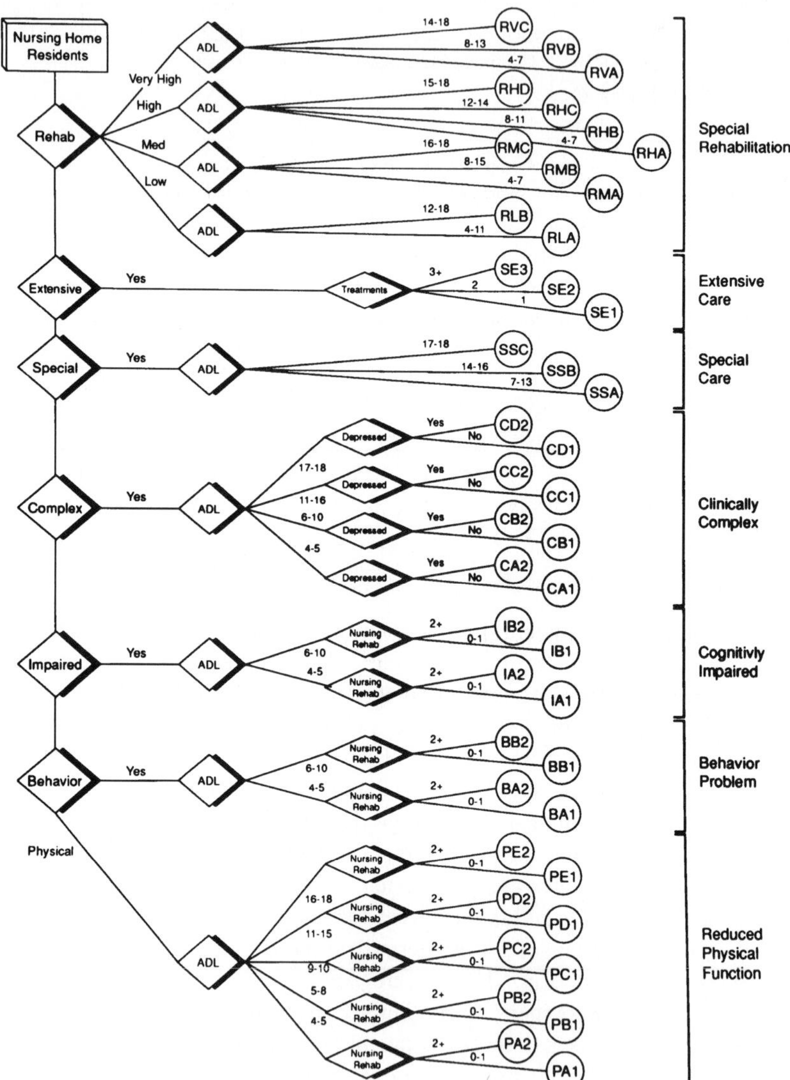

Figure 1-10 The Resource Utilization Groups, (RUG-III) case-mix classification system. RUGs will be generated from items in the minimum data set (MDS) and used as a basis for case-mix reimbursement. (Figures supplied by Dr Brant Fries.)

RUG system is the incentive it provides to keep NH residents sicker and more dependent so as to achieve higher reimbursement. Appropriate incentives for rehabilitation approaches must therefore be built in. One appealing alternative to a case-mix reimbursement system has been developed by Dr Robert Kane: reimbursement based on NH performance in relation to projected outcomes for different types of residents. This system requires a sophisticated ability to accurately predict the clinical course of NH residents (which has been done in a relatively large sample) but offers the advantage of providing an incentive to maintain or improve the resident's status—in contrast to the potentially negative incentive in the RUG system.

We would be remiss if we did not mention one other strategy to deal with the frightening projected growth in the costs of NH care: support for biomedical and health services research. This type of research would require only a minuscule fraction of the cost of NH care. Only through research will disorders such as Alzheimer's disease, osteoporosis and incontinence—which account for so much morbidity and expenditure at the end of life—be prevented or cured and cost-effective methods of managing conditions affecting NH residents be developed.

SUGGESTED READINGS

American Health Care Administration: *Long Term Care Data Book.* Washington, DC, American Health Care Associates, 1988.

Fries BE, Schneider D, Foley WJ, Favazzi M, Burke R, and Cornelius E: Refining A Case-Mix Measure for Nursing Homes: Resource Utilization Groups (RUG-III). *Medical Care* 32:668–680, 1994.

Harrington C, Cassel C, Estes CL, et al: A national long-term care program for the United States. *JAMA* 266:3023–3029, 1991.

Holtzman J and Lurie N: Causes of increasing mortality in a nursing home population. *J Am Geriatr Soc* 44:258–264, 1996.

Kane RA and Kane RL: *Long Term Care: Principles, Programs, and Policies.* New York, Springer, 1987.

Kane RL, Finch M, Blewett L, et al: Use of post-hospital care by Medicare patients. *J Am Geriatr Soc* 44:242–250, 1996.

Kemper P and Murtaugh CM: Lifetime use of nursing home care. *N Engl J Med* 324:595–60, 1991.

Schneider EL and Guralnik JM: The aging of America: Impact on health care costs. *JAMA* 263:2335–2340, 1990.

Vladeck BC: Long term care for the elderly: The future of nursing homes. *West J Med* 150:215–220, 1989.

Weiner J: Financing long-term care: A proposal by the American College of Physicians and the American Geriatrics Society. *JAMA* 271:1525–1529, 1994.

CHAPTER

TWO

THE NURSING HOME ENVIRONMENT AND THE GOALS OF NURSING HOME CARE

The nursing home (NH) is often pictured as a sterile one- or two-story building with a small reception area and business office near the entrance, long corridors with shiny waxed floors, 25 to 50 residents' rooms, each with two or three hospital-type beds crowded in it, and a few scattered, cramped nursing stations. Nursing home residents are generally thought of as old, female, wheelchair-bound, and demented.

Although these stereotypical images are common, NHs and their residents are much more heterogeneous than is often believed by physicians whose contact with them is limited. The purpose of this chapter is to provide a brief overview of NHs and NH residents and to outline the basic goals of NH care, so that physicians will have a broader context within which to view their own NH practice.

NURSING HOMES

Nursing homes in this country have evolved over the last century from publicly run facilities housing the indigent and chronically ill. Three major factors have lead to the development of today's NH: (1) legislation in the 1950s (Hill-Burton) that provided public funding for the construction of NHs, (2) the institution of Medicare and Medicaid in the 1960s, and (3) the strict federal and state regulations that currently control NH care.

Unfortunately for the physical environment of today's NH, all three of these factors have led to an emphasis on "nursing" rather than "home." The growth of subacute care in NHs has reinforced this emphasis. As a result, relatively few facilities offer a homelike atmosphere for those chronically ill residents who may live several of the last years of their lives in an NH. Nursing homes are too commonly structured like small hospitals. Long corridors restrict many residents' access to social life. Rooms tend to be cramped, offering little privacy and little if any space for personal effects. A growing number of architects have developed considerable interest and expertise in the design of NHs that combine homelike environments, creative space management, safety, accessibility, and color designs for physically and cognitively impaired residents while also meeting federal, state, and local requirements. Consultation from this type of expert should be sought whenever a NH is going to be renovated or rebuilt or when a new facility is in its initial planning phases.

Table 2-1 illustrates the distribution of NHs and NH beds by ownership, certification, and bed size. Note that most facilities are small (over one-half have 100 or fewer beds), and that a majority of beds in are for-profit NHs.

Figure 2-1 illustrates the general organizational structure of a typical community-based NH, though there is considerable variability in this structure depending on ownership, facility size, and other factors. At the facility level, the two key individuals are the administrator and the director of nursing. As discussed in Chapter 6, the typical medical director is usually not based in the facility and has little influence on the process of care. Many NHs have full-time social workers and activities therapists, while others obtain these services by contractual, part-time arrangements. Rehabilitation therapists (physical, occupational, speech) and respiratory therapy as well as pharmacy, clinical laboratory, and radiology services are generally provided by contract with professionals, who often provide services to many NHs simultaneously. In hospital-based NHs,

Table 2-1 Selected characteristics of nursing homes[a]

Total number of nursing homes	15,142
Total number of licensed nursing home beds	1,658,310
% of nursing homes in for-profit	73%
% of nursing homes non-profit or church-related	22%
% of nursing homes government-run	4%
% of beds licensed as skilled	45%
Nursing home size (in number of licensed beds)	
50–100	48%
101–150	32%
151–200	13%
201 +	7%
% of nursing homes Medicare certified	68%
% of nursing home revenue from Medicaid	56%

[a]Data adapted from Marion Merrell Dow Managed Care Digest, Long Term Care Edition, 1994.

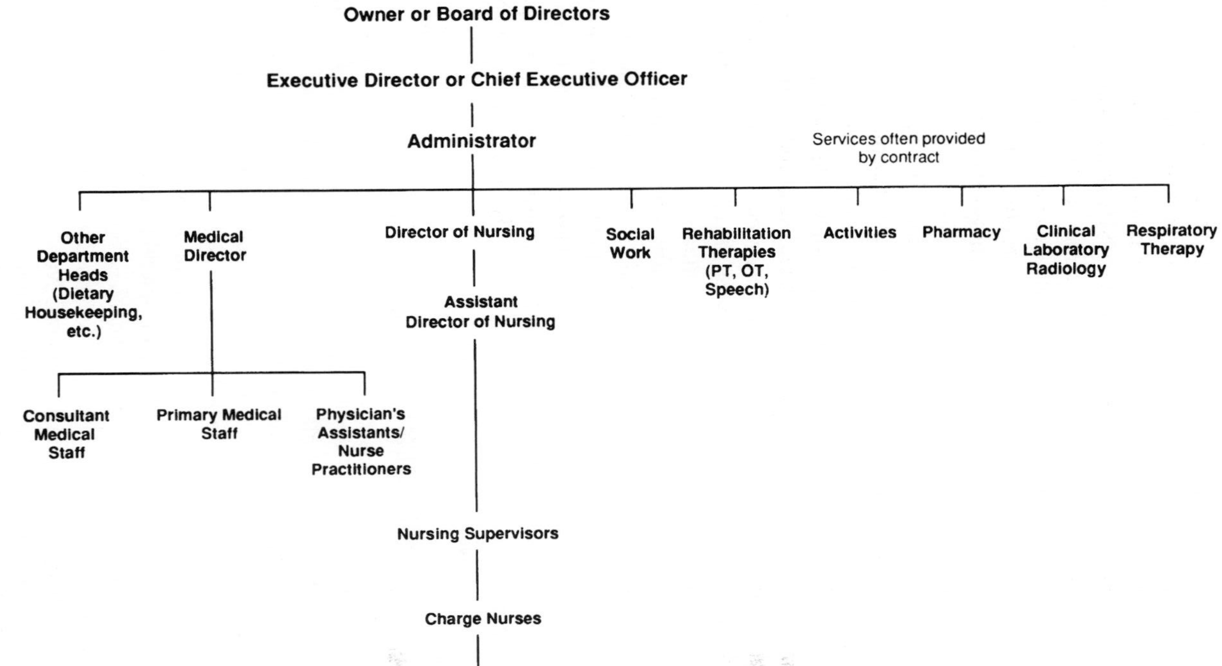

Figure 2-1 Organizational structure of a typical community-based nursing home.

administrative oversight and health care services are generally provided by staff who are hired by and report to the acute hospital.

Several emerging trends are worthy of brief mention. First, many large, for-profit chains of multiple NHs have developed. Currently, the nation's 32 largest chains account for 3162 NHs, or 21 percent of all NHs and 22 percent of NH beds. While there are potential disadvantages to this trend, it may offer a unique opportunity to implement many standardized medical care and quality assurance protocols. Second, the number of continuing-care retirement or life care communities, both private and nonprofit, is growing rapidly. Each of these communities has a NH. This structure affords the opportunity to develop an efficient continuum of long-term-care services for a defined population and to maximize the quality of the NH because of the vested community oversight. Third, many hospitals are using unfilled beds to create hospital-based NHs ("transitional care" or "subacute care" units; see Chapter 6). Although structurally even farther away from a "home" than the typical NH, these facilities play an important role in providing optimal and efficient care to subacutely ill patients who have been rapidly discharged from the acute hospital—or in the case of HMOs patients may have bypassed the acute hospital stay altogether. Ready access to many of the ancillary services that are difficult to obtain in community NHs may be critical in these residents. (These issues are discussed further in Chapter 5.) Finally, some NHs are becoming affiliated to academic institutions. Multidisciplinary educational and research programs can provide a wealth of opportunity to modify the process and even the structure of NH care and can certainly contribute to improving and enlivening the NH environment. Education and research programs are discussed in Chapter 26.

NURSING HOME RESIDENTS

Table 2-2 shows some basic demographic characteristics of NH residents compared to the community-dwelling geriatric population. **Figure 2-2** rather dramatically illustrates the degree of functional impairment of the NH population as opposed to elderly people in the community. In addition to these impairments in basic activities of daily living, less than half of NH residents are ambulatory, and the prevalence of dementia exceeds 50 percent in most NHs.

Despite the extremely high prevalence of functional disability and dementia, NH residents are actually quite a heterogeneous population. It is critical to recognize this heterogeneity if we are to develop appropriate goals and approaches to the care of individual residents. Nursing home residents can be broadly characterized on the basis of their length of stay: "short" (i.e., 1 to 6 months) versus "long." Short stayers can be subdivided into two groups: residents who enter the NH for short-term rehabilitation after an acute illness (e.g., hip fracture, stroke) and those who are medically unstable or terminally ill,

Table 2-2 Demographic characteristics of nursing home residents vs community dwelling residents age 65 and older

	Nursing home residents	Community dwelling residents
Age		
65–74 years	16	62
75–84	39	31
85 +	45	8
Sex		
Male	25	41
Female	75	59
Race		
White (including Hispanics)	93	91
Black and other	7	9
Marital status		
Married	12	55
Widowed	69	34
Divorced or separated	5	6
Never married	14	4

Source: After Kane RL, Ouslander JG and Abrass IB: *Essentials of Clinical Geriatrics*, 2d ed. McGraw-Hill, New York, 1994.

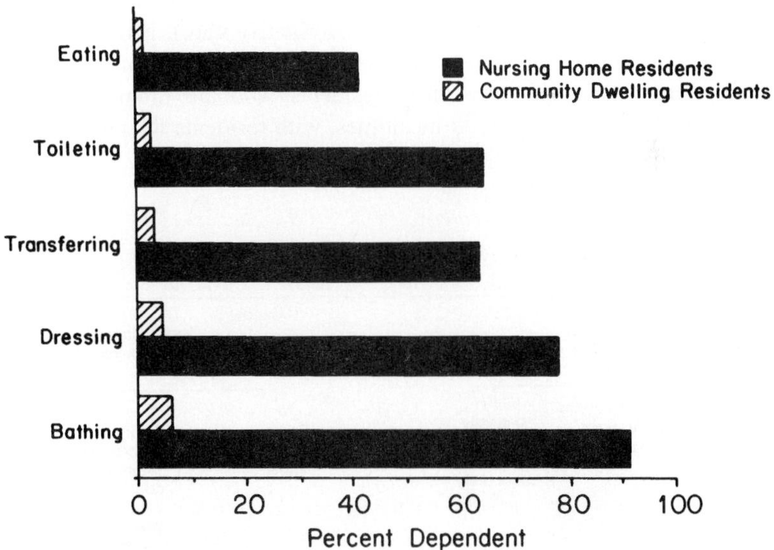

Figure 2-2 Ability to perform basic activities of daily living among nursing home residents versus community-dwelling elderly. (After Kane RL, Ouslander JG, and Abrass IB: *Essentials of Clinical Geriatrics*, 2d ed. New York, McGraw-Hill, 1994.)

who are either quickly discharged to an acute care hospital or die in the NH. These types of residents represent a growing segment of the NH population because of the continued growth of subacute care (see Chapter 6). Long stayers can be subdivided into three groups: those with primarily cognitive impairment (e.g., the ambulatory, wandering resident with Alzheimer's disease), residents with primarily physical impairments (e.g., severe arthritis or end-stage heart or lung disease), and those with both cognitive and physical impairments.

Figure 2-3 illustrates this subgrouping of the NH population. Obviously residents may move from one subgroup to another when acute illnesses intervene, chronic illness develops or progresses, or cognitive function declines. **Figures 2-4 to 2-9** illustrate case examples of each subgroup of residents.

The conceptualization of NH residents in this manner has important implications for the goals of NH care, quality assurance, and even the structure of the NH environment. The goals of caring for a previously healthy resident who is undergoing rehabilitation after a hip fracture are obviously very different from those of caring for one with advanced dementia and related behavioral disorders or another with a terminal malignancy. Similarly, from the perspective of quality assurance, processes and outcomes of care that are relevant for one subgroup of residents may be inappropriate or irrelevant to another subgroup. From a structural standpoint, many NHs attempt to separate different subgroups of residents geographically. This approach, when it is feasible, offers many potential advantages: the physical environment can be modified for certain types of residents (e.g., wanderers), the staff can be trained and develop expertise in managing specific types of care (e.g., terminal or hospice-type care, subacute care, or rehabilitative care), and residents may be more comfortable when they are around others like themselves. This is especially true for cognitively intact residents who are often distressed by constant interaction, especially at mealtimes, with residents who have dementia and associated behavioral disorders.

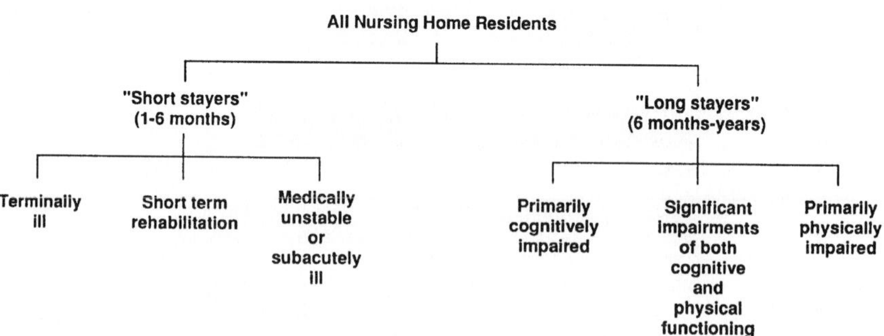

Figure 2-3 Basic types of nursing home residents. Residents frequently go from one subgroup to another. See text and Figs 2-4 to 2-9 for examples. (After Kane RL, Ouslander JG, and Abrass IB: *Essentials of Clinical Geriatrics*, 2d ed. New York, McGraw-Hill, 1994.)

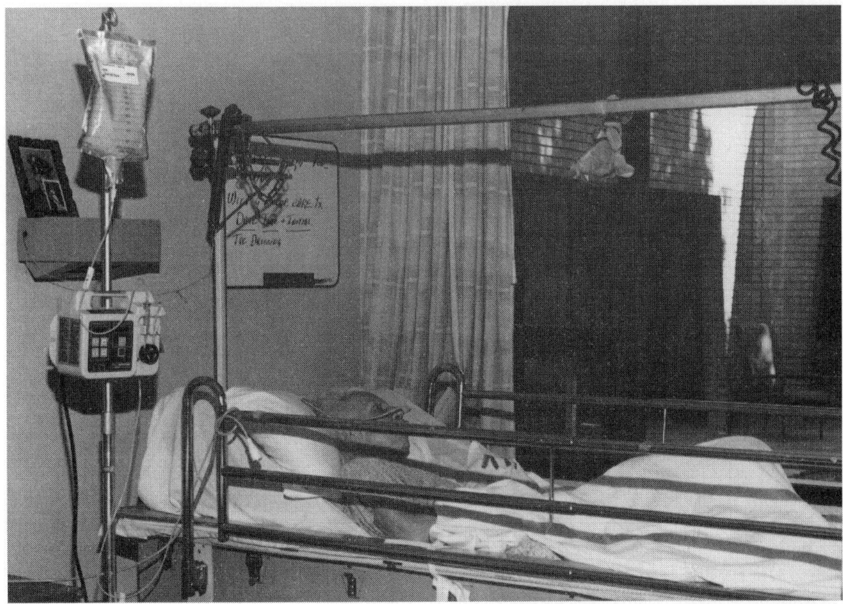

A

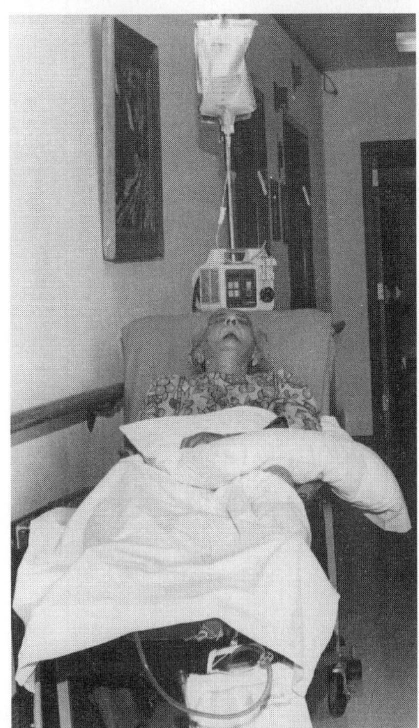

B

Figure 2-4 Examples of short-staying nursing home residents—terminally ill. A. A 93-year-old woman who suffered a massive stroke; she requires enteral feeding, oxygen, suctioning, and an air-fluidized mattress for the management of a deep pressure sore. B. An 88-year-old woman with end-stage renal failure (not on dialysis), severe multi-infarct dementia, and heart failure requiring enteral feeding, an indwelling catheter to monitor urinary output, and frequent doses of diuretics to manage respiratory distress.

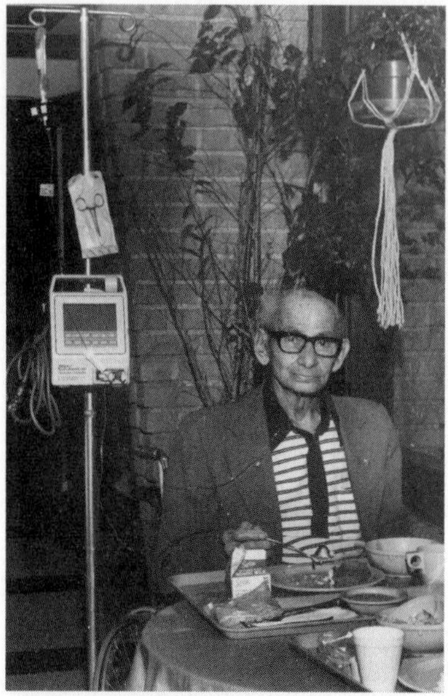

Figure 2-5 Example of a short-staying nursing home resident—subacutely ill. An 86-year-old man who developed subacute bacterial endocarditis and required 6 weeks of parenteral antibiotic therapy via a subclavian catheter.

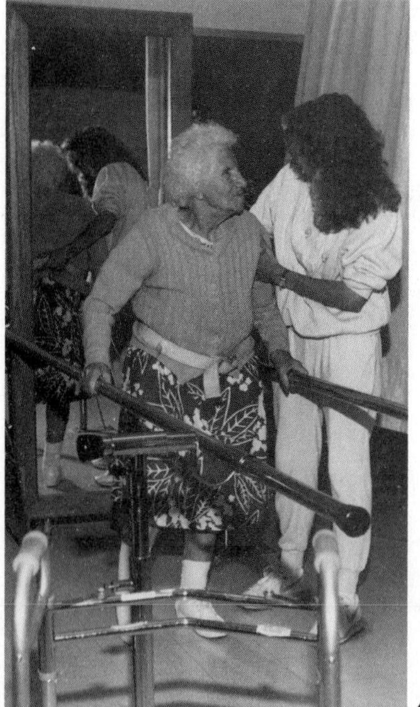

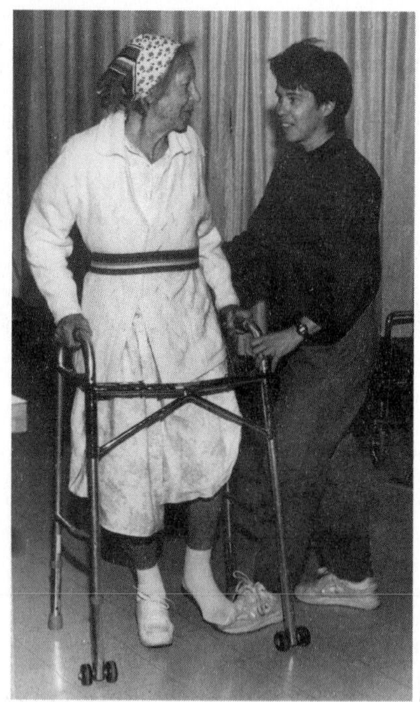

Figure 2-6 Examples of short-staying nursing home residents—short term rehabilitation. A. A 92-year-old woman undergoing gait retraining after a subcapital hip fracture and hemiarthroplasty. B. An 84-year-old woman getting physical therapy with partial weight bearing after an intertrochanteric hip fracture and surgical pinning of the fracture.

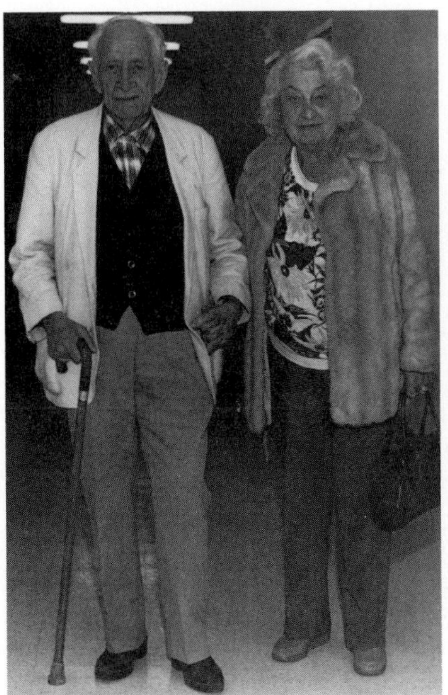

A

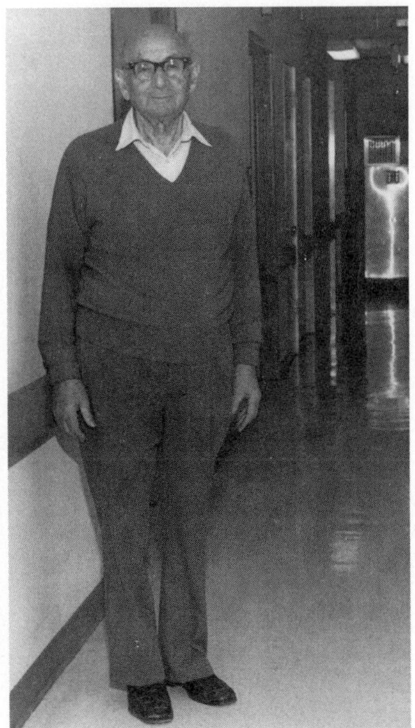

B

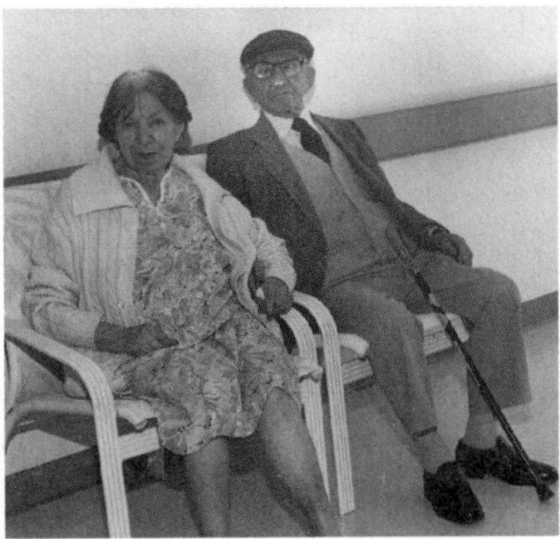

C

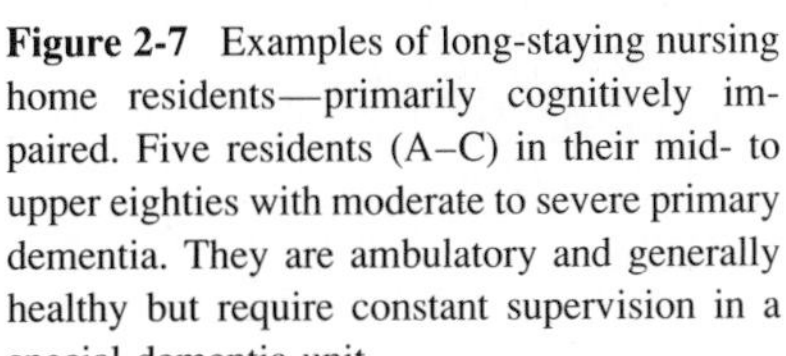

Figure 2-7 Examples of long-staying nursing home residents—primarily cognitively impaired. Five residents (A–C) in their mid- to upper eighties with moderate to severe primary dementia. They are ambulatory and generally healthy but require constant supervision in a special dementia unit.

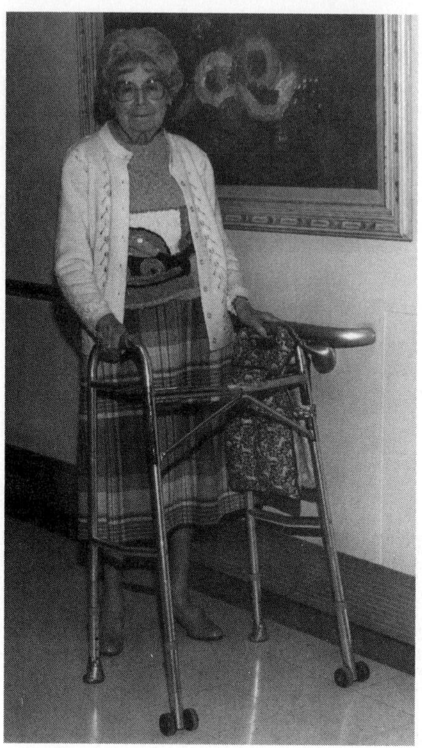

Figure 2-8 Example of a long-staying nursing home resident—primarily physically impaired. An 89-year-old woman with degenerative joint disease, osteoporosis, atherosclerotic cardiovascular disease, and recurrent syncope who requires periodic nursing observation and assistance with dressing and bathing.

GOALS OF NURSING HOME CARE

Table 2-3 outlines broad goals for the care of NH residents. Physicians who care for NH residents must recognize the importance of focusing on functional abilities, autonomy, quality of life, comfort, and safety as goals of medical care. While optimal medical care is clearly essential to these types of outcomes, especially among residents undergoing subacute care, the vast majority of NH residents would rather be safe, comfortable, maximally independent, and able to participate in decisions about their lives and their health care than have the most advanced high-tech medical care available. This implies that primary care physicians must be sensitive to the nonmedical complaints of their residents (e.g., as to difficulties with roommates or other residents, the quality of their food, inability to leave the facility or to obtain clothing or other personal items). Although it may not be the primary physician's responsibility to deal in detail with these complaints, he/she should listen to them and try to communicate the expressed concerns to appropriate members of the interdisciplinary team as well as to help the medical director to change or create policies and procedures fostering an improved quality of life for the residents.

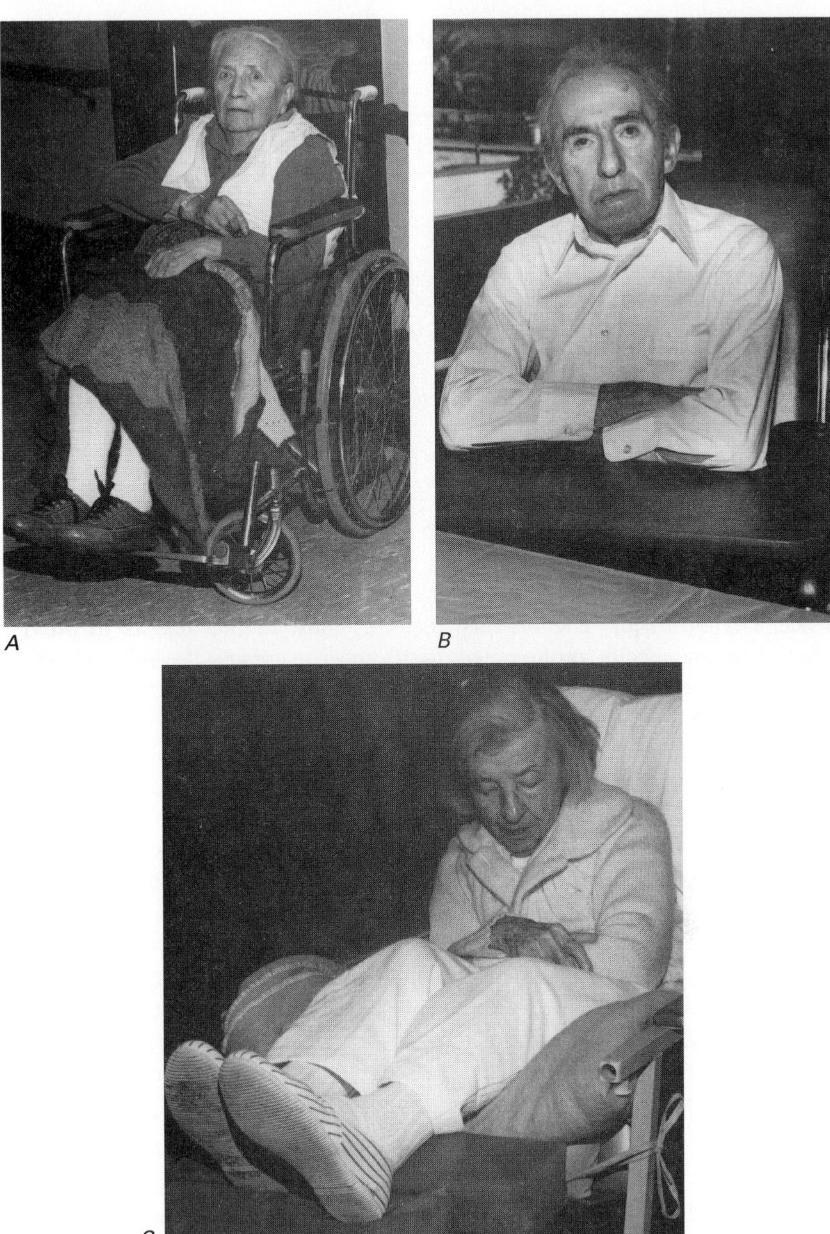

Figure 2-9 Examples of long-staying nursing home residents with impairments of both physical and cognitive functioning. A. A 92-year-old woman with severe congestive heart failure, degenerative joint disease of the lumbosacral spine, and moderately advanced Alzheimer's disease. B. An 87-year-old man with severe Parkinson's disease and dementia. C. A 79-year-old woman with a rapidly progressive dementia, depression, and frequent agitated and disruptive behaviors who is non-ambulatory due to gait apraxia.

Table 2-3 Goals of nursing home care

1. Provide a safe and supportive environment for chronically ill and dependent people
2. Restore and maintain the highest possible level of functional independence
3. Preserve individual autonomy
4. Maximize quality of life, perceived well-being and satisfaction with care
5. Provide comfort and dignity for terminally ill residents and their loved ones
6. Provide coordinated, interdisciplinary care to subacutely ill residents who plan to return home or to another lower level of care
7. Stabilize and delay progression, whenever possible, of chronic medical conditions
8. Prevent acute medical and iatrogenic illnesses, and identify and treat them rapidly when they do occur

Source: After Kane RL, Ouslander JG, Abrass IB: *Essentials of Clinical Geriatrics*, 2d ed. McGraw-Hill, New York, 1989.

The goals of medical care per se are, insofar as is possible, to identify, stabilize, and delay progression of chronic medical conditions and to prevent acute medical and iatrogenic conditions—identifying and treating them rapidly when they do occur. The primary focus of most of this text is to provide physicians and health professionals with specific, practical, and—whenever possible—scientifically based strategies for managing these medical aspects of care among NH residents.

At one NH in St Louis (NMC Maryland Heights), a similar program involving the introduction of large animals (donkey, goats, geese, pot belly pigs, dogs, chickens, and rabbits) as well as giving individual birds (parakeets) to residents who wished to have them (**Fig. 2-10**). In addition residents, developed their own vegetable garden. In this program, individual residents have had a marked improvement in their mood, and the birds appeared to have a major therapeutic effect. Overall the careful introduction of animals and plants into a nursing home, preserving resident autonomy appears to be an excellent addition to complete NH care. Another component is the involvement of residents in meal preparation. Many of the residents have spent a large proportion of their lives in kitchens, and for those who saw this as a pleasure and took pride in their cooking, continued access to the condition may improve quality of life.

INNOVATIVE STRATEGIES TO ENHANCE THE NURSING HOME ENVIRONMENT

Nursing homes often have a sense of institutionalized sameness to them. To reintroduce the feeling of home residents and families can be encouraged to individually decorate their rooms. This can introduce a pride in ownership as well as a sense of being at home. The presence of objects chosen by residents often

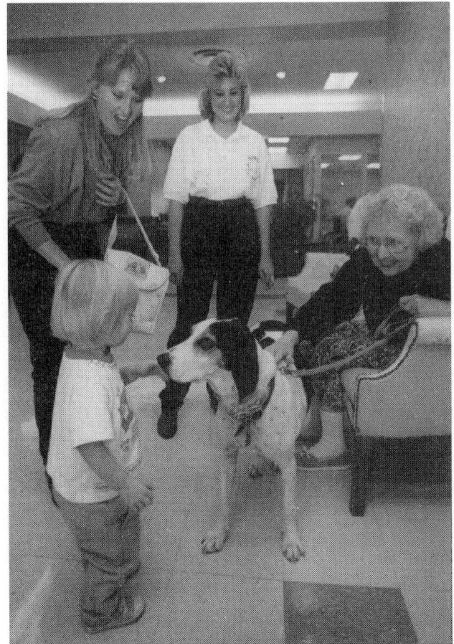

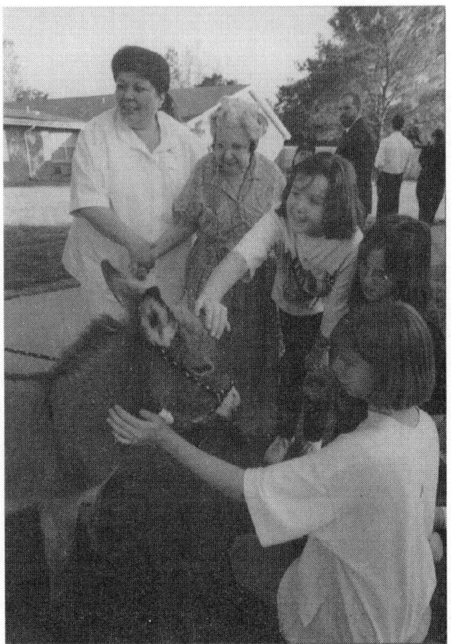

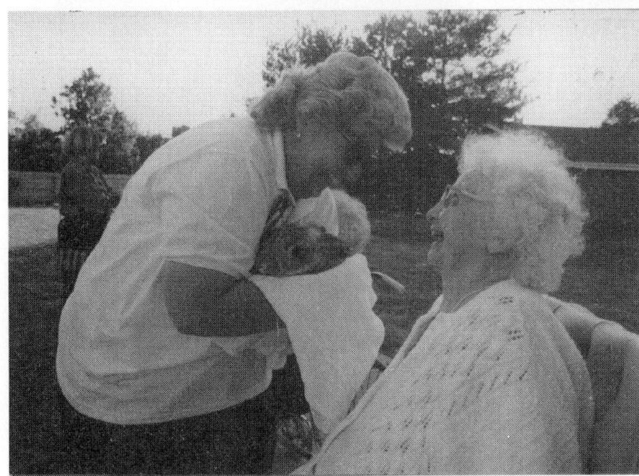

Figure 2-10 Nursing home residents enjoying interactions with various animals.

gives clues to the resident's personality and makes an excellent discussion point during the physician's visit.

There are now a number of architects who specialize in NH design. Most of these are moving away from the sterile institutionalized environment towards a more homely environment. In particular they are removing the nursing stations from view, provide lounge space instead of being shared by resident's and staff and utilizing alcoves in the hallways for medicine carts and work space for the nursing staff. The introduction of skylight windows in the roof of common areas leads to decreased dependence on artificial lighting. The introduction of aviaries, aquariums, jukeboxes, pianos, and pianolas break the monotony of the

Table 2-4 Components of the Eden alternative

- Introduction of a variety of plants within the NH
- Introduction of a variety of animal species in the NH environment
- Empowerment of employees and development of caring teams
- Introduction of children (e.g. after-school care and summer camp) into the NH

environment. While many of these features are easier to include in new homes, some of them can relatively easily be included into older homes as well.

William H. Thomas, MD has created an innovative approach to NH care in which he has worked with the NH staff to develop a NH habitat which includes animals, plants, and many visits by children, together with a team approach to care. His uncontrolled study suggests that the "Eden alternative" resulted in a decrease in the use of psychotropic medicines, a decrease in infections, a decrease in death and a decrease in staff turnover. **Table 2-4** lists the full components of Eden alternative.

SUGGESTED READINGS

Kane RA and Kane RL: *Long Term Care: Principles, Programs, and Policies*. New York, Springer, 1987.

Marion Merrell Dow Managed Care Digest Series, Institutional Digest, 1995 (Marion Merrell Dow, Kansas City, MO).

Ouslander JG: Medical care in the nursing home. *JAMA* 262:2582–2590, 1989.

Thomas WH: *The Eden Alternative: Nature, Hope and Nursing Homes*. Eden Alternative Foundation. Sherburne, New York, 1995.

CHAPTER
THREE

PREADMISSION ASSESSMENT

The decisions involved in placing an individual in a long-term care institution are complex and frequently associated with significant emotional distress. In this chapter, residential care (e.g., board and care, assisted living) and nursing homes (NHs) will be discussed as one continuum of long-term care. The purpose of this chapter is to review briefly the main reasons for institutionalization and the goals and objectives of preadmission assessment. Preadmission to the subacute/transitional care unit is discussed in Chapter 6.

THE NEED FOR NURSING HOME CARE

A vast body of literature exists on the physical, psychological, social, and economic factors associated with the need for institutional care of the elderly and the disabled. It is commonly believed that disability and diminished social support are the predominant factors leading to institutionalization of the frail elderly. It is also recognized that relocation to a different environment, especially a NH, is associated with some adverse effects—commonly referred to as relocation trauma.

Candidates for long-term care are generally dependent on the assistance of others for substantial periods of time. This assistance addresses the health, personal care, and social needs of individuals who lack some capacity for self-care (in Chapter 1, **Table 1-1** describes in more detail characteristics of individuals who are in need of NH admission). Most long-term care in the United States is provided by a host of individuals referred to as "informal support."

These persons may be family, friends, or neighbors. When this system fails to provide for the needs of persons with disability, a formal long-term care system is needed. It is estimated that about 15 percent of the elderly have significant disability. For each person in a NH today, there are between one and three equally disabled persons living in the community. A variety of community-based long-term care services are available, although they are generally not reimbursed by third-party payers and in many areas are fragmented and difficult to coordinate (in Chapter 1, **Table 1-2** lists examples of community resources for long-term care). NH placement becomes inevitable when community-based long-term care alternatives fail, are inappropriate, not feasible, or not desired by the individual or the caregivers. Public demand for more NH beds is growing due to demographic and economic factors (see Chapter 1). The Prospective Payment System, implemented in 1983, and more recently the increasing role of managed care have also placed pressure on acute care hospitals to shorten the average length of stay, resulting in a shift toward more skilled nursing placements.

Candidates for NH care need to be carefully assessed prior to admission in order to determine their needs and to advise them and their families on the most appropriate level of care. Studies in the United States and elsewhere have shown that careful assessment in community-based geriatric assessment clinics prevents inappropriate NH placement. In addition to determining care needs, a comprehensive geriatric assessment before NH admission can help prevent the underdiagnosis and underreporting of treatable illness and functional disabilities in elderly people. There is also a lack of emphasis on geriatric preventive measures such as vaccination against influenza and pneumococcal infection, screening for impaired vision and hearing, dental care, and assessment of ambulation. These, as well as more traditional preventive measures such as periodic screening for cancer, thyroid disease, and cognitive and affective disorders, can be accomplished when a preadmission assessment is being performed. New regulations, resulting from the Omnibus Budget Reconciliation Act (OBRA), 1987, also require screening for mental illness and/or mental retardation within 72 h of NH admission.

From the societal perspective, the preadmission assessment provides a gatekeeping function. In life care communities, the assessment is critical to

Table 3-1 Objectives of preadmission geriatric assessment

Determine psychosocial and functional status
Identify active medical problems
Screen for cognitive impairment and mental health problems
Determine the appropriate level of care
Determine capacity to make decisions for health care
Determine program eligibility for third party reimbursement
Act as gatekeeper for appropriate use of long-term-care services
Develop a multidisciplinary approach to the individual's care needs

ensure proper utilization of resources and cost-effectiveness of services, which, in turn, guarantee the financial viability of the institution. **Table 3-1** summarizes the objectives of the preadmission assessment. The product of this assessment should be a multidisciplinary plan of care.

TIMING AND SITE OF ASSESSMENT

The timing of preadmission assessment is dictated by events that lead to increased dependence on services. This often occurs following a major illness that requires acute hospitalization. The site of the evaluation may vary. Patients awaiting discharge from the acute care hospital might be screened during their hospital stay by a registered nurse or geriatric nurse practitioner. In hospitals where a geriatrician is available, a gerontological consultation may be very helpful in the discharge planning.

Several states have developed specific preadmission assessment procedures, which are conducted by a registered nurse or a case manager and focus on the patient's functional and psychosocial needs. Such assessments are carried out in hospitals, rehabilitation units, clinics, and in the home setting.

THE PROCESS OF PREADMISSION ASSESSMENT

Depending on the setting, the assessment team may include only one person (a case manager, with social work or nursing background, for example), or as many as described in **Table 3-2.** It is our belief that an appropriate preadmission assessment can be performed only under the supervision of a physician interested and trained in geriatric medicine. For NHs or long-term care programs that do not have geriatricians available, interested internists or family physicians may acquire the skills required for this kind of assessment through programs sponsored by universities or other geriatric educational centers.

It is important to assign specific tasks to each team member, to conduct the assessment efficiently, and to be sensitive to the patient's anxieties and potential to fatigue easily. **Table 3-3** describes the team members and the tasks they are responsible for. The sequence of the various assessments may vary, but geriatric

Table 3-2 Individuals involved with preadmission assessment

Clerical personnel
Social worker/case manager
Rehabilitation therapists (physical therapist, occupational therapist)
Geriatric nurse practitioner, physician assistant, or registered nurse with geriatric assessment skills
Physician/geriatrician

Table 3-3 Examples of team assignments and instruments for preadmission assessment

Discipline	Tasks	Instrument/approach
Clerical worker	Determining financial eligibility for state or federal programs, information on methods of payment programs, identify responsible party and primary physician	Nonstructured or structured interview
Social worker	Interview for background, roommate compatibility, personal preferences Assess instrumental activities of daily living (IADL) Screen for affective disorders	Interview, Lawton IADL Scale Geriatric Depression Scale
Occupational therapist	Assess basic activities of daily living	Katz ADL or direct observation (when applicable)
Physical therapist[a]	Gait and balance assessment	Tinetti Gait and Balance Scale or "Get up and walk and sit down" test
Nurse practitioner	Mental status exam Vision and hearing screen Review medical records	Folstein MMSE, Jaeger card, Welch Allyn Audioscope, or clinical method
Physician	History and physical exam	Systematic, focus on function Utilize structured forms

[a]If rehabilitation therapists are not available, these tasks may be performed by a trained nurse practitioner or registered nurse.

medicine evaluation should be the last appointment, when information gathered by other team members is available. The administrative interview is critical for establishing eligibility for federal or state programs, determining availability of funds, and identifying the responsible party. The social worker may play a dual role in certain situations. Usually the social worker will gear the interview to leisure activities and social preferences. Social workers can also screen for cognitive and affective disorder by administering a depression scale and standardized mental status exam (examples are included in Chapters 11 and 12).

Table 3-4 lists commonly used instruments and their characteristics. The choice of specific assessment tools is based on their validity, reliability, and the time it takes to administer them. Sometimes the choice is a compromise between the three characteristics. All assessment tools should be relevant to the patient and the environment he or she is going to live in.

The assessment instruments listed in **Table 3-4** include both self-report and performance-based assessments. The time and economic advantage of

Table 3-4 Instruments and procedures applicable to the preadmission assessment

	Function assessed	Administration	Strengths	Weaknesses	Comments
Katz ADL Scale	Basic self-care abilities	By patient or interviewer, based on judgment and report	Simple assessment of basic skills, useful in rehabilitation setting	Limited range of activities assessed, rating subjective	Not sensitive to small changes (see Chap. 22)
Instrumental ADL	More complex activities, food preparation, shopping, housekeeping, handling the phone, medications	By patient or interviewer, based on judgment and report	Assesses functions important for independent living	Rating subjective	Higher functions, not sensitive to small changes (see Table 3-5)
Tinetti Gait and Balance Scale	Performance-based testing of mobility	By observation of performance	Provides information about risk of falls; can identify specific abnormalities	No standard cutoff score	Sensitivity not determined (see Chap. 14)
Folstein Mini Mental State Examination (MMSE)	Memory, orientation, attention, constructional ability	By interviewer	Fairly quick and sensitive	Will not detect mild disability	Test score <24 considered abnormal but not necessarily indicative of dementia (see Chap. 9)
Geriatric Depression Scale (GDS)	Symptoms of depression	By patient	Quick, reliable, avoids an excess of somatic questions	Not evaluated for specificity among medically ill; use limited in presence of severe dementia	Score >14 on the long form or >5 on the short form indicates depression (see Chap. 10)
Cornell Scale	Symptoms of depression	By interviewer to patient and caregiver	Useful in patients with or without dementia; range of questions suited for elderly patients	Not widely tested, requires two interviewers	See Suggested Readings

using self-administered scales is counterbalanced by the fact that patients tend to rate their abilities higher than trained observers would. Family members tend to rate a patient's function lower. The cognitively intact elderly are, however, more accurate than family members and physicians. The rationale for administering an instrumental activities of daily living (IADL) scale is that some patients may be capable of living at home if most of these functions are preserved. **Table 3-5** illustrates the Lawton IADL scale, which can be used for this purpose. Where it is clear from the beginning that a patient's NH placement is inevitable, a basic ADL assessment, such as the Katz ADL scale, is more relevant for determining the areas in which assistance is needed (see Chapter 26). The use of a performance-based gait and balance scale provides a description of function related to ambulation. It is useful in the sense that it helps describe any specific abnormalities and also yields a score that can be followed over time (see Chapter 18). The Folstein Mini Mental State Exam (MMSE) is useful because of its brevity, its relatively good sensitivity for significant abnormalities, and its excellent test-retest reliability. All depression scales have limitations. The geriatric depression scale (GDS) was originally designed for self-administration; the validity of an interviewer-administered GDS has not yet been examined. In a recent study comparing case finding tools for depression in the NH, the 15-item GDS agreed with the criterion standard of depression, thus making it the preferred tool to screen for depression in the NH. The Cornell Scale has some promise, since it can be administered relatively easily and is suitable for the cognitively impaired as well. Other functional tests have been described—such as the timed hand-function test developed by Mark Williams—that correlate highly with the need for long-term care services and institutionalization in particular.

These assessment tools are useful for establishing baseline characteristics, screening for undetected problems, and helping to set rehabilitational goals. In certain situations, such as life care communities, identifying persons at risk for needing more long-term care services may be another goal of these assessments. Following administration of these assessments, a detailed history, review of any pertinent records, and a physical examination are necessary. **Table 3-6** describes the focal points of the history and physical examination. Recent studies have shown that brief measures of health and self-reported physical functioning in very old persons have acceptable validity. In one study, self-reported mental health problems and objective upper extremity functioning predicted a change in level of care. Another study showed that a diagnosis of dementia, an abnormal Katz ADL score, and hearing loss were all predictors of transfer to the NH. Upper- and lower-extremity strength and performance, hand-grip strength, and mental status have been found to predict stability versus chronic deterioration in a cohort of frail older persons. The physical exam should particularly focus on factors that might impair functioning. Certain arm functions are important in performing activities; distal functions such as manual dexterity affect writing or using eating utensils. Proximal functions are involved in transfers from sitting to

Table 3-5 Instrumental activities of daily living (IADL) scale (self-rated version)[a]

Item	Score
Ability to use telephone	
Operate telephone on own initiative, looks up and dials numbers, etc.	1
Dials a few well-known numbers	1
Answers telephone, but does not dial	1
Does not use telephone at all	0
Shopping	
Takes care of all shopping independently	1
Shops independently for small purchases	0
Needs to be accompanied on any shopping trip	0
Completely unable to shop	0
Food preparation	
Plans, prepares, and serves adequate meals independently	1
Prepares adequate meals if supplied with ingredients	0
Heats, serves, and prepares meals, or prepares meals, but does not maintain adequate diet	0
Needs to have meals prepared and served	0
Housekeeping	
Maintains household alone or with occasional assistance (e.g., "heavy work domestic help")	1
Performs light daily tasks such as dishwashing, bedmaking	1
Performs light daily tasks but cannot maintain acceptable level of cleanliness	1
Needs help with all home maintenance tasks	1
Does not participate in any housekeeping tasks	0
Laundry	
Does personal laundry completely	1
Launders small items–rinses stockings, etc.	1
All laundry must be done by others	0
Mode of transportation	
Travels independently on public transportation or drives own car	1
Arranges own travel via taxi, but does not otherwise use public transportation	1
Travels on public transportation when accompanied by another	1
Travel limited to taxi or automobile with assistance of another	0
Responsible for own medications	
Is responsible for taking medication in correct dosages at correct time	1
Takes responsibility if medication is prepared in advance in separate dosages	0
Is not capable of dispensing own medication	0
Ability to handle finances	
Manages financial matters independently (budgets, writes checks, pays rent, bills, goes to bank), collects and keeps track of income	1
Mananges day-to-day purchases, but needs help with banking, major purchases, etc.	1
Incapable of handling money	0
SCORE______	/8

[a] This instrument is a component of the Philadelphia Geriatric Multilevel Assessment Instrument.

Source: Lawton MP, Moss M, Fulcomer M, Kleban MH: A research and service-oriented multilevel assessment instrument. *J Gerontol* 37:91–99, 1982.

standing or lying to sitting, raising the arm to comb hair or brush teeth, and putting on a shirt. Falls and immobility often arise from the accumulated effects of multiple disabilities, which may include sensory and cognitive impairments as well as dysfunction of the legs. A patient who has had recent trips or falls should be evaluated by being watched as he or she rises from a chair, walks about 10 ft,

Table 3-6 Key components of the preadmission geriatric evaluation

History
- Reasons for seeking admission
- Medical problems (active and chronic)
- Past medical history
- Preventative measures: vaccination, eye, dental, and foot care
- Medication history (including over-the-counter drugs)
- Review of symptoms

Physical Examination
- In addition to traditional system approach, focus on the following:
  - Nutritional status (weight/height)
  - Orthostatic changes in blood pressure
  - Functional muscle strength
  - Proximal and distal functions

Functional Assessment (see Tables 3-4 and 3-5)
- Corroborate responses with patient appearance, question family members if accuracy is uncertain

Mobility
- Ask patient to get out of chair, walk, turn around, and sit down
- Judgment based on direct observation
- Tinetti Gait and Balance Scale (see Table 3-4 and Chap. 14)

Cognitive Assessment
- Administer MMSE; if score <24, search for causes of cognitive impairment (see Table 3-4 and Chap. 9)
- Ask "Do you often feel sad or depressed?" If answer is yes, administer Geriatric Depression Scale (see Table 3-4 and Chap. 10)

Hearing
- Screen utilizing Welch Allyn Audioscope testing threshold of 20, 25, and 40 dB at 500, 1000, 2000, 4000 Hz (see Chap. 15)
- Whisper a short easily answered question such as "What is your name?" in each ear while your face is out of direct view

Vision
- Utilize Jaeger card at 14 in. while patient wears his or her corrective lenses (inability to read greater than 20/40 is abnormal) or
- Have patient read something to test ability to see well enough to read

and returns and sits down as well as by a means of full neurological and musculoskeletal examination (see Chapter 18). Walking speed may be a good discriminator for level of functioning. The walking speed of NH residents is typically <0.6 m/s, and is associated with an increased rate of falls, while a walking speed between 0.7–1.0 m/s is characteristic of well-functioning board and care residents.

The score on the MMSE should be interpreted cautiously. It may be affected by level of education and, to a lesser degree, by impairments in hearing and vision. A score of less than 24 in a resident who has had at least a high school education

Table 3-7 Assessing capacity of decision-making

Determine whether residents:
- Understand relevant information
- Manipulate information rationally
- Communicate choices

should lead to further investigation, but does not necessarily make the diagnosis of dementia. Among residents with less than a high school education, 18 is a better cutoff score. NH residents with mental status scores at the borderline of normal may appear to function well because of assistance in daily activities that is being given by a spouse or other person. If this help is lost, the patient's functional disabilities related to mental impairment may become more prominent. This has significance in a board and care facility, where regulations require that residents have the capacity to respond to emergencies. Thus, the discovery of mental impairment on the MMSE does not necessarily call for an immediate intervention but should alert the caregiver and prompt reevaluation if a source of support is lost. The short portable mental state questionnaire (SPMSQ) is a 10-item test that may serve as an alternative to the MMSE. This instrument is, however, less sensitive. Depression can be screened by a single, simple question: "Do you often feel sad or depressed?" However, this can also serve as an introduction to a more detailed investigation. Patients who respond affirmatively should be tested with the GDS (see Chapter 14). The capacity to make decisions is assessed utilizing a clinical approach described in **Table 3-7,** and the determination should indicate whether or not the resident is capable of making decisions of all levels of complexity, capable of participating in decision-making with recommendations to involve the designated proxy for more complex decisions, or lacks the capacity requiring proxy involvement in all decisions (see also Chapter 27).

A comprehensive preadmission assessment can become the cornerstone of the patient's care plan in the NH. The physician can summarize the multidisciplinary preadmission assessment in a dictated report. The report should be clear,

Table 3-8 Format of preadmission consultation/evaluation

Patient identification
Reason for consultation/evaluation
Primary care physician
Referral source
Summary of assessments
  Active medical problems
  Functional problems
    Rehabilitation potential
    Capacity to make health care decisions
  Psychosocial problems

Recommendations/plans
  Limit to five focusing on management
Data base following traditional format
  Present history
  Past medical history
  Symptom review
  Results of functional status assessments
  Physical examination

SECTION I. DISEASE DIAGNOSES

Check only those diseases that have a relationship to current ADL status, cognitive status, mood and behavior status, medical treatments, nursing monitoring, or risk of death. (Do not list inactive diagnoses)

1.	DISEASES	*(If none apply, CHECK the NONE OF ABOVE box)*			
		ENDOCRINE/METABOLIC/ NUTRITIONAL		Hemiplegia/Hemiparesis	v.
				Multiple sclerosis	w.
		Diabetes mellitus	a.	Paraplegia	x.
		Hyperthyroidism	b.	Parkinson's disease	y.
		Hypothyroidism	c.	Quadriplegia	z.
		HEART/CIRCULATION		Seizure disorder	aa.
		Arteriosclerotic heart disease (ASHD)	d.	Transient ischemic attack (TIA)	bb.
				Traumatic brain injury	cc.
		Cardiac dysrhythmias	e.	**PSYCHIATRIC/MOOD**	
		Congestive heart failure	f.	Anxiety disorder	dd.
		Deep vein thrombosis	g.	Depression	ee.
		Hypertension	h.	Manic depression (bipolar disease)	ff.
		Hypotension	i.		
		Peripheral vascular disease	j.	Schizophrenia	gg.
		Other cardiovascular disease	k.	**PULMONARY**	
		MUSCULOSKELETAL		Asthma	hh.
		Arthritis	l.	Emphysema/COPD	ii.
		Hip fracture	m.	**SENSORY**	
		Missing limb (e.g., amputation)	n.	Cataracts	jj.
		Osteoporosis	o.	Diabetic retinopathy	kk.
		Pathological bone fracture	p.	Glaucoma	ll.
		NEUROLOGICAL		Macular degeneration	mm.
		Alzheimer's disease	q.	**OTHER**	
		Aphasia	r.	Allergies	nn.
		Cerebral palsy	s.	Anemia	oo.
		Cerebrovascular accident (stroke)	t.	Cancer	pp.
				Renal failure	qq.
		Dementia other than Alzheimer's disease	u.	*NONE OF ABOVE*	rr.
2.	INFECTIONS	*(If none apply, CHECK the NONE OF ABOVE box)*			
		Antibiotic resistant infection (e.g., Methicillin resistant staph)	a.	Septicemia	g.
				Sexually transmitted diseases	h.
		Clostridium difficile (c. diff.)	b.	Tuberculosis	i.
		Conjunctivitis	c.	Urinary tract infection **in last 30 days**	j.
		HIV infection	d.	Viral hepatitis	k.
		Pneumonia	e.	Wound infection	l.
		Respiratory infection	f.	NONE OF ABOVE	m.
3.	OTHER CURRENT OR MORE DETAILED DIAGNOSES AND ICD-9 CODES	a. ______	| | | |•| |		
		b. ______	| | | |•| |		
		c. ______	| | | |•| |		
		d. ______	| | | |•| |		
		e. ______	| | | |•| |		

Figure 3-1 MDS section on diagnosis.

summarizing the problems in a concise, organized manner, with no more than five recommendations. Recommendations should preferably focus on management rather than diagnostics. The report should include statements regarding the patient's prognosis, rehabilitation potential, and capacity for making health care decisions. **Table 3-8** presents a suggested format for the report. The report is meant to serve the primary care physician as well as the NH staff.

SECTION J. HEALTH CONDITIONS

1.	PROBLEM CONDITIONS	***(Check all problems present in last 7 days** unless other time frame is indicated)*			
		INDICATORS OF FLUID STATUS		Dizziness/Vertigo	f.
				Edema	g.
		Weight gain or loss of 3 or more pounds within a 7 day period	a.	Fever	h.
				Hallucinations	i.
				Internal bleeding	j.
		Inability to lie flat due to shortness of breath	b.	Recurrent lung aspirations in **last 90 days**	k.
		Dehydrated; output exceeds input	c.	Shortness of breath	l.
				Syncope (fainting)	m.
		Insufficient fluid; did **NOT** consume all/almost all liquids provided during **last 3 days**	d.	Unsteady gait	n.
				Vomiting	o.
		OTHER		*NONE OF ABOVE*	p.
		Delusions	e.		
2.	PAIN SYMPTOMS	*(Code the **highest level of pain** present in the **last 7 days**)*			
		a. FREQUENCY with which resident complains or shows evidence of pain 0. No pain ***(skip to J4)*** 1. Pain less than daily 2. Pain daily		**b. INTENSITY** of pain 1. Mild pain 2. Moderate pain 3. Times when pain is horrible or excruciating	
3.	PAIN SITE	***(If pain present, check all sites** that apply **in last 7 days**)*			
		Back pain	a.	Incisional pain	f.
		Bone pain	b.	Joint pain (other than hip)	g.
		Chest pain while doing usual activities	c.	Soft tissue pain (e.g., lesion, muscle)	h.
		Headache	d.	Stomach pain	i.
		Hip pain	e.	Other	j.
4.	ACCIDENTS	***(Check all that apply)***			
		Fell in **past 30 days**	a.	Hip fracture in **last 180 days**	c.
		Fell in **past 31-180 days**	b.	Other fracture in **last 180 days**	d.
				NONE OF ABOVE	e.
5.	STABILITY OF CONDITIONS	Conditions/diseases make resident's cognitive, ADL, mood or behavior patterns unstable—(fluctuating, precarious, or deteriorating)			a.
		Resident experiencing an acute episode or a flare-up of a recurrent or chronic-problem			b.
		End-stage disease, 6 or fewer months to live			c.
		NONE OF ABOVE			d.

Figure 3-2 MDS section on health problems.

SECTION P. SPECIAL TREATMENTS AND PROCEDURES

1. SPECIAL TREATMENTS, PROCEDURES, AND PROGRAMS

a. SPECIAL CARE—*Check treatments or programs received during the last 14 days* [Note—count only post admission treatments]

TREATMENTS			
Chemotherapy	a.	Ventilator or respirator	l.
Dialysis	b.	**PROGRAMS**	
IV medication	c.	Alcohol/drug treatment program	m.
Intake/output	d.	Alzheimer's/dementia special care unit	n.
Monitoring acute medical condition	e.	Hospice care	o.
Ostomy care	f.	Pediatric unit	p.
Oxygen therapy	g.	Respite care	q.
Radiation	h.	Training in skills required to return to the community (e.g., taking medications, house work, shopping, transportation, ADLs)	r.
Suctioning	i.		
Tracheostomy care	j.		
Transfusions	k.	*NONE OF ABOVE*	s.

b. THERAPIES - *Record the number of days and total minutes each of the following therapies was administered (for at least 15 minutes a day) in the* ***last 7 calendar days*** *(Enter 0 if none or less than 15 min. daily)* **[Note—count only post admission therapies]**

(A) = # of days administered for **15 minutes or more**
(B) = total # of minutes provided in **last 7 days**

	DAYS (A)	MIN (B)
a. Speech - language pathology and audiology services		
b. Occupational therapy		
c. Physical therapy		
d. Respiratory therapy		
e. Psychological therapy (by any licensed mental health professional)		

2. INTERVENTION PROGRAMS FOR MOOD, BEHAVIOR, COGNITIVE LOSS

(Check all interventions or strategies used in last 7 days—no matter where received)

Special behavior symptom evaluation program	a.
Evaluation by a licensed mental health specialist in **last 90 days**	b.
Group therapy	c.
Resident-specific deliberate changes in the environment to address mood/behavior patterns—e.g., providing bureau in which to rummage	d.
Reorientation—e.g., cueing	e.
NONE OF ABOVE	f.

3. NURSING REHABILITATION/RESTORATIVE CARE

Record the NUMBER OF DAYS each of the following rehabilitation or restorative techniques or practices was ***provided to the resident for more than or equal to 15 minutes per day in the last 7 days*** *(Enter 0 if none or less than 15 min. daily.)*

a. Range of motion (passive)		f. Walking	
b. Range of motion (active)		g. Dressing or grooming	
c. Splint or brace assistance		h. Eating or swallowing	
TRAINING AND SKILL PRACTICE IN:		i. Amputation/prosthesis care	
d. Bed mobility		j. Communication	
e. Transfer		k. Other	

4. DEVICES AND RESTRAINTS

(*Use the following codes for* ***last 7 days:***)
0. Not used
1. Used less than daily
2. Used daily

Bed rails	
a. —Full bed rails on all open sides of bed	
b. —Other types of side rails used (e.g., half rail, one side)	
c. Trunk restraint	
d. Limb restraint	
e. Chair prevents rising	

Figure 3-3 MDS section on treatments.

SECTION Q. DISCHARGE POTENTIAL AND OVERALL STATUS

1.	DISCHARGE POTENTIAL	a. Resident expresses/indicates preference to return to the community 0. No 1. Yes	
		b. Resident has a support person who is positive towards discharge 0. No 1. Yes	
		c. Stay projected to be of a short duration—discharge projected **within 90 days** (do not include expected discharge due to death) 0. No 2. Within 31-90 days 1. Within 30 days 3. Discharge status uncertain	
2.	OVERALL CHANGE IN CARE NEEDS	Resident's overall self sufficiency has changed significantly as compared to status of **90 days ago** (or since last assessment if less than 90 days) 0. No change 1. Improved—receives fewer supports, needs less restrictive level of care 2. Deteriorated—receives more support	

Figure 3-4 MDS section on discharge potential.

It is always important to remember that even in cases where the assessment team is employed by the institution, the team is ethically obligated to provide any useful information to the patients and their caregivers in the event that the individual is not admitted to the institution.

MINIMUM DATA SET (MDS)

Physician input is essential for data in the MDS, which needs to be completed within 14 days of NH admission. **Figure 3-1** illustrates Section I on diagnoses. **Figure 3-2** illustrates Section J on signs and symptoms. **Figure 3-3** lists the recommended interventions and disposition. Physician determination of discharge potential is useful for discharge planning (**see Fig. 3-4**).

SUGGESTED READINGS

Alexopoulos GS, Abrams RC, Young RC, Shamoian CA: Use of the Cornell Scale in nondemented patients. *J Am Geriatr Soc* 36:230–236, 1988.

Applebaum, PS, Grisso, T: Assessing patients' capacities to consent to treatment. *N Engl J Med* 319:1635–1638, 1988.

Applegate WB, Blass JP, Williams TF: Instruments for the functional assessment of older patients. *N Engl J Med* 322:1207–1212, 1990.

Lachs MS, Feinstein AR, Cooney LM, et al: A simple procedure for general screening for functional disability in elderly patients. *Ann Intern Med* 112:699–706, 1990.

Munso-Ashman J: Geriatric assessment—An Australian idea. *Soc Sci Med* 29:939–942, 1989.

Osterweil D, Martin M, Syndulko K: Predictors of skilled nursing placement in a multilevel long-term-care facility. *J Am Geriatr Soc* 43:108–112, 1995.

Siu AL, Hays RD, Ouslander JG, et al: Measuring functioning and health in the very old. *J Gerontol:Med Sci* 48:M10–M14, 1993.

Williams ME, Hornberger JC: A quantitative method of identifying older persons at risk for increasing long term care services. *J Chronic Dis* 37:705–711, 1986.

CHAPTER
FOUR

HEALTH MAINTENANCE, SCREENING, AND PREVENTIVE PRACTICES

This chapter provides several recommendations for practices related to health maintenance, screening, and prevention in the nursing home (NH) setting. These recommendations must be prefaced by several general comments. First, with few exceptions, the efficacy and cost-effectiveness of the recommendations presented herein have not been well studied. For the most part, they reflect the authors' opinions and judgments on the basis of current knowledge, best standards of care, practicality, and cost. Second, not all of the practices recommended are relevant for all NH residents. As discussed in Chapter 2 and depicted in Figs. 2-3 through 2-9, NH residents are heterogeneous. Thus, for example, recommendations for health maintenance and screening are generally not relevant for residents who are in the NH for short-term rehabilitation or terminal care. Third, while some of the practices recommended are mandated by federal and/or state guidelines, they are time-consuming and inadequately reimbursed. It is therefore critical that these practices be incorporated, to the extent possible, in the general context of medical practice in the NH and, where relevant, in the policies and procedures of the facility.

Before outlining the specific practices, we present a brief overview of the general context of medical care in the NH. It is within this context that the recommended medical practices should be implemented.

THE GENERAL CONTEXT OF MEDICAL PRACTICE IN THE NURSING HOME

Physicians whose practice is primarily in the NH are the exception rather than the rule. Most physicians visit NHs on a monthly basis—more often if they care for

Table 4-1 Summary of federal regulations relevant to primary care physicians in nursing homes

Regulation	Interpretation
A physician must personally approve in writing a recommendation that an individual be admitted to a facility. Each resident must remain under the care of a physician	A physician's "personal approval" of an admission recommendation must be in written form. The physician's admission orders will be accepted as "personal approval" of the admission.
Physician supervision The facility must ensure that: (1) The medical care of each resident is supervised by a physician; and (2) Another physician supervises the medical care of residents when their attending physician is unavailable.	"Supervising the medical care of residents" means participating in the resident's assessment and care planning, monitoring changes in resident's medical status, and providing consultation or treatment when called by the facility. It also includes, but is not limited to, prescribing new therapy, ordering a resident's transfer to the hospital, conducting required routine visits or delegating and supervising follow-up visits to nurse practitioners or physician assistants.
Physician visits The physician must: (1) Review the resident's total program of care, including medications and treatments at each required visit (2) Write, sign, and date progress notes at each visit; and (3) Sign and date all orders.	The intent of this regulation is to have the physician take an active role in supervising the care of residents. This should not be a superficial visit, but should include an evaluation of the resident's condition and a review of and decision about the continued appropriateness of the resident's current medical regime. Total program of care includes all care the facility provides residents to maintain or improve their highest practicable mental and physical functional status, as defined by the comprehensive assessment and plan of care. Care includes medical services and medication management, physical, occupational, and speech/language therapy, nursing care, nutritional interventions, social work and activity services that maintain or improve psychosocial functioning. The physician records resident's progress and problems in maintaining or improving their mental and physical functional status. The physician need not review the total plan of care at each visit, but must review the total plan of care at required visits. In cases where facilities have created the option for a resident's record to be maintained by computer, rather than hard copy, electronic signatures are acceptable.

<table>
<tr>
<td></td>
<td>Physician orders may be transmitted by facsimile machine if the following conditions are met:
• The physician should have signed and retained the original copy of the order from which the facsimile was transmitted and be able to provide it upon request. Alternatively, the original may be sent to the facility at a later time and substituted for the facsimile.
• The facility should photocopy the faxed order since some facsimiles fade over time. The facsimile copy can be discarded after facility photocopies it.
• A facility using such a system should establish adequate safeguards to assure that it is not subject to abuse.
• It is not necessary for a physician to re-sign the facsimile order when he/she visits the facility.</td>
</tr>
<tr>
<td>Frequency of physician visits
(1) The resident must be seen by a physician at least once every 30 days for the first 90 days after admission, and at least once every 60 days thereafter
(2) A physician visit is considered timely if it occurs not later than 10 days after the date the visit was required
(3) All required physician visits must be made by the physician personally, except if NPs, PAs, or clinical nurse specialist are approved by the State to perform selected visits.
(4) At the option of the physician, required visits in SNFs, after the initial visit, may alternate between personal visits by the physician and visits by a PA, NP or clinical nurse specialist.</td>
<td>“Must be seen” means that the physician must make actual face-to-face contact with the resident. There is no requirement for this type of contact at the time of admission, since the decision to admit an individual to a nursing facility (whether from a hospital or from the individual’s own residence) generally involves physician contact during the period immediately preceding the admission.

After the initial physician visit in SNFs, where States allow their use, a qualified NP, PA, or clinical nurse specialist may make every other required visit (See Chapter 9).

In a NF, the physician visit requirement, in accord with State law, may be satisfied by NP, PA, or clinical nurse specialist.

The timing of physician visits is based on the admission date of the resident. Visits will be made within the first 30 days, and then at 30-day intervals up until 90 days after the admission date. Visits will then be at 60-day intervals. Permitting up to 10 days slippage of a due date will not affect the next due date. The regulation states that the physician (or his/her delegate) must visit the resident at least every 30 or 60 days. There is no provision for physicians to use discretion in visiting at intervals longer than those specified.

Policy that allows an NP, PA, or clinical nurse specialist to make every other required visit, and that allows a 10-day slippage in the time of the visit, does not relieve the physician of the obligation to visit a resident when the resident’s medical condition makes that visit necessary.</td>
</tr>
</table>

Table 4-1 (*Continued*)

	It is expected that visits will occur at the facility rather than the doctor's office unless office equipment is needed or a resident specifically requests an office visit. If the facility has established policy that residents leave the grounds for medical care, the resident does not object, and this policy does not infringe on his/her rights, there is no prohibition to this practice. The facility should inform the resident of this practice. When a PA, NP, or clinical nurse specialist performs a delegated physician visit, and determines that the resident's condition warrants direct contact between the physician and the resident, the physician must follow-up promptly with a personal visit.
Availability of physicians for emergency care The facility must provide or arrange for the provision of physician services 24 hours a day, in case of an emergency.	If a resident's own physician is unavailable, the facility should attempt to contact that physician's designated referral physician before assuming the responsibility of assigning a physician. Arranging for physician services may include assuring resident transportation to a hospital emergency room/ward or other medical facility if the facility is unable to provide medical care at the facility.

a substantial number of residents in a particular facility. Thus, if standard approaches to health maintenance, screening, and prevention are to be implemented consistently, the facility must develop appropriate policies, procedures, and documentation practices and convey them to the primary medical staff. This is one of the critical responsibilities of the medical director, as discussed in Chapter 6. Examples of specific policies and documentation formats are presented in the Appendix.

Table 4-1 outlines federal regulations relevant to the primary care physician role in NHs. **Table 4-2** outlines the areas covered by the federally mandated Minimum Data Set (MDS) and resident assessment protocols (RAPs).

Table 4-3 outlines key aspects of the various types of medical assessments performed by primary care physicians in NHs. Physicians assess NH residents in four general contexts: (1) an initial assessment within the first few days of NH admission; (2) periodic assessments, generally performed monthly; (3) assessment of acute or subacute changes in status on an as-needed basis; and (4) a major reassessment of long-staying residents, generally done annually.

The initial assessment has several important objectives (**Table 4-3**). Because NH residents are frequently admitted and readmitted to the NH from an acute care hospital, previous hospital histories and physicals and/or discharge summaries are commonly used in the admission assessment. Because these hospital summaries too often omit data that are critical to the NH plan of care, we recommend that a separate assessment be documented, including such information as the resident's chronic medical conditions, psychosocial status and functional capabilities. In addition, we recommend that a medical face sheet be completed (or revised in the case of a readmission), which summarizes critical information in an easily readable format. Examples of an admission assessment data base and Medical Face Sheet are included in the Appendix. As discussed in Chapter 26, these documents can be incorporated into a standard computer format for easy updating; they can also be linked to a data base for quality-assurance purposes. An extremely important component of the initial assessment process is the determination and documentation of treatment status decisions, including decisions about the intensity of care to be given should the resident become acutely ill. This is a complex yet important area that is discussed in detail in Chapter 27. The Appendix includes examples of policies, procedures, and documentation formats relevant to this process. The time necessary to complete the initial assessment will depend on the admitting physician's prior knowledge of the resident. If, as is often the case, there is a change in physician, information from prior physicians and acute care hospitalizations are critical and should be requested from appropriate sources. Since many NH residents cycle between an acute care hospital and the NH, it may not be necessary to repeat the entire initial assessment data base at the time of readmission. A concise readmission note and updating of the medical face sheet will generally suffice after a brief hospital stay. Strategies for communication and documentation between the hospital and the NH are discussed further in Chapter 5.

Table 4-2 Areas covered by the Minimum Data Set and resident assessment protocols[a]

Sections of the Minimum Data Set	Problems addressed by resident assessment protocols	Discipline(s) responsible for completion[c]
Demographic and background information (includes advanced directives)		Medical record staff, nursing
Cognitive patterns[b]	Delirium	Nursing
	Cognitive loss or dementia	Social work
Communication/hearing patterns	Communication	Nursing, audiology, and speech therapy
Vision patterns	Visual function	Nursing, optometry
Physical functioning[b]	Activities of daily living, functional rehabilitation potential, falls	Occupational therapy
		Physical therapy
Continence[b]	Urinary incontinence/indwelling catheter	Nursing
Psychosocial well-being	Psychosocial well-being (feelings about self and social relationships)	Nursing
		Social work, psychology
Mood and behavior[b]	Mood state (depression, anxiety)	Nursing
	Behavior problems (wandering, verbal abuse, physical aggression)	Social work
		Psychology
Activity pursuit patterns	Activity (inactivity, lack of participation)	Activities
Disease diagnoses[b]		Nursing
Health conditions		Nursing
Oral/nutritional status[b]	Nutritional status	Nursing
	Feeding tubes	Dietary
	Dehydration/fluid maintenance	
Oral/dental status	Dental care	Dental
Skin condition	Pressure ulcers	Nursing
Medication use[b]	Psychotropic drug use	Nursing, psychology, psychiatry
Special treatments and procedures (dialysis, intravenous medications, restraints)	Physical restraints	Nursing

[a]The Minimum Data Set must be completed within 14 days of admission. Selected items of the Minimum Data Set are intended to trigger use of one or more resident assessment protocols to assess specific problems in residents (see text).

[b]Area must be updated quarterly.

[c]The physician should be involved in the assessment of all problems identified on the Minimum Data Set that trigger use of a resident assessment protocol (see text).

Table 4-3 Important aspects of various types of medical assessment in the nursing home

Type of Assessment	Timing	Major objectives	Important aspects
Initial	Within 48 hours of admission	Verify medical diagnoses Document baseline physical findings, mental and functional status, vital signs, and skin condition Attempt to identify potentially remediable, previously unrecognized medical conditions Get to know the resident and family (if this is a new resident) Establish goals for the admission and a medical treatment plan	A thorough review of medical records and physical examination are necessary Relevant medical diagnoses and baseline findings should be clearly and concisely documented in the medical record Medication lists should be carefully reviewed and only essential medications continued Requests for specific types of assessment and inputs from other disciplines should be made An initial medical problem list should be documented (see example of Medical Face Sheet in Appendix) Treatment status (i.e., No CPR, etc.) should be documented (See Chapter 27 and Appendix)
Periodic	Usually monthly	Monitor progress of active conditions Update medical orders Communicate with resident and nursing home staff	Progress notes should include clinical data relevant to active medical conditions and focus on changes in status (**See Table 4-2**) Unnecessary medications, orders for care, and laboratory tests should be discontinued Mental, functional, and psychosocial status should be reviewed with nursing staff and changes from baseline noted The medical problem list should be updated

Table 4-3 (*Continued*)

Type of Assessment	Timing	Major objectives	Important aspects
As needed	When acute changes in status occur	Identify and treat causes of acute changes	On-site clinical assessment by the physician (or nurse practitioner or physician's assistant), as opposed to telephone consultation, will result in more accurate diagnoses, more appropriate treatment, and fewer unnecessary emergency room visits and hospitalization Vital signs, food and fluid intake, and mental status often provide essential information Infection, dehydration, and adverse drug effects should be at the top of the differential diagnosis for acute changes in status Treatment status (i.e., No CPR, etc.) should be reviewed if appropriate
Major reassessment	Annual	Identify and document any significant changes in status and new potentially remediable conditions, including review of the most recent MDS and RAPs which have been triggered	Targeted physical examination and assessment of mental, functional, and psychosocial status and selected laboratory tests should be done (**See Table 4-6**)

Table 4-4 "SOAP" format and key data for medical progress notes on nursing home residents

Subjective	New complaints
	Symptoms related to active medical conditions
	Reports from nursing staff
	Progress in rehabilitative therapy
Objective	General appearance
	Weight
	Vital signs
	Physical findings relevant to new complaints and active medical conditions
	Reports of other interdisciplinary team members (if relevant)
	Laboratory data
	Consultant reports
Assessment	Presumptive diagnosis(es) for new complaints or changes in status
	Stability of active medical conditions
	Response to interventions, especially psychotropic medications and rehabilitative therapy
Plans	Changes in medications or diet
	Nursing interventions (e.g., monitoring of vital signs, skin care)
	Assessments by other disciplines (e.g., physical therapists, consultants)
	Laboratory studies
	Discharge planning (if relevant)

See Appendix for an alternative standardized format for routine medical progress notes.

We recommend that NH residents generally be reassessed on a monthly basis. **Table 4-4** outlines a "SOAP" (subjective, objective, assessment, plans) format and key data for routine medical progress notes on NH residents. The Appendix includes an alternative standardized format for a routine progress note. If legibility is a problem, these notes can be dictated. Software is now available that can be used to format the progress notes and make the process more efficient for physicians who favor computers. Particular attention should be paid to the monitoring practices discussed below and to discontinuing or modifying outdated orders. Physicians' order sheets should be printed in an organized format to facilitate efficient but thorough review. Physicians need to be aware that in most nursing homes physician orders are transcribed to a medication administration sheet. Regular review of the nurses' medical sheet is essential as it may vary substantially from the order sheet. Routine rounds are best made with a nurse who knows the residents well. Nurse's notes and medication records should be reviewed. In our experience, monthly visits that encompass these recommended procedures on relatively stable residents take 15 to 25 minutes per resident. We also recommend that, on a periodic basis—quarterly, for example—interdisciplinary rounds be conducted with nursing, social service, and other staff to facilitate review of residents' progress. This will also enhance communication about residents whose status has changed or who have particularly difficult and complex problems.

Acute and subacute changes in status occur commonly among NH residents. They are relevant to the focus of this chapter in that many of these changes will result in new problems (which should be added to problem lists), new medications, a reevaluation of treatment status (i.e., CPR, etc.), and conditions that require monitoring, as described below. Since assessment of these acute or subacute changes is often done by telephone, it is important for the physician to document important events the next time they are in the facility. The management of acute and subacute conditions in the NH is discussed further in Chapters 5, 6 and 9.

The value of the annual history and physical examination in the NH population has been questioned. We suggest there are several important reasons to recommend some type of annual reassessment for long-staying NH residents. First, most of these residents do not undergo a thorough physical examination on routine visits. Thus, an annual physical examination is important to detect and document changes and conditions that may require intervention. Second, it affords an opportunity to thoroughly reassess the resident's functional status and to screen for changes in cognitive, affective, and social status that may require intervention. Third, an annual panel of screening tests is probably warranted in most NH residents and can be performed or ordered at the time of the annual reassessment. Recommendations for these screening practices are outlined below. A suggested format for documenting the annual review is included in the Appendix.

MONITORING

Table 4-5 lists examples of practices we recommend for periodic monitoring in selected residents. These practices focus on the management of common chronic medical conditions in the NH population, such as diabetes, cardiovascular disorders, arthritis, and anemia. Because many serious problems can develop insidiously and are commonly asymptomatic, we recommend these practices as an adjunct to the monthly visit. Examples of these problems include weight loss, dehydration, hyper- and hypoglycemia, hypo- or hypernatremia, azotemia, upper gastrointestinal bleeding from nonsteroidal anti-inflammatory drugs (NSAIDs), anemia, behavioral changes including depression and agitation, and drug toxicity. Appropriate policies on monitoring should help identify these conditions before serious consequences occur and can be a key component of a medical quality assurance program.

SCREENING

Recommendations for screening practices vary considerably among different patient populations and are highly debated in the medical literature. Very few

Table 4-5 Examples of periodic monitoring practices in selected nursing home residents

Practice	Recommended frequency[a]	Comments
All residents:		
Vital signs, including weight	Monthly	More often if unstable or subacutely ill
Diabetics:		
Fasting and postprandial glucose and/or glycosylated hemoglobin	Monthly	More often if unstable Fingerstick tests may also be useful if staff can perform reliably
Residents on diuretics or with renal insufficiency (creatinine > 2 mg/dl, or BUN[b] > 35 mg/dl):		
Electrolytes, BUN creatinine	Every 2–3 months	Nursing home residents are more vulnerable to dehydration, azotemia, hyponatremia, and hypokalemia
Residents on non-steroidal antiinflammatory (NSAID) drugs:		
Hemoglobin/hematocrit, stool for occult blood	Every 1–2 months	Bleeding frequently asymptomatic
Anemic residents who are on iron replacement or who have hemoglobin < 10 g:		
Hemoglobin/hematocrit	Monthly until stable, then every 2–3 months	Iron replacement should generally be discontinued once hemoglobin value stabilizes
Blood level of drug for residents on specific drugs, e.g.:		
Digoxin Dilantin Lithium Quinidine Procainamide Theophylline Nortriptyline	Every 3–6 months	More frequently if drug treatment has just been initiated or dosage adjusted

[a]Data for the efficacy and timing of these practices are limited.
[b]BUN, blood urea nitrogen.

Table 4-6 Examples of screening practices in the nursing home

Practice	Frequency	Comments
History and physical examination	Yearly	Generally required, but yield of routine annual history and physical is debated Focused exam probably beneficial, including assessment of mental status, skin condition, rectal exam, breast exam, and, pelvic exam in selected women
Weight	Monthly	Generally weight loss should prompt a search for treatable medical, psychiatric, and functional conditions (See Chapter 14)
Functional status assessment, including gait and cognitive function, basic activities of daily living, and screening for depression	Yearly	Functional status assessed periodically by staff Systematic global functional assessment should be done at least yearly in order to document changes in status, detect potentially treatable conditions or prevent complications (See Appendix for examples of assessment techniques)
Visual testing	Yearly	Assess acuity, and identify correctable problems
Hearing testing	Yearly	Identify correctable problems
Dental	Yearly	Assess status of any remaining teeth, fit of dentures, and identify any pathology
Podiatry	Yearly	More frequently in diabetics and residents with peripheral vascular disease Identify correctable problems and ensure appropriateness of shoes
Tuberculosis	On admission and yearly	All residents and staffshould be tested Booster testing is recommended for the first test in nursing home residents (See Chapter 19)
Laboratory tests Stool for occult blood Complete blood count Fasting glucose Electrolytes Renal function tests Albumin, calcium, phosphorus Thyroid function tests	Yearly	These tests appear to have reasonable yield in the nursing home population
Chest radiograph	On admission if recent radiograph not available	May be helpful as baseline
Electrocardiogram	On admission if recent tracing not available	May be helpful as baseline
Mammography	Yearly	May benefit some women; those at high risk and those who would receive curative therapy if cancer discovered

studies have addressed the cost-effectiveness of screening in the NH population, and no specific recommendations for screening in the NH have been put forth by any organization.

Table 4-6 lists recommendations for what we believe to be reasonable screening practices in the NH setting. Obviously these recommendations apply only to the long-staying subgroup of NH residents. The assumptions underlying these recommendations are as follows: (1) even among very old NH residents with varying degrees of physical functional and cognitive impairments, remediable conditions can be identified, such as depression and incontinence; (2) screening for conditions such as weight loss, inadequate dentition, podiatric problems, and gait instability may lead to interventions that will prevent complications from malnutrition and falls; (3) the identification of depression, visual and auditory disturbances, and dental problems is critical for maximizing quality of life; (4) screening for tuberculosis may prevent outbreaks in a susceptible resident population and among staff who in many areas are immigrants from other countries; and (5) selected laboratory tests may be beneficial but should be limited to those tests whose abnormal results would lead to a specific intervention (e.g., further evaluation of anemia, institution of thyroid replacement therapy). Note that annual chest radiographs and electrocardiograms are not recommended; there are no data to support their inclusion and they are very expensive, especially when the national costs of such recommendations are calculated.

The Appendix contains a sample format for documenting the results of the annual review. Examples of commonly used assessments for functional and mental status, depression, and gait are included in relevant chapters throughout the text.

PREVENTION

While it may seem unusual to think of preventive practices in the NH, there are actually several that are relevant in this setting. Examples are listed in **Table 4-7**. Many preventive practices relate to infections and infection control, topics covered in more detail in Chapter 19. Because of the extreme immobility of many NH residents, body repositioning and range-of-motion exercises are important aspects of care to prevent pressure sores, contractures, and aspiration. The monitoring of environmental safety and the ongoing evaluation of accidents are critical quality assurance functions in every facility. This type of surveillance is designed to prevent, to the extent possible, unnecessary accidents and injuries among residents, staff, and visitors. Computer databases which allow regular review of trends in accidents such as falls can enhance the preventive potential of this type of monitoring.

Table 4-7 Examples of preventive practices in the nursing home

Practice	Frequency[a]	Comments
Influenza vaccine	Yearly	All residents and staff with close resident contact should be vaccinated
Antiviral agents amantadine/ rimandidine	Within 24–48 hours of outbreak of suspected influenza A	Dose should be reduced to 100 mg per day in elderly; further reduction if renal failure present Unvaccinated residents and staff should be treated throughout outbreak (See Chapter 19)
Pneumococcal vaccine	Once	Efficacy in nursing home residents has not been well studied
Tetanus booster	Every 10 years, or every 5 years with tetanus-prone wounds	Many elderly people have not received primary vaccinations; they require tetanus toxoid, 250–500 units of tetanus immune globulin, and completion of the immunization series with toxoid injection 4–6 weeks later and then 6–12 months after the second injection (See Chapter 19)
Tuberculosis prophylaxis	Skin test conversion in selected residents	Residents with pulmonary disease, diabetes, end-stage renal disease, hematological malignancies, steroid or immunosuppressive therapy, or malnutrition should be treated (See Chapter 19)
Antimicrobial prophylaxis for residents at risk	Generally recommended for dental procedures, genitourinary procedures, and most operative procedures (See Chapter 19 for details)	Chronically catheterized residents should not be treated with continuous prophylaxis (See Chapter 19)
Body positioning and range of motion for immobile residents	Ongoing	Frequent turning of very immobile residents is necessary to prevent pressure sores Semi-upright position is necessary for residents with swallowing disorders or enteral feeding to help prevent aspiration Range of motion to immobile limbs and joints is necessary to prevent contractures
Infection control procedures and surveillance (See Chapter 19)	Ongoing	Policies and protocols should be in effect in all nursing homes Surveillance of all infections should be continuous to identify outbreaks and patterns
Environmental safety	Ongoing	Appropriate lighting, colors, and the removal of hazards for falling are essential in order to prevent accidents Routine monitoring of potential safety hazards and accidents may lead to alterations which may prevent further accidents

[a]Data for the efficacy and timing of these practices are limited.

SUGGESTED READINGS

American Geriatrics Society Clinical Practice Committee: *Position statement on screening for cervical carcinoma in the elderly.* New York, American Geriatrics Society, 1993.

American Geriatrics Society Clinical Practice Committee: *Position statement on screening for breast cancer in elderly women.* New York, American Geriatrics Society, 1993.

Applegate WB, Blass JP and Williams TF: Instruments for functional assessment of older patients. *N Engl J Med* 322:1207–1214, 1990.

Balducci L, Schapira DV, Cox CE, Greenberg HM and Hyman GH: Breast cancer of the older woman: An annotated review. *J Am Geriatr Soc* 39:1113–1123, 1991.

Domoto K, Ben R, Wei JY, et al: Yield of routine annual laboratory screening in the institutionalized elderly. *Am J Public Health* 75:243–245, 1985.

Elon R and Pawlson GL: The impact of OBRA on medical practice within nursing facilities. *J Am Geriatr Soc* 40:958–963, 1992.

Fleming KC, Evans JM, Weber DC, and Chutka DS: Practical functional assessment of elderly persons: A primary-care approach. *Mayo Clin Proc* 70:890–910, 1995.

Gambert SR, Duthie EH, and Wiltzius F: The value of the yearly medical evaluation in a nursing home. *J Chronic Dis* 35:65–68, 1982.

Irvine PW, Carlson K, Adcock M, et al: The value of annual medical examinations in the nursing home. *J Am Geriatr Soc* 32:540–545, 1984.

Joseph C and Lyles Y: Routine laboratory assessment of nursing home patients. *J Am Geriatr Soc* 40:98–100, 1992.

Lachs MS, Feinstein AR, Cooney Jr, LM, Drickamer MA, et al: A simple procedure for general screening for functional disability in elderly patients. *Ann Int Med* 112:699–706, 1990.

Levenstein MR, Ouslander JG, Rubenstein LZ, et al: Yield of routine annual laboratory tests in a skilled nursing home population. *JAMA* 258:1909–1941, 1987.

Morris JN, Hawes C, Fries BE, Phillips CD, et al: Designing the national resident assessment instrument for nursing homes. *Gerontologist* 30:293–307, 1990.

Mulrow CD and Lichtenstein MJ: Screening for hearing impairment in the elderly: Rationale and strategy. *J Gen Int Med* 6:249–258, 1991.

Ouslander, JG and Osterweil D: Physician evaluation and management of nursing home residents. *Ann Intern Med* 121:584–592, 1994.

Patriarca PA, Arden NH, Koplan JP, and Goodman RA: Prevention and control of type A influenza infections in nursing homes. *Ann Intern Med* 107:732–740, 1987.

Siu A: Screening for dementia and its causes. *Ann Int Med* 115:122–132, 1991.

Wolf-Klein GP, Holt T, Silverstone FA, et al: Efficacy of routine annual studies in the care of elderly patients. *J Am Geriatr Soc* 33:325–329, 1985.

Woolf SH, Kamerow DB, Lawrence RS, Medalie JH, and Estes EH: The Periodic Health Examination of Older Adults: The recommendations of the U.S. Preventive Services Task Force. Part II Screening Tests. *J Am Geriatr Soc* 38:933–942, 1990.

Zimmerman DR, Karon SL, Arling G, et al: Developments and testing of nursing home quality indicators. *Health Care Financing Review* 16(No. 5):107–127, Summer 1995.

CHAPTER

FIVE

THE NURSING HOME–ACUTE CARE HOSPITAL INTERFACE

The interface between the nursing home (NH) and the acute care hospital is a dynamic one. Statistics are changing rapidly because of the growth of subacute care and a resultant increase in the severity of illness in the NH population. The acute care hospital, in part because of Medicare's 3-day-stay hospital requirement, is the source of many NH admissions. Viewed from the hospital's perspective, over 6 percent to 10 percent of hospitalized geriatric patients are discharged to a NH. The proportion is higher among women, those above age 80, patients with both physical and mental diagnoses, and patients who were admitted to the hospital from a NH. From the NH's perspective, approximately half of the residents admitted come from an acute care hospital. Once in the NH, approximately half stay just a few (1 to 6) months. Of those residents discharged alive, approximately half go to an acute care hospital. Many NH residents frequently bounce back and forth between one or more NHs and the acute care hospital. Reported hospitalization rates per NH bed per year during the 1980s varied from 0.21 to 0.55. **Figure 5-1** illustrates this dynamism of the NH–acute care hospital interface by depicting the natural history of a cohort of NH residents discharged after their first NH admission.

Transfer of a NH resident to an acute care hospital is a costly process. The costs are high not only in terms of the dollars spent (on transporting the resident to the acute care hospital, emergency room evaluation, hospital admission, and readmission to the NH) but also because hospitalization is often physically uncomfortable and emotionally traumatic for the NH resident and his or her loved ones. In addition, NH residents admitted to an acute care hospital are at

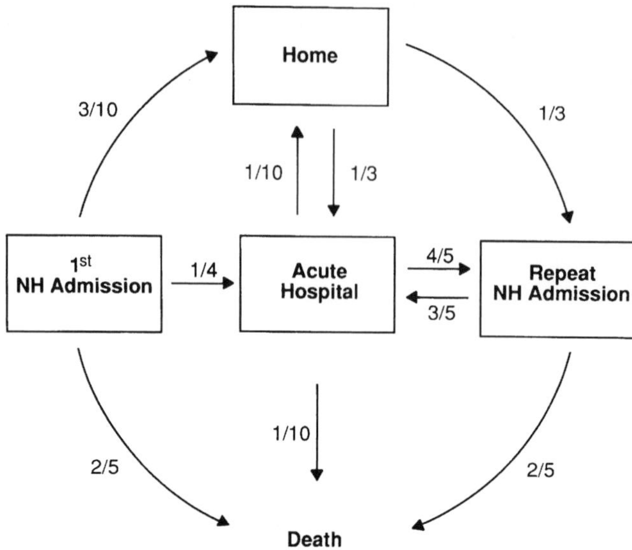

Figure 5-1 An example of the dynamic nature of the NH–acute hospital interface. The diagram represents the natural history of a cohort of NH residents after discharge from their first NH stay. Fractions represent approximate proportion moving from one status to another; not shown are about 5 percent of discharges that went from their first NH to another NH. (After Kane RL, Ouslander JG, and Abrass IB: *Essentials of Clinical Geriatrics*, 2d ed. New York, McGraw-Hill, 1989. Data source: Lewis MA, Cretin S, and Kane RL: The natural history of nursing home patients. *Gerontologist* 25:382–388, 1985.)

relatively high risk for iatrogenic complications such as delirium (e.g., "sundowning"), adverse drug reactions, falls, pressure sores, and complications from diagnostic and surgical procedures. The decision to hospitalize a NH resident is a complex one involving a myriad of considerations. The clinical status of the resident is, of course, paramount. Acute medical conditions must be treated unless an explicit decision has been made not to do so. Even in the latter instance, hospitalization may be necessary to provide optimal palliative and comfort care. Hospital-based NHs and many community facilities with "subacute" units are prepared to care for many of the common acute illnesses that frequently result in hospitalization, including infections, dehydration, gastrointestinal disorders, hip fractures, and decompensated chronic cardiac or pulmonary disease (**Table 5-1**). Most NHs, however, have limited capabilities in this regard. Factors such as financial incentives, the availability of ancillary services and trained nurses, the capability to provide on-site medical and mental health assessment and treatment, and ethical considerations all play a role in the hospitalization of NH residents. **Table 5-2** summarizes these factors and their implications. The purpose of this chapter is to briefly discuss several of the key

Table 5-1 Conditions most commonly responsible for the hospitalization of nursing home residents[a]

	% of residents hospitalized
Infection	10–49
Dehydration	<17>
Cardiovascular	10–16
Gastrointestinal	13–17
Fracture	7–9
Behavioral disorders[b]	5–10

[a]Based on the results of several published studies.
[b]Includes depression, delirium, disruptive behaviors.

issues surrounding the NH–hospital interface. The extreme variability in the relationship between NHs and their affiliated acute care hospitals makes specific recommendations difficult to offer. Several general recommendations are presented that might improve the appropriateness, process, and outcomes of the hospitalization of NH residents.

ECONOMIC CONSIDERATIONS

Outside of capitated systems of care, financial incentives strongly favor hospitalizing a NH resident who becomes acutely or subacutely ill. Reimbursement for adequate physician supervision and for the NH to provide subacute care is generally very limited. Hospital-based NHs get higher rates and can, to some extent, take advantage of economies of scale; community-based NHs with Medicare "distinct part" units can get higher reimbursement for subacute care. Such care within the NH may, however, result in logistically complex and emotionally disruptive movement of residents. At the same time, acute care hospitals with empty beds are more than willing to accept admissions from NHs, especially if the NH is willing and able to accept the patient back before he or she becomes a "DRG outlier" (a patient who has a length of stay substantially longer than the average for the admission DRG). Physicians are also reimbursed more for providing hospital as opposed to NH care.

One pilot demonstration project in Monroe County, New York, tested a Medicare "sudden decline" benefit. The benefit was instituted rapidly and provided reimbursement to both the NH and the physician to manage acute illness in the NH. The results of this demonstration project were promising, a larger randomized trials of such a strategy is underway to clearly demonstrate the cost-effectiveness of this approach.

Table 5-2 Factors surrounding the hospitalization of nursing home residents

Factors	Implications	Potential Strategies to Reduce Hospitalization	Caveats
Financial incentives	Physicians, NHs, and acute hospitals each potentially benefit financially by hospitalizing NH residents outside of capitated systems of care	Reasonable reimbursement for NHs and physicians to care for selected acutely ill residents in the NH setting Capitated systems of care provide a financial incentive to utilize the less costly NH environment	Acute hospitals with empty beds and substantial admissions from NHs may lose revenue The cost effectiveness of enhanced reimbursements for acute care in the NH has not been studied Criteria must be established so that residents who do require acute care are hospitalized
Availability of ancillary services	In order to effectively manage some acute illnesses in the NH, a variety of ancillary services, such as radiographs, blood drawing, respiratory therapy, must be available	Contract arrangements with local providers or acute hospitals for radiographs, blood drawing, laboratory testing, pharmacy supplies, respiratory therapy, etc.	These services may not be available locally to many NHs
Medical staff organization	Physicians are rarely present and often unwilling to visit the NH regularly Medical directors frequently have only minimal involvement in the NH and inadequately supervise the medical care	Use nurse practitioners or physicians' assistants for the initial assessment and ongoing monitoring of acute problems (see Chapter 9) Establish a small, committed medical staff that visits the facility at least biweekly Hire and adequately reimburse a medical director with training and/or special interest in geriatrics and long-term care administration	Limited reimbursement for nurse practitioner and physician assistant services may be inadequate to cover their costs Few physicians are willing to commit a substantial amount of time to NH care Relatively few physicians are committed to a career in geriatrics

Limitations in nursing care	Licensed nursing staff in many NHs are too few in number and/or inadequately trained to monitor acutely ill residents	Provide inservice training in the assessment and management of acute illnesses, especially parenteral fluid and antibiotic administration Establish designated areas for subacute care with specially trained staff within larger NHs Develop policies and procedures for notification of physicians for acute problems (see Appendix)	There are shortages of nursing staff in many areas, and qualified nurses often choose to work in other settings Caring for acutely ill may detract from the care of other residents Criteria must be established so that residents who do require acute care are hospitalized
Lack of psychiatric care	Acute problems often involve psychological factors and psychiatric conditions	Develop a relationship with a psychiatrist, and/or psychologist with special interest in geriatrics Develop in-service programs for medical, nursing and social service staff on the assessment and treatment of common psychiatric disturbances Develop and monitor standards for medical documentation Carefully develop and utilize intra-facility transfer forms (see Appendix)	There are very few psychiatrists and psychologists with training and/or interest in geropsychiatry Current constraints in Medicare limits reimbursement for psychiatric care in NHs

Table 5-2 (*Continued*)

Factors	Implications	Potential Strategies to Reduce Hospitalization	Caveats
Limited documentation	NH medical records are often superficial and inaccurate	Consider the use of computers to maintain files of key medical information for use by on-call physician	The NH record becomes discontinuous because of regulations on documentation Some NHs use more than one acute hospital, making standardized documentation difficult Not all physicians are familiar with personal computers
Lack of protocols	Policies and procedures for preventing complications that could lead to acute illness are not well developed	Develop sound policies and procedures for infection control, catheter care, periodic screening and monitoring, and oral/enteral feeding to prevent aspiration (See Chapters 4, 14, 19)	The effectiveness of these types of protocols has not been proved in NH settings
Ethical dilemmas	Many severely ill NH residents and/or their loved ones do not want intensive treatment or any treatment at all that will prolong life	Encourage NH residents to complete advance directives Establish an ethics committee Develop, implement, and monitor policies for cardiopulmonary resuscitation, hospitalization, etc (See Chapter 27)	Many NH residents do not have decision-making capacity or a suitable proxy Religious and cultural beliefs may make policy development and implementation difficult

Financial incentives outside of capitated systems of care will continue to favor hospitalization. Thus, it is critically important for NHs to establish good working relationships with one or more acute care hospitals. The hospital can identify one discharge planner to oversee readmission to the NH, so that he or she can become familiar with the facility's staff and capabilities. Where feasible, NHs might arrange for acute care diagnostic and therapeutic services to be provided by the hospital facilities and staff (see section on "Ancillary Services", below). As discussed later in this chapter, this type of relationship can also foster the development of better interfacility communication and documentation procedures.

ANCILLARY SERVICES

The ability of a NH to provide acute and subacute care is critically dependent on the availability of several ancillary services. These include a clinical laboratory and blood drawing service that can process tests rapidly, an on-site or portable radiology service as well as a radiologist to provide immediate interpretations, respiratory therapy for inhaled bronchodilator treatments and the monitoring of oxygen delivery, and a pharmacy that can provide medications (especially antibiotics) in a timely manner. Most facilities are too small to provide these services on site. In many areas, these types of services are readily available by contract. In most large metropolitan areas, for example, there are services that will even provide on-site noninvasive vascular exams for deep vein thrombosis or abdominal ultrasonography. In rural areas these contracted services maybe difficult to find. Where they are available, they may be very costly. As already mentioned, it may be mutually beneficial for an NH to make arrangements with a local acute care hospital to provide some or all of these services. Making appropriate arrangements for the ancillary services listed above is a key responsibility of the NH medical director (see Chapter 6).

ORGANIZATION OF MEDICAL STAFF

The manner in which most medical care is provided to NH residents tends to foster the use of the emergency room and acute care hospital. Physicians are rarely based in NHs, and in most NHs a physician is available on site for very limited periods of time. Physicians who provide primary care to NH residents generally have busy office practices or other responsibilities at some distance from the NH. Thus, even if adequate reimbursement were available for the on-site assessment of an acute problem, logistical considerations often make it difficult for the physician to do so. In addition, medical directors, also, are generally not available on site and provide minimal supervision of medical staff activities. As a result, most acute problems are handled over the telephone and are often dealt with by transferring the patient to an emergency room for evaluation.

There are at least two alternatives to this approach. Some NHs are large enough and located in areas where there are enough physicians to organize adequate medical coverage to see the NH's residents more frequently, or a practice that may even be based in part at the facility. The second alternative is the use of physician's assistants (PAs) and/or nurse practitioners (NPs). Medicare now provides reimbursement for NPs and PAs in NHs. Reimbursement will still generally not be adequate to cover the full-time salary of a NP or PA, and when direct reimbursement to the NP or PA is requested, the physician is not reimbursed for the visit. Thus, creative strategies to supplement direct reimbursement—by shared funding by the NH and a physician group and/or an acute care hospital—are necessary in order to make this a viable option. The role of PAs and NPs in the NH is discussed further in Chapter 9.

NURSING CARE

The shortage of licensed nurses willing to work in NHs has been a major barrier to providing high quality care in this setting. Typically there is one licensed vocational nurse (LVN or LPN) for every 30 or so residents and one registered nurse for every 50 to 100 residents providing direct care during daytime hours. The vast majority of hands-on care is provided by nurses' aides, who are neither trained nor skilled in the assessment of acute or subacute illnesses. In many cases, nurse registries play an important role in the NH. The use of registry nurses poses several problems. In addition to the fact that they do not have a vested interest in the NH, registry nurses do not generally get to know the NH residents over time. Unlike the situation in an acute care hospital, this lack of familiarity with the chronically ill may make it more difficult for the registry nurse to recognize the subtle changes that often indicate the onset of an acute illness. Further, registry nurses are generally not familiar with the NH's policies and procedures, which may interfere with their ability to assess and manage acute illnesses in the NH setting.

Even when a NH is blessed with a stable group of licensed nurses, the management of acute illnesses may be problematic. Nurses who work in NHs choose to do so in preference to working in acute care hospitals. They may, therefore, be less likely to be interested and skilled in the management of acute illnesses than they are in rehabilitation and chronic care. When acutely or subacutely ill NH residents are managed in the NH, it takes limited licensed staff time away from the care of the majority of residents who are chronically ill. Thus, it may be difficult to monitor vital signs frequently and to oversee the parenteral administration of fluids and medications without cutting back on other nursing care activities for less seriously ill residents.

Nursing homes that choose to manage some acute and subacute illnesses may assist their nursing staff in several ways. First, as already mentioned, PAs and NPs are extremely helpful in the assessment and treatment of acute and subacute illnesses in the NH. Second, NHs that are large enough may choose to create a "distinct part" unit in which all subacutely ill residents are managed. This may create some logistical complexities because of intrafacility room changes, but it can facilitate the training of selected nursing staff members to provide this type of care and offers the possibility of gaining higher per diem rates for Medicare bed days. Third, specific policies and procedures focusing on the assessment and management of acute and subacute conditions should be developed. One example is a policy and procedure for physician notification and physician responsiveness. We have developed such a policy, which is shown in the Appendix. It details the conditions that require immediate versus nonimmediate notification of the primary care physician; this provides the nursing staff with reasonable guidelines and assurance that their calls will be responded to appropriately. It also eliminates the need for many unnecessary telephone communications.

PSYCHIATRIC CARE

The high prevalence of psychiatric disorders among NH residents has been increasingly recognized. Behavioral disorders associated with dementia and/or depression are very common (see Chapters 9 and 10). Psychiatric disorders may account for as many as 10 percent of transfers to acute care hospitals and probably contribute to many more. At the same time, psychiatric care in the NH is quite limited. Mental health professionals must become more involved with NH care, and reimbursement for their services should be set at an adequate level. We recommend that all NHs arrange for consultations and follow-ups with a psychiatrist and/or clinical psychologist who is interested and skilled in the management of common psychiatric disorders in the geriatric population. In addition, some social workers and nurses have special training in geriatric psychiatry and can provide valuable clinical skills as well as assistance in the development and implementation of appropriate policies and procedures related to psychiatric conditions. There is also a need to improve the prescription and monitoring of psychotropic medications. At present, this is handled largely by primary care physicians with limited knowledge of psychopharmacology. It should, however, be recognized that many psychiatrists over-utilize psychotropic medications. A NH physician with an interest and knowledge of geriatrics may perform better in this area, and should evaluate the psychiatrist's recommendation as they would any other consultant recommendation. The use of psychotropic medications is discussed in detail in Chapter 23.

DOCUMENTATION

The frequent transfer of NH residents to acute care hospitals and back creates many problems with documentation and information transfer. Even when a NH has an ongoing relationship with only one such hospital, medical records become discontinuous and often omit information on chronic problems that are essential to the resident's care. Hospital discharge and NH admission or readmission frequently result in an inefficient transfer of critical information. Physicians orders, for example, are frequently written on a transfer form, retranscribed by a NH nurse, then reverified by telephone with the primary care physician.

Several documentation procedures can improve the efficiency and accuracy of information transfer at the NH–acute hospital interface. These include: (1) a standard packet of information that accompanies the resident when transferred from NH to acute care hospital, including medical and administrative face sheets, recent orders, medical/nursing progress notes, laboratory results and information on advance directives; (2) a standard nursing assessment focusing on activities of daily living and nursing needs that accompanies the resident when transferred from acute hospital to NH; (3) an abbreviated hospital discharge summary (which can also serve as the required NH admission documentation) that contains information critical to the immediate care plans (a standard discharge summary that includes the necessary information can also serve this purpose if it can be transcribed before hospital discharge); and (4) physician's orders for the NH that are written by the physician and transferred to the NH at the time of acute hospital discharge. Examples of forms for these documentation practices are included in the Appendix. Some physicians and NHs use fax transmissions to handle some of these communications. The increasing use of computers may also facilitate communication. (See Chapter 4, Table 4-1 for HCFA regulations related to fax orders and electronic signatures.)

ETHICS

A chapter on the NH–acute hospital interface would not be complete without at least brief mention of ethical issues that frequently arise at the time of interfacility transfer. A more complete overview of ethical issues is provided in Chapter 27.

Ethical concerns are common both at the time of transfer from hospital to NH as well as at the time of transfer from NH to hospital. In the former situation, the patient's decision-making capacity and autonomy become critical. Is it the individual's desire to be transferred to a NH? Is he or she capable of making independent decisions in this regard? Are family members acting in the patient's best interest? Are viable alternatives to NH admission available? With regard to a transfer from the NH to the acute care hospital, the resident's desires for intensive medical treatment are a critical concern. Situations clearly arise in which the best interests of the resident are not served by transferring him or her to a hospital for specific and/or intensive treatment (e.g., surgery, intravenous antibiotics, etc.). Instead, palliative and comfort care in familiar surroundings may be a more desirable option for all concerned. Because many NH residents are already incapable of making decisions at the time of NH admission, the use of advance directives must also be incorporated into the practice of geriatric medicine in ambulatory care settings. We recommend that all NHs develop policies and procedures for the use of advance directives and standardized documentation practices that will help ensure that the resident's desires for intensive treatment under specific conditions are honored. Examples of such policies and procedures and documentation formats are included in the Appendix.

SUGGESTED READINGS

Barker WH, Zimmer JG, Jackson Hall W, Ruff BC, et al: Rates, patterns, causes, and costs of hospitalization of nursing home residents: A population-based study. *Am J Public Health* 84:1615–1620, 1994.

Campion EW, Bang A, and May MI: Why acute care hospitals must undertake long-term care. *N Engl J Med* 308:71–75, 1983.

Freiman MP, and Murtaugh CM: Interactions between hospital and nursing home use. *Pub Health Reports* 110:546–554, 1995.

Gordon WZ, Kane RL, and Rothenberg R: Acute hospitalization in a home for the aged. *J Am Geriatr Soc* 33:519–523, 1985.

Irvine PW, Van Buren N, and Crossley K: Causes for hospitalization for nursing home residents: The role of infection. *J Am Geriatr Soc* 32:103–107, 1984.

Kane RL, Matthias R, and Sampson S: The risk of placement in a nursing home after acute hospitalization. *Med Care* 21:1055, 1983.

Kayser-Jones JS, Wiener CL, and Barbaccia JC: Factors contributing to the hospitalization of nursing home residents. *Gerontologist* 29:502–510, 1989.

Lewis MA, Cretin S, and Kane RL: The natural history of nursing home patients. *Gerontologist* 25:382–388, 1985.

Lewis MA, Kane RL, Cretin S, et al: The immediate and subsequent outcomes of nursing home care. *Am J Public Health* 75:758–762, 1985.

Murtaugh CM, and Freiman MP: Nursing home residents at risk of hospitalization and the characteristics of their hospital stays. *Gerontologist* 35:35–43, 1995.

Rubenstein LZ, Ouslander JG, and Wieland D: Dynamics and clinical implications of the nursing home-hospital interface. *Clin Geriatr Med* 4:471–491, 1988.

Sager MA, Leventhal EA, and Easterling DV: The impact of Medicare's prospective payment system on Wisconsin nursing homes. *JAMA* 257:1762–1766, 1987.

Tresch DD, Simpson WM, and Burton JR: Relationship of long-term and acute care facilities: The problem of patient transfer and continuity of care. *J Am Geriatr Soc* 33:819–826, 1985.

Zimmer JG and Watson NM: Physician response to notification of acute problems in the nursing home. *J Am Geriatr Soc* 39:348–352, 1991.

Zimmer JG, Eggert GM, Treat A, et al: Nursing homes as acute care providers: A pilot study of incentives to reduce hospitalizations. *J Am Geriatr Soc* 35:124–129, 1987.

CHAPTER

SIX

SUBACUTE CARE

Service innovation in long term care has been motivated by changes in technology applied to older patients and new market opportunities. These have led to the emergence of dedicated units providing specialized care ranging from rehabilitation to subacute care. The most rapid growth in the nursing home (NH) industry has in fact been in the number of skilled nursing beds dedicated to care for post-hospitalized patients, usually with subacute problems, rehabilitation needs or a combination of both. One prominent development leading to this growth was implementation of Medicare's Prospective Payment System (PPS) for hospitals. By creating incentives to shorten hospital stays, the PPS increased demand for post discharge treatment. Other market place forces have also contributed, especially expansion of managed care organizations seeking less costly alternatives for beneficiaries with chronic illness (such as AIDS or head trauma), and those with Medicare risk contracts caring for the elderly patients with chronic illness who admit some of these patients directly to subacute care without acute hospitalization. It has been suggested that subacute care NHs are becoming the primary care hospitals of the future. Changes in technology and treatment options offered to older Americans such as coronary bypass grafting and cancer chemotherapy, have also increased survival from previously fatal illnesses and increased the demand for subacute care. Medicaid NH reforms in some states have created staffing standards and payment incentives to admit patients with heavier care needs. This trend has created challenges for NH physicians and medical directors previously caring for chronic, stable conditions. However, there are some potential advantages of care in a subacute unit versus an acute hospital for geriatric patients (**Table 6-1**).

Table 6-1 Potential advantages of subacute care over acute hospitals for geriatric patients

1. Decreased costs
2. More focused on rehabilitation
3. Residents eat in the dining room
4. Residents take part in activities outside of formal therapy
5. Nursing is more focused on functional status
6. Nursing has greater expertise in preventing and treating pressure sores
7. Physical restraints are rarely used
8. Nutrition and food intake have a high priorty
9. No loss of rehabilitation time during transfer between different levels of care
10. More comprehensive assessment including psychosocial issues

The scope of this chapter is to review the admission criteria and the process of care involved in skilled nursing facilities caring for subacute and rehabilitative patients. These units may be a part of an acute hospital transitional care unit (TCU) or situated within a designated area of a regular community nursing facility (Distinct Part) or be a whole nursing facility dedicated to the care of subacute and patients with rehabilitation needs.

DEFINITION OF SUBACUTE CARE

Subacute is a payer designation and not a formal licensing level of care. The Joint Commission on Accreditation of Health Care Organizations (JCAHO), recognizing this trend, has defined subacute care as follows: "Subacute care is comprehensive inpatient care designed for someone who has an acute illness, injury, or exacerbation of a disease process. It is goal oriented treatment rendered immediately after, or instead of, acute hospitalization to treat one or more specific active complex medical conditions or to administer one or more technically complex treatments, in the context of a person's underlying long-term conditions and overall situation. Generally, the individual's condition is such that the care does not depend heavily on high-technology monitoring or complex diagnostic procedures. Subacute care requires the coordinated services of an interdisciplinary team including physicians, nurses, and other relevant professional disciplines, who are trained and knowledgeable to assess and manage these specific conditions and perform the necessary procedures. Subacute care is given as part of a specifically defined program, regardless of the site. It is generally more intensive than traditional nursing facility care and less than acute care. It requires frequent (daily or weekly) recurrent patient assessment and review of the clinical course and treatment plan for a limited (several days to several months) time period, until the condition is stabilized or a predetermined treatment course is completed." This definition has also been adopted by the American Health Care Association (AHCA).

PATIENT CHARACTERISTICS

Subacute patients are typically admitted for a short stay of 7–21 days and are expected to return home or to residential care homes after a specific, planned treatment. Compared to the average NH population, these patients tend to be younger, less likely to be cognitively impaired, generally enter the subacute unit on more medications, and are more likely to have problems amenable to rehabilitation. Importantly, they are also more likely to be rehospitalized. They do tend to be elderly with typically at least 75 percent older than 65 years. Most are Medicare insured, and are referred by the acute hospital after at least a 3-day qualifying stay. Shorter average lengths of stay in acute hospitals (which declined from 10.1 days in 1980 to 8.8 days in 1992) are creating a marked increase in acuity of these NH residents. Managed capitated care programs admit patients of all ages to the subacute units. Approximately 4–16 percent of acute hospital admissions are potential candidates for a subacute unit. Typical diagnoses are hip fractures, strokes, acute compression fractures and other fractures, pressure ulcers and vascular conditions, cardiac and pulmonary disorders, postoperative conditions with deconditioning, and cancer. Patients' needs are complex, requiring intensive and frequent involvement by multiple disciplines, such as nursing, rehabilitation, other ancillary services as well as close monitoring by the physician and pharmacist. The goals of treatment for these sicker patients are often the same as those in the acute care unit, and include rapid identification and treatment of new problems, as well as improving function to the highest possible level. These goals differ in many aspects from the goals of nursing home care where the focus is on preventive and supportive care, alleviation of pain and suffering, and provision of comfort and dignity for the terminally ill. Therefore the physician and facility must use a more expeditious process for the subacute patient, focusing on the acute illness, rehabilitation and an early discharge back to the community or former living arrangement. Patients may have primarily rehabilitation needs, medical needs, or a combination of both. If the need is primarily rehabilitative, the patient should have a tolerance for skilled therapy of up to 3 h/day. Patients often start with low endurance, but then improve enough to be discharged to a lower level of care. Patients may have a level of acuity similar to that in the acute hospital but without the need for high technology diagnostic services or intensive monitoring.

THE SUBACUTE PROCESS OF CARE

Subacute care is generally initiated by identifying patients in the acute hospital who may benefit from additional care before returning home. This can be

Table 6-2 Admission criteria to subacute units

Intravenous antibiotics
Physical therapy 6–7 times/week
Occupational therapy 5 times/week
Weaning oxygen with blood gas measurements 3 times/week
Tracheal suctioning at least 2 times/shift
Respiratory therapy treatment 3 times/day or more frequently
Capillary blood glucose monitoring 2 times/day with insulin coverage
Injectable medications every 8 hours or 2 times/day
Wound care (sterile) daily
Tube feeding
Lab monitoring every 2–3 days
Renal dialysis with monitoring
Bladder training
Pain management (parenteral)
Skilled nursing observation of congestive heart, liver, or renal failure
Physician visits at least weekly

accomplished prospectively upon admission to the acute hospital by targeting certain diagnostic groups for early admission to the subacute unit utilizing clinical pathways, or when the patient's diagnostic work-up has been completed and intensive monitoring is no longer required. Alternatively, targeting could address premorbid functional status as a predictor for length of inpatient stay. Mobility impairment, impaired cognition, and decreased functional status are indicators for considering subacute care relatively early in the process. An example would be a patient admitted from a residential care facility with pneumonia. This patient is more likely to become deconditioned and require rehabilitation before being able to return to the prior dwelling. At this point, an evaluation is done using screening criteria, such as those in **Table 6-2**. This table lists the services that are available and covered by Medicare at the skilled nursing facility level, and may serve as inclusionary criteria for admission.

The range of treatments provided by subacute units varies. These may include hospital-based, specialized programs such as ventilator weaning, burn care, cancer chemotherapy, and pain management. The more professionally and technically complex the services are, the more competitive and lucrative the unit becomes.

Clearly defining the goals of care for the individual patient is critical for both patient care and appropriate discharge planning. The role of the subacute unit representative evaluating the appropriateness for transfer is, among others, to review patients' needs for care and to assure that the referring physician has a clear plan for this admission and that the patient or his/her proxy is informed as well. Assuring patients' and family participation in the process of care and decisions is critical for the success of the care and discharge plan. Discussions regarding advance directives and intensity of treatment in the subacute unit should preferably take place before the transfer.

Admission Process

The admission process varies, depending on the location of the subacute unit. First, the unit coordinator reviews the patient's chart in the acute hospital or utilizes a screening form obtaining the relevant information via phone or fax from the acute unit manager. This is to ensure that the patient's needs can be met and that the needs meet payor specifications (Medicare, other). The physician should consult with the coordinator on the appropriateness of the transfer and be involved in providing the necessary documentation for a smooth transfer. A more detailed description of the pre-admission process is discussed in Chapter 3.

For managed care patients who may come to the subacute directly from the emergency department or from home, the preadmission assessment needs to focus on the acuity of the patient's illness and whether she or he needs cardiac monitoring or more hours of care than are usually available on the subacute unit. Examples of patients who can be successfully treated in a subacute care unit without hospital admission include those with pneumonia, urinary tract infections, deep vein thrombosis, pressure ulcers, severe malnutrition and increasing fraility with the new onset falls. The potential advantages of sucacute units over an acute care setting for these types of patients are summarized in **Table 6-1.**

Interdisciplinary Team Conferences

The role of the interdisciplinary team in nursing homes is discussed in some detail in Chapter 10. In subacute care, weekly team conferences to review the plan of care and monitor progress are good practice. Members of the team include representatives from disciplines such as nursing, rehabilitation services, dietary, activities, social services and medicine. In hospital-based subacute units, the pharmacy and the medical director may participate as well. We recommend physician participation on a weekly basis in units with a high turnover of patients who tend to require close medical supervision. The unit nurse manager or supervisor should act as the meeting facilitator. Depending on the size of the unit and number of new admissions, a protocol may be necessary in which patients are only reviewed at set intervals. The facilitator should keep the meeting on track, allowing only new and relevant information to be presented. Relevant information from each discipline is presented both to ensure proper utilization and to discuss problems and issues that may affect patient care, progress or outcomes. An example of a form for briefly summarizing in the weekly interdisciplinary team conference is included in the Appendix.

Discharge planning is a critical function of the interdisciplinary team. It should start at the time of admission, and be updated based on input from all members of the team. Major factors involved in discharge planning are the living environment, amount of social support, amount of assistance required, financial assets, nature of illness, and patients' progress. While instrumental activities of daily living (IADLs) are important to independent living, independence in basic activities of daily living (ADLs) is of particular importance to discharge to the community. All of these factors are discussed and final discharge plans are often arrived at during team meetings. The goal is to optimize the patient's function while ensuring appropriate availability of support and utilization of resources in as low a level of care as possible.

DOCUMENTATION

Although more useful for long stay patients, completion of the Minimum Data Set (MDS) within 7–14 days of admission to the subacute is still required (at the time of this writing). Different disciplines complete designated sections of the MDS. In subacute care, physician input is critical. The MDS is not as useful in care planning in the subacute care units because of brief lengths of stay and rapid changes in patient status. Although federal regulations call for completion of the MDS within 14 days, team members should begin the evaluation upon admission in order to address the assessments directly related to the problem/diagnosis leading to admission to the subacute care unit.

Within 48 h of the time of admission to the subacute unit, the attending physician is responsible for completing a history and physical (critical elements of which are listed in **Table 6-3**). On each subsequent visit, physician documentation must address the patient's progress and responses to therapy and skilled care needs, as well as interim medical problems. At the time of discharge

Table 6-3 Key elements of the admission medical assessment to subacute care

Admitting diagnosis(es)
History of present illness
Summary of acute hospital course (if applicable)
Past medical/surgical history
Physical examination
Special focus on systems relating to reason(s) for subacute care
Allergies
Functional status
Interdisciplinary team assesses for Minimum Data Set
Mental status
Interdisciplinary team assesses for Minimum Data Set
Relevant laboratory/imaging results
Major studies during acute hospital stay should be included
Treatment plan
Rehabilitation potential
Discharge plan

Table 6-4 Key elements of the discharge medical summary from subacute care

Dates of admission and discharge
Reason(s) for admission to subacute care unit
Course in medical and rehabilitation unit
Final diagnoses
Discharge functional status
Relevant laboratory/imaging results
Discharge location–Support–home care, etc.
Discharge medications
Follow-up plans
Next physician appointments
Visiting nurse/home care/other support services

an abbreviated discharge summary needs to be completed, which should include at least the elements listed in **Table 6-4**.

ROLE OF PHYSICIANS

In subacute care physicians need to focus not only on subacute medical problems, but also on restoration of function and/or enhancement of self-sufficiency, to enable the patient to successfully remain at home. This is especially challenging with conditions such as stroke and other neurologic disorders, renal failure, cancer, AIDS, or severe cardiopulmonary disorders. Because of the hybrid nature of treatment goals and the more dynamic nature of the process of care, the physician must approach patients in a more expeditious manner than in long-term patients, simultaneously focusing on both the acute illness and related rehabilitation needs. Efforts must also emphasize preventing rehospitalization. The subacute nature of illness in the patients necessitates the physician providing more hands-on medical care and team leadership than the traditional nursing facility. Visits need to be more frequent (1–2 per week) for problem assessments and intervention. Physicians must be prepared for this challenge by acquiring knowledge about the nursing home environment and regulations, and by developing skills in managing common geriatric syndromes.

In the subacute care units, physicians are required to see their patients as often as necessary to provide essential medical care, but not less than once every 30 days. We recommend that subacute patients be seen at least once or twice per week. **Table 6-5** summarizes American Medical Association (AMA) guidelines for physician responsibilities in subacute care.

Appropriate documentation specifying the reasons for subacute care, the goals of the stay, and potential for rehabilitation is critical for maintaining high standards of care and assuring appropriate reimbursement for both the facility

Table 6-5 Guidelines for physician responsibilities in subacute care[a]

1. Physicians are responsible to their patients for delivery of care in all subacute care settings, 24 hours a day, 7 days a week.
2. Patients who might benefit from subacute care should be admitted to and discharged under the orders of the physician who is responsible for the continuous medical management needed to meet the patient's needs and safety and maintaining quality of care.
3. Physicians are responsible for coordinating care for their patients with other physicians including medical directors, primary care physicians, and appropriate specialists, to optimize the quality of care in subacute settings.
4. Physicians are responsible for supervision and coordination of the medical care for their patients and providing leadership for all other health care providers in subacute care.
5. Physicians should guide procedures for their patients performed within integrated practices and direct other health care providers, consistent with federal and state regulations.
6. Physicians are responsible for:
   (a) Fulfilling their roles and identifying the medical skills needed to deliver care in subacute facilities and for creating and developing continuing medical education to meet the special needs of patients in subacute care.
   (b) Identifying and appropriately utilizing subacute care facilities in their communities.
   (c) Oversight of physician credentialing in subacute settings.
   (d) Promoting medical staff organization and by-laws that may be needed to support peer evaluations.
   (e) Planning care of their patients with acute and chronic conditions in subacute care, as well as pursuing efforts to restore and maintain functions for quality of life.
7. Subacute units and or programs need physician medical directors to assure quality of medical care, provide peer group liaisons, and coordinate and supervise patients and families input and needs.
8. Physicians provide a plan of care for medically necessary visits after completing an initial assessment within 24 hours of admission that identifies the medical services expected during subacute care.
9. Attending physicians should:
   (a) Make an on-site visit to review the interdisciplinary care plan within 72 hours of admission.
   (b) Determine the number of medically necessary follow up visits; these may occur daily but never less often than weekly.
   (c) Document active involvement of physicians in interdisciplinary care and all major components of the patient care plan including completing a progress note for each patient visit.
10. Physicians should implement these guidelines through organized medical staff by-laws in subacute settings to assure quality patient care.

[a]AMA Board of Trustees Report 21–1–95.

and the physician. It is important to appropriately document visits following Health Care Financing Administration (HCFA) guidelines. These include two out of three components under one of the following codes—99311, 99312, or 99313 (**see Table 6-6**). Furthermore, visits for new problems requiring a more thorough evaluation that lead to a new diagnosis or a permanent change in condition need to be appropriately coded utilizing five digit codes, and should carry procedure

Table 6-6 Billing codes for subsequent nursing facility care relevant for subacute care[a]

Code	Components (Need 2 of 3)	Examples
99311	1. Problem-focused interval history 2. Problem-focused examination 3. Medical decisions of low complexity	Follow-up visit following successful treatment for cellulitis
99312	1. Expanded problem-focused interval history 2. Extended problem-focused examination 3. Medical decision-making of low to moderate complexity	Visit to determine the need for physical restraints in a patient having falls, requiring no change in the medical care plan
99313	1. Detailed interval history 2. Detailed physical examination 3. Medical decision-making of moderate to high complexity	Visit to evaluate acute confusional state with revision of the medical plan of care

[a]Major changes may require higher codes. See Chapter 1.

codes 99303 or 99302 for those requiring a change of care plan and a new MDS. Billing should be based on the complexity of the decisions involved, not on the time spent making them. It is important to dispel the myth prevalent among some physicians that Medicare approves only one visit every 30 days or up to 12 visits. This limit has been eliminated with the new HCFA Physician Payment Reform for Physician Evaluation and Management Services. HCFA has accepted the notion that services should be reimbursed based on the effort and complexity. Patients should be seen as often as needed, even daily, and visits should be supported by appropriate documentation (see Chapter 1).

THE ROLE OF THE MEDICAL DIRECTOR IN THE SUBACUTE UNIT

The role of the medical director in nursing homes is discussed in detail in Chapter 7. In many states, subacute care facilities are governed by the same rules that govern free-standing skilled nursing facilities. The medical director essentially functions as the subacute units chief of staff, assisting in the development of, and monitoring compliance with, its policies and procedures, and educating the staff about the special regulations of long-term care facilities that apply to subacute units. Specific responsibilities of the TCU medical director are outlined in **Table 6-7**. The subacute unit medical director has responsibility for developing medical policies and procedures appropriate for subacute care, which should meet or exceed the standards of practice at affiliated acute hospitals. Many subacute units

Table 6-7 Subacute care unit medical director responsibilities

1. Oversee and ensure quality medical care
2. Ensure appropriateness of subacute unit admissions
3. Ensure appropriate utilization of therapies, diagnostic studies, etc.
4. Education of medical staff
5. Education of subacute unit interdisciplinary team staff
6. Ensure compliance with state and federal rules and regulations
7. Develop, implement and monitor policies and procedures relevant to medical aspects of subacute care
8. Informal communication with primary care physicians
9. Formal consultation on appropriateness for admission and/or geriatric care issues
10. Serve as liaison to acute hospital Department of Medicine, medical staff committees, administration

are seeking JCAHO accreditation, and this process will involve strong medical leadership. Credentialing of physicians has become an issue, especially for managed care programs, and has not been fully addressed in most states. Guidelines and standards for subacute care for credentialing, infection control, and other practices have been published by the JCAHO (see "Suggested Readings").

The most important role of the medical director is ensuring quality medical care for all subacute patients. This is done on both a systems and an individual review basis. The medical director can also regularly review the care of patients in the unit by attending the weekly interdisciplinary team conferences. When issues of care or utilization arise, the medical director may contact the attending physician for appropriate action. The medical director participates in quality assurance and pharmacy meetings, and reviews particular medical aspects of care such as pharmacy, radiology and laboratory services. The medical director also contributes to the development of written patient care policies covering such areas as admission, transfer, and discharge policies, physician services, nursing services, dietary services, diagnostic services, medical records, etc. These policies are developed with input from a patient care policy committee, which is composed of the medical director, administrator, director of nursing, pharmacist, activities director, and representatives from other disciplines as appropriate. Policies are reviewed at least yearly under the direction of the committee.

The subacute unit medical director may participate in the admission process in several ways. On a systems level he or she may contribute to the development of policies and specific admissions criteria, development and promotion of special treatment programs, and outcomes assessment to measure the effects of care in different patient subpopulations.

The medical director is the liaison between the subacute unit and the hospital medical staff. He or she does this through direct communication, and by other means, such as geriatric consultations. An appropriately trained medical director may guide and educate physicians on recommended methods of practice and documentation. He or she is also the subacute unit's liaison with hospital management via regular meetings, assisting in the development and review of policies and procedures, and by input to the budget process. In hospital-based units oversight and quality improvement activities are often integrated into the general acute hospital processes for continuous quality improvement.

Education of hospital medical staff is another important task for the subacute unit medical director. This can be done formally and informally. Formal education can be accomplished through conferences focusing on topics relevant to subacute care. A potential barrier to physicians' appropriate use of subacute units is a lack of understanding of their purpose, unique capabilities, and types of patients they serve. Informal education is accomplished by spontaneous discussions with physicians as well as by formal consultation on a case-by-case basis.

STRATEGIES TO IMPROVE SUBACUTE CARE

Strategies for improving care in subacute units are outlined in **Table 6-8**. Because subacute units are characterized by different dynamics from typical nursing homes and acute care hospitals, issues such as communication and the interdisciplinary team approach to discharge planning are critical for success. Strategies to maintain continuity of care and efficient communication between the acute hospital and subacute units are also critical, and are discussed in Chapter 5.

A critical component of improving subacute care is the medical records' procedure to assure transfer of appropriate information. Since discharge from the hospital may be associated with the disruption of medical records due to delays in transcribing of discharge summaries, an effective strategy includes providing subacute unit staff with a brief transfer note in addition to admission orders. This approach assures communication of essential information to initiate the subacute care admission process. Information includes active diagnoses/problems, most recent diagnostic studies, rehabilitation potential and prognosis. Communication about advance directives and a summary of decisions on the intensity of treatment discussed in the acute hospital will facilitate compliance with the patient's or family's wishes. Similarly, a concise discharge summary facilitates the transfer of information to the patient's primary care physician (if different from the subacute attending), and documents the course and status at the time of discharge from the subacute unit (**see Table 6-4**).

The second strategy consists of a procedure for writing and signing subacute unit admission orders before the actual transfer takes place. This prevents unnecessary delays in service upon admission to the unit and unnecessary phone calls to the admitting physicians to verify over-the-phone orders. Third, a clear policy on when to call the physician is needed. This includes guidelines on what information to make available to the attending physician and what notifications

Table 6-8 Strategies to improve care in subacute units

Goals	Strategies
Strengthen the role of the medical director	Formal training in geriatric medicine and medical administration Medical Director's Certification (CMD) from the American Medical Directors Association (AMDA)
Develop a systematic approach to assessment	Incorporate specific admission criteria, assessment of functional/mental status, decision-making capacity, and social supports
Improve hospital–SNF communication	Abbreviated hospital discharge summary Physician admitting orders written upon discharge from acute hospital Relevant information transferred from hospital medical record
Minimize ethical dilemmas	Utilize advance directives and prospective decision-making practices
Improve documentation	Utilize standardized forms
Improve response time	Round at least once or twice per week Utilize nurse practitioner/physician assistant
Improve staff–physician communication	Policy on when to call the physician Utilize standardized procedures Weekly interdisciplinary conference summary Use fax and e-mail
Avoid polypharmacy	Easy-to-read drug regimen report Participation of pharmacist in weekly inter-disciplinary conference

may wait until the next business day. An example of such a policy and a related communication form are included in the Appendix.

Standardized procedures, protocols and implementation parameters further reduce unnecessary phone calls, freeing staff and physicians for a meaningful exchange of clinical information. Standardized procedures is an approach in which registered nurses can fulfill functions that traditionally are not delineated in the nurses' licensing privileges and, therefore, require a policy and protocol to allow registered nurses, physician assistants, nurse practitioners or clinical nurse specialists to diagnose and intervene in certain conditions such as skin tears, constipation, pressure ulcers and others.

Utilization of nurse practitioners (NP) and physician assistants (PA) is a fourth strategy to improve subacute care. The role of NPs. and PAs is discussed in detail in Chapter 9. In subacute units, nurse specialists (NS) and PAs may be especially helpful in providing frequent monitoring of subacutely ill patients. This strategy has been adopted by several managed care organizations. These practitioners' privileges can be further expanded under standardized procedures.

The fifth strategy for improving care involves the interdisciplinary team weekly conference, which serves as a forum for communicating clinical information. To facilitate the flow of relevant information to the attending physician, who may not attend the conference, a written summary can be used (an example is included in the Appendix). The key to effective communication is to focus on meaningful information. In our experience, the weekly "team conference summary" has been well received by staff and physicians alike since it has filled a gap, especially in reporting progress in functioning, psychosocial status, nutrition and discharge planning. The form can become part of the medical record and a copy can be forwarded to the attending physician via mail, fax or e-mail. All these, of course, cannot substitute for physician-to-physician and physician-to-nurse direct communication regarding particularly challenging patients.

A major incentive for physicians to use subacute units is the demonstration of good patient outcomes and patient satisfaction. It has been shown that the acuity level of patients in successful units increases with time, as physicians become more comfortable with the quality of care and the ability to take care of medically complex patients. The medical director plays a key role in promoting high quality care, which will translate into more appropriate subacute utilization, and more cost-effective care in an era of growing cost containment.

SUGGESTED READINGS

American Health Care Association: *Subacute Care in Freestanding Skilled Nursing Facilities*, Washington, DC, AHCA, 1994.

Smith RL, Osterweil, D: The medical director in hospital-based transitional care units. *Clin Ger Med* 11: 73–89, August, 1995.

The Joint Commission for the Accreditation of Healthcare Organizations: *Accreditation Protocol for Subacute Programs*, Oakbrook Terrace, Illinois, JCAHO, 1996.

American Medical Directors Association: *Position Statement on the Role of the Medical Director of a Subacute Care Program.*

CHAPTER
SEVEN

THE ROLE OF THE MEDICAL DIRECTOR

The importance of the medical director to the quality of medical care in the nursing home (NH) cannot be overemphasized. Until recently, medical directorship in most NHs has largely been relegated to physicians with little if any training in geriatrics, long-term care, or administration; unfortunately, this responsibility has often been carried out in a perfunctory manner meeting only minimal requirements and standards.

Better defining the role of the medical director as well as strengthening and setting high standards for it is critical to improving NH care. The purpose of this chapter is to provide a brief overview of the role of the NH medical director. Those interested in more detailed information should read the books of Steven Levenson listed in the suggested readings. Many of the ideas set forth in this chapter are derived from his work and are included with his kind permission. In addition, NH medical directors should be encouraged to join the national association as well as such state or local organizations as may exist. The current address of the American Medical Directors Association (AMDA) is 10480 Little Patuxent Parkway, Suite 760, Columbia, Maryland 21044; (410) 740–9743 or (800) 876–AMDA. AMDA offers a series of course work in medical direction leading to certification as a certified medical director (CMD).

OVERVIEW OF THE ROLE

The specific role, responsibilities, and authority of the medical director will vary depending on a number of factors, such as those listed in **Table 7-1**. Politics are local, and the ratio of responsibility to authority will depend on a number of these

Table 7-1 Factors influencing the role of the medical director

1. Facility ownership
   (private, non-profit, government)
2. Location
   (free-standing, hospital based, component of a life care community)
3. Facility size
4. Administrative structure
5. Relationship of facility to other health care providers
6. Local demand for NH beds
7. Medical staff organization and structure
   (formal hospital-like staff; full time versus part time; open versus closed)
8. Availability of primary and consultant physicians
9. Availability of ancillary services
   (laboratory, X-ray, etc.)

factors. The medical director of a nonproprietary facility in an area of high bed demand—with readily accessible ancillary services, an adequate supply of primary and consultant physicians, and an organized medical staff structure—will have considerable authority and leverage with respect to the medical staff. On the other hand, the medical director of a small proprietary facility in a rural community—with limited demand for NH beds, a relatively sparse physician population, and poor access to ancillary services—will have considerable responsibility but limited authority and leverage over the medical staff.

Whatever the local politics, medical directors should arrange for explicit terms of agreement with the NH owners or board of directors. Important aspects of such terms are listed in **Table 7-2**. The amount of time to be committed will vary depending on the size of the facility and whether or not the medical director

Table 7-2 Important aspects of a medical director's agreement with the nursing home

1. Date and term of agreement
2. Terms of relationship (employee, contractor, etc.)
3. Line of reporting and authority
4. Job description (including privileges, rights, responsibilities, duties)
5. Hours per week, including a description of what is included in compensable time
6. Terms of compensation, including:
   Fringe benefits
   Professional liability coverage
   Rights to retain income from patient care and other revenues
7. Resources and support provided by the facility
8. Terms of renewal and termination of agreement

After Levenson S (ed): *Medical Direction in Long Term Care: A Guidebook for the Future.* Durham, North Carolina, Carolina Academic Press, 1993.

Table 7-3 Key responsibilities of the nursing home medical director

1. Organize comprehensive medical services
2. Ensure that primary and consultant physicians and other health professionals fulfill their obligations to residents and the facility
3. Collaborate with administrators and other department heads to develop and implement appropriate policies and procedures
4. Monitor and attempt to continually improve the quality of medical services
5. Act as a spokesperson for the facility to other health care agencies and the community
6. Oversee an employee health program
7. Assist in the development, organization and presentation of educational activities for staff, residents and families
8. Facilitate appropriate research

also serves as a primary care physician. Even in the smallest facilities, the medical director should be present at least twice a month to meet with facility staff, solve problems, and carry out mandatory activities such as utilization review and quality assurance.

Facilities of 100 to 200 beds should probably have a quarter-time medical director; those with more than 200 beds should have at least a half-time medical director. There are advantages and disadvantages to being a medical director who also serves as a primary care physician. The advantages are that he or she will be present in the facility more often and will get to know the staff, process, and quality of care well. The disadvantage is a potential conflict of interest between the roles of medical director and primary care physician. As discussed below, one of the key responsibilities of the medical director is to ensure the quality of medical care; if the medical director provides primary care to a substantial proportion of the residents, a "fox guarding the chicken coop" situation can arise. The best strategy may be for the medical director to serve as primary care physician to a modest proportion of the facility's residents (e.g., 25 percent or less). Compensation for medical directors varies considerably; hourly rates range from $25 to $100 per hour and annual salaries for half- to full-time range from $45,000 to over $100,000. In general, medical directors have been undercompensated. A reasonable compensation rate considering the complexities of the role of the medical director is $20,000 per 100 beds. Such a rate is presently rarely achieved.

Table 7-3 outlines the key responsibilities of the NH medical director. Each of these responsibilities is briefly discussed in the sections that follow. Unique considerations for medical directors of subacute care units are discussed briefly at the end of the chapter.

ORGANIZATION OF MEDICAL SERVICES

The diversity and complexities of medical conditions among NH residents as well as requirements for certain types of care (e.g., dental, podiatric) demand that

Table 7-4 Types of medical services needed for nursing home residents

Primary physicians who visit the facility at least monthly[a]
Consultant physicians, e.g.:
Cardiology
Dermatology[a]
Gastroenterology
Geriatric medicine
Gynecology
Nephrology
Neurology
Neurosurgery
Oncology/hematology
Ophthalmology
Otolaryngology
Proctology
Psychiatry[a]
Pulmonary
Radiology
Rheumatology
Surgery (general)
Urology
Vascular surgery
Dentistry[a]
Podiatry[a]
Wound care specialist[a]
Audiology
Optometry[a]
Psychologist[a]
Consultant pharmacist[a]
Pharmacy services available on a daily basis
Diagnostic services
Clinical laboratory
X-ray
Other
Ultrasonography
Noninvasive cardiovascular studies
(Holter monitor, vascular doppler, etc.)
Pulmonary function
Social work
Rehabilitation therapies
Physical
Occupational
Speech
Prosthetics
Respiratory therapy

[a]Regular visits to the facility (at least monthly) are desirable.

a wide variety of medical services be available. **Table 7-4** lists the types of services that NH residents should have access to. It is a fundamental responsibility of the medical director to ensure that the NH can provide or arrange for these types of services. The precise nature of these arrangements will vary considerably depending on the size and resources of the NH and the availability and accessibility of these services in the surrounding community.

With respect to primary care physicians, NHs are generally not large enough to have a full-time medical staff. Most NHs have a loosely organized panel of primary-care physicians who admit and care for residents in the facility. Frequently there are dozens of physicians involved in a single NH. This situation can create significant communication problems for the nursing staff and makes the oversight role of the medical director very difficult. Increasingly, NH residents receive their primary care from a physician and/or nurse practitioner employed by a health maintenance organization (HMO) or employed by a physician group that contracts with an HMO—further complicating the oversight function of the medical director. In many areas there is no easy solution; there are not enough primary care physicians who have the time or interest to care for large numbers of NH residents. In addition, the NH may be dependent upon many physicians to admit their patients in order to fill the beds. The result is a large number of primary care physicians. Each of these cares for only a small proportion of the facility's residents, is physically present in the NH for very short periods of time, and is busy elsewhere with other activities when not in the NH. Whenever practical, NHs and medical directors should attempt to minimize the number of primary care physicians involved. While it is neither legal nor ethical to not allow NH residents their choice of a primary care physician, it may be both feasible and in the best interests of all concerned to strive to limit the number of primary care physicians involved in a particular NH. In some areas, this can be accomplished by arranging for a small group of physicians to provide most of the primary care and, if acceptable to all concerned, transferring the care of residents to this group at the time of NH admission. In some areas this type of arrangement has evolved naturally. The fewer physicians involved, the easier it will be to develop and adhere to policies, procedures, and high standards of care and the easier it will be for NH staff to develop a good rapport with the medical staff. Whatever specific arrangements are developed, the NH should have some type of written agreement from the primary care physicians that acknowledges their responsibilities to their residents as well as to the facility.

In most communities, consultant physicians in the various specialties—as well as dentistry, podiatry, audiology, and optometry—are available. Large NHs, especially those associated with other levels of care (e.g., life care communities), have developed specialty clinics that are held at the NH site. Though this requires space, some equipment, and NH staff time to assist with the clinics, it can save the time and energy that would be required to transport residents to and from offices outside the NH. The medical director is responsible not only for ensuring that residents have access to these specialists but also for assuring the quality of care such consultants provide, developing appropriate documentation and communication practices, and assisting the consultants in adhering to the NHs policies and procedures with respect to resident care.

The medical director is also responsible for helping the NH to obtain and assure the quality of other resident care services. A well-organized pharmacy and experienced pharmacy consultants are critical to high-quality medical care in the NH. Many pharmacies have developed a NH specialty or are totally dedicated to providing services for NHs. The medical director must work closely with the pharmacy as well as the nursing staff to ensure the appropriate prescription and delivery of drugs. This is generally accomplished through a pharmacy committee. The ready availability of several types of diagnostic services (listed in **Table 7-4**) is also critical to high-quality medical care. Some bioclinical laboratories, like pharmacies, have developed a specialty in providing services to NHs. These types of laboratories can be especially helpful because of their familiarity with the process of care in the NH, and many provide both in-service training and assistance with infection control. Portable radiology services are generally available in most areas. In some cities, services that perform other diagnostic testing, such as ultrasonography and noninvasive cardiovascular studies, will come to the NH. These services are essential for the NH's ability to assess and manage acute and subacute conditions without transferring the resident to an emergency room. It may be practical and administratively and financially advantageous in some settings for the NH to contract for these services with a local acute care hospital that looks after the NH's residents when they become acutely ill. Whatever specific arrangements are made, the medical director is responsible for developing policies and procedures relating to the communication and documentation of results of diagnostic tests and for monitoring the utilization of the diagnostic services. Ancillary services that are critical for the quality of life of NH residents, such as dentistry, podiatry, and optometry, must be provided. Finally, several types of therapies are essential for NH residents. In addition to the traditional physical, occupational, and speech therapies and the related prosthetic services (e.g., braces, splints, special shoes, prostheses, etc.), respiratory therapy can be extremely valuable in managing subacutely ill residents. Respiratory therapists can help the nursing staff to oversee oxygen therapy, provide respiratory treatments (e.g., nebulized bronchodilators), monitor oxygenation, perform pulmonary function tests and test arterial blood gases, and assist in obtaining sputum specimens. Services for counseling by a psychologist or licensed social worker are reimbursed by Medicare and should be utilized as they can markedly decrease the use of psychotropic drugs and improve the resident's quality of life. Although the medical director may not be responsible for overseeing these therapeutic services, he or she must work with the director of nurses and administrator to assure their availability, quality, and appropriate utilization.

POLICY AND PROCEDURE DEVELOPMENT

The medical director must work collaboratively with the administrator, director of nursing, and other NH staff to develop, implement, and oversee adherence to appropriate policies and procedures. Obviously, just because policies and procedures exist does not ensure that they will be followed or that a high quality of care is being provided. But written policies and procedures offer several important advantages. First, they help to establish and communicate the medical director's and NH's expectations of the medical staff and services. Second, they assist in the development of specific standards of care. Third, they document these expectations and standards in writing, making it difficult for medical or other staff to evade responsibility for knowing what is expected of them. Finally, written policies and procedures are helpful in demonstrating to regulatory bodies that the facility has thought through specific approaches to various areas of care.

A wide variety of policies and procedures relating to medical care and the role of the medical director should be developed. **Table 7-5** lists several specific examples. As indicated in the table, many of these policies and procedures are discussed in other chapters. Specific examples of selected policies and procedures are included in the Appendix.

QUALITY ASSURANCE

The medical director is responsible for monitoring and continually attempting to improve the quality of medical services. Quality assurance is a complex activity, and quality assurance programs in NHs are generally not well developed. The Omnibus Budget Reconciliation Act (OBRA) 1987 mandates that there be an active quality assurance program in every NH. In this chapter, we will provide a brief overview of quality assurance as it relates to medical care in the NH and the role of the medical director. More detailed discussion of quality assurance based on principles of total quality management and continuous quality improvement can be found in Chapter 8.

Quality assurance in general focuses on three aspects of care: structure, process, and outcome. In a NH, this requires a multidisciplinary and interdisciplinary approach; all levels of staff—including the administrator, the directors of the medical and nursing departments, social services, pharmacy, dietary, housekeeping, and maintenance—must be involved. Structural considerations target the adequacy and safety of the physical environment. Most quality assurance activities tend to focus on the process of care. Assessing process is tedious and, in fact, sometimes boring; it has been overemphasized to the point of creating a lot of unnecessary paperwork that probably detracts from rather than enhances the quality of care. But some focus on process is necessary, especially in the NH, where standards of care are generally low and

Table 7-5 Examples of policies and procedures

1. General policies
   - Medical department and staff organization
   - Job descriptions (e.g., physician's assistants, nurse practitioners, assistant medical director)
2. Admissions, discharges, transfers
3. Standards for primary and consultant physicians
4. Communications with nursing and other staff
   - Physician notification for acute and subacute changes in resident status
   - Physician responsiveness
5. Documentation
   - Admission database
   - Periodic progress notes
   - Medical record organization
   - Physician orders
   - Incident reports
6. Laboratory services and other diagnostic testing
7. Health maintenance (See Chapter 4)
   - Screening
   - Monitoring
   - Preventive practices
8. Infection control and the use of antimicrobials (See Chapter 19)
9. Medication prescribing (See Chapter 23)
   - General
   - Psychotropics
   - Antimicrobials
10. Specific medical care issues[a], e.g.,
    - Pressure sores
    - Incontinence management
    - Indwelling catheter use and care
    - Assessment of cognitive and affective status
    - Rehabilitation, including gait and mobility assessment
    - Nutrition and hydration
    - Enteral feeding
11. Ethical issues (See Chapter 27)
    - Assessment of decision making capacity
    - Determination of treatment status (i.e., DNR orders, etc.)
12. Employee health
    - Preemployment examinations
    - Annual examinations
    - Accidents, injuries, worker's compensation

[a]Policies and procedures related to clinical conditions should be consistent with the Minimum Data Set (MDS), resident assessment protocols (RAPs), and quality of care standards contained in OBRA 1987.

Table 7-6 Basic approaches to quality assurance[a]

1. Develop, approve and adopt broad principles, goals and objectives for a quality assurance program
2. Select important aspects of care and areas of interest
3. Develop standards key indicator measuring tools
4. Collect and organize the data
5. Analyze and summarize the data
6. Identify problems and trends
7. Develop strategies to deal with problems and trends
8. Provide feedback to staff
9. Implement policies and procedures to correct problems
10. Re-evaluate and provide feedback on problem resolution

[a]See Chapter 8 for a more complete discussion of quality assurance.

many procedures, such as simple medical documentation, are done poorly. Surveyors have begun to emphasize the importance of assessing outcomes of care. In general, outcomes relevant to medical care include physiologic status, ability to perform the activities of daily living, pain, cognition, affect, social activities and interactions, satisfaction with care and environment, and quality of life. The technology to assess some of these outcomes (e.g., physiologic status, cognition) is reasonably well developed, but for others (e.g., pain, quality of life) is far from adequate. Much more research is needed to develop valid and reliable measures of outcomes that are important for NH residents. In addition, because of the heterogeneity of the NH population, "good" outcomes must be viewed in the context of the overall goals of care for individual residents. For example, a good outcome for a resident admitted to the NH for rehabilitation after a hip fracture (independent ambulation and discharge home) may be inappropriate and irrelevant to a resident admitted to the NH with a terminal malignancy or end-stage dementia whose family can no longer care for him or her at home.

Table 7-6 presents a basic approach to standard quality assurance activities. In general, quality assurance involves selecting areas of interest to assess, developing standards for performance on outcomes, designing methods of measurement, collecting and analyzing data, identifying problems and solutions, and monitoring. In the NH, these activities are usually carried out through various committees. Most facilities have several committees that address quality assurance issues, including pharmacy and infection control. The pharmacy committee oversees the prescription, administration, documentation, and monitoring of drug therapy in the facility. Many strategies can be helpful in improving drug therapy in the NH; they are discussed further in Chapter 23. The infection control committee is responsible for reviewing surveillance data on infections that occur in the facility and for developing, implementing, and monitoring policies and procedures related to infectious diseases. Infections and infection control are discussed in detail in Chapter 19. Some examples of quality assurance activities related to medical conditions might include: (1) identifying residents with low hemoglobin levels and determining if they have been evaluated appropriately; (2) determining if depression has been identified and treated; (3) examining the appropriateness of drug prescription (e.g., antimicrobials, psychotropics); and (4) determining if recurrent fallers receive appropriate evaluation.

COMMUNITY RELATIONS

The medical director should act as a spokesperson for the NH to the community. Nursing homes often have a bad reputation both within and outside the medical community. The medical director has a responsibility to attempt to improve the image of the NH through informal and formal discussions with colleagues, health care agencies, and the general public. The NH's essential role in society and families' appropriate expectations for care in the NH should be emphasized. Invitations to visit the facility might be extended to interested parties so that they can get a better understanding of the type and quality of care provided in the NH. The medical director should also represent the facility to other health care providers in the community. This involves not only those listed in **Table 7-4** but also local acute care hospitals, home care agencies, and other providers of long-term health care services. Appropriate policies and procedures for resident care should be mutually agreed upon (see **Table 7-5**), and strategies for effective communication and documentation should be developed. Some relevant examples that may be helpful to medical directors are provided in the Appendix.

EMPLOYEE HEALTH

The medical director is generally responsible for overseeing an employee health program for the NH. This basically involves three activities: (1) an initial health assessment (i.e., a preemployment history and physical examination); (2) periodic reassessment (usually an annual one is required); and (3) evaluation of injuries and in some cases worker's compensation claims. Some medical directors incorporate the NH's employee health program into their own general practice, while others arrange for other physicians to do the examinations. Nurse practitioners and physician's assistants can play an important role in the employee health program. worker's compensation issues are often handled by outside entities, either through a union or other arrangements made by the facility. In many areas of the country, a large proportion of NH staff, especially nurses' aides, comprises recent immigrants and/or individuals of relatively low socioeconomic status. In addition, many licensed nurses have been recruited from abroad. These characteristics of NH staff give rise to a whole set of health issues of which the medical director must be aware. These range from immunization status to the potential for communicable disease to alcohol and drug abuse. If the medical director is not familiar with these areas, he or she should seek consultation from others who can help in setting policies and procedures for the facility's employee health program.

EDUCATION AND RESEARCH

Teaching programs and research are critical to improving NH care. An increasing number of schools for health professionals are establishing affiliations with local NHs for teaching and research purposes. The medical director should facilitate the development of such affiliations and, where appropriate, become a faculty member at the school. In addition to teaching programs related to academic institutions, the medical director should be involved in the education of all levels of NH staff as well as that of residents and their families. The nature of research in the NH will increasingly involve more NHs in order to obtain adequate sample sizes, especially for clinical studies addressing issues important to typical community NHs. The support of medical directors will therefore become increasingly important to the success of NH research. Specific strategies to enhance the success of academic programs in the NH setting are discussed further in Chapter 28. The medical director must also continually educate himself or herself to keep current in geriatric medicine and administrative and regulatory issues related to long-term care. Yearly attendance at either the AMDA national meeting or the national meeting of the American Geriatrics Society is encouraged. *Nursing Home Medicine* (the official AMDA publication) and the *Journal of the American Geriatrics Society* carry many articles relevant to nursing home administration and direct resident care.

MEDICAL DIRECTION IN SUBACUTE CARE UNITS

The rapid growth of subacute care (see Chapter 6) has created a new area of responsibility for medical directors. Medical directors of NHs may or may not also serve as the medical director of the subacute program within their facility. A large number of acute care hospitals have converted unused beds into subacute or "transitional care" units which need medical direction. **Table 7-7** outlines several key aspects of medical directorship of subacute care units. Readers are referred to Chapter 6 and the AMDA position statement referenced in the "Suggested Readings" for further information.

Table 7-7 Key aspects of medical directorship of subacute care programs[a]

Qualifications

1. Understanding of quality indicators for common conditions and services in subacute care.
2. Knowledge and skill working in an interdisciplinary environment
3. Knowledge of various payment sources for subacute care services
4. Understanding the continuum of care and the place of subacute care in that continuum

Functions

1. Responsible for overall coordination of medical care
2. Ensure adequate physician performance, including appropriate credentialing and participation in interdisciplinary care process
3. Ensure overall program provides safe, effective, and efficient care
4. Help establish and ensure quality improvement mechanisms to determine outcomes and improve care
5. Help create an effective continuum of care that links various care sites, including communication and information channels
6. Represent the medical staff to the NH or hospital administration and board regarding the subacute care program
7. Educate physicians, other health providers, administration, patients and families about the goals, objectives and services of the subacute care program

[a]After AMDA position statement (see "Suggested Readings"). Only functions unique or specific to subacute care are listed.

Table 7-8 Criteria for admission to assisted living facilities

1. Residents must be able to mentally and physical negotiate a path to safety unassisted. They may use assistive devices to help them such as a can, walker or wheelchair. They must be able to open the exit door with an understanding that the door goes to the outside of the building.
2. Residents must have a mental understanding of a "fire" or "emergency".
3. Residents must understand the boundaries of the care facility (i.e., they cannot be wanderers).
4. If residents use a wheelchair they must be able to transfer from that wheelchair to a bed or a chair unassisted.
5. If incontinent, the resident must be mentally capable of responding to a bowel and bladder training program.
6. The resident must be able to self-feed.
7. The resident cannot have a communicable disease.
8. The resident should be mentally stable and not a danger (or extreme nuisance) to self or others.
9. The resident may only smoke in restricted areas.
10. The resident will have all medicine dispensed for them unless they have a doctor's order for self-medication.
11. The resident may receive assistance with bathing and/or dressing.
12. The resident should display some dependence in instrumental activities of daily living.

MEDICAL DIRECTION IN LIFECARE FACILITIES

Free-standing apartment or housing complexes for seniors have become relatively common. Many of these now have a medical director who has responsibility for determining if an individual is capable of maintaining his/her free-living status (see **Table 7-8**), monitoring employee health and overssing policies and procedures concerning potential infectious disease epidemics. These medical directors often provide care for those elderly in their complexes who are to frail to travel to their own doctor. Many of these complexes also offer an assisted living section where persons can have their medications given to them and receive assistance with some of their activities of daily living such as bathing.

SUGGESTED READINGS

American Medical Directors Association: *Position on the medical director's role and responsibilities*. Available from AMDA, 10480 Little Patuxent Parkway, Suite 760, Columbia, Maryland 21044.

American Medical Directors Association: *Position statement on the role of the medical director of a subacute care program*. Available from AMDA, 10480 Little Patuxent Parkway, Suite 760, Columbia, Maryland 21044.

Blumenthal D: Total quality management and physicians' clinical decisions. *JAMA* 269:2775–2778, 1993.

Institute of Medicine. *Improving the Quality of Care in Nursing Homes*. National Academy Press, Washington, DC, 1986.

Johnson-Pawlson J: *Quest for Quality. A Continuous Quality Improvement Program for Long Term Care Facilities*. Washington, DC, American Health Care Association, 1991.

Joint Commission of Accreditation of Healthcare Organizations: *1996 Comprehensive Accreditation Manual in Long Term Care*. Chicago, Illinois, JCAHO, 1996.

Karuza J and Katz PR: Physician staffing patterns correlates of nursing home care: An initial inquiry and consideration of policy implications. *J Am Geriatr Soc* 42:787–793, 1994.

Levenson SA (ed): *Medical Direction in Long Term Care: A Guidebook for the Future*. Durham, North Carolina, Carolina Academic Press, 1993.

Levenson SA and Tarnove L (eds): *Medical Director's Policy and Procedure Manual*. Baltimore, Maryland, National Health Publishing, 1990.

Ouslander JG and Tangalos E (eds): Medical Direction in Long Term Care. *Clin Ger Med* 11(3), August, 1995.

CHAPTER

EIGHT

TOTAL QUALITY MANAGEMENT

Quality improvement processes in nursing homes (NHs) have played an important role in enhancing the care and quality of life of residents. The understanding and involvement of physicians in the facilities' quality improvement programs is a key to their success. The importance of the physician in the success of quality assurance was cast in a negative light by Merry who suggested that the physician can often act as the "natural killer cell" of the system.

The original concepts for quality control processes were developed by Florence Nightingale in her 1859 book entitled *Notes on Nursing*. She developed standards for nursing care and suggested actions that would bring about change to conform to these standards. The concepts on which modern quality improvement programs are based were developed by an American, W. Edwards Deming, who revolutionized the quality of products produced by Japan by the application of his principles. His system consists of statistical analysis of outcomes to pinpoint problems in the process and identify those problems most commonly associated with poor outcomes. This strategy was coupled to a process of continuous quality improvement in which workers continuously identify and correct problems, focusing on the areas where the highest rate of deficiencies was identified. The Deming approach has marked similarities to modern geriatric principles in which an interdisciplinary team identifies and corrects problems in a group of individuals at high risk. **Table 8-1** provides a comparison between total quality management (TQM) techniques and conventional quality assurance approaches. Principles of TQM have been successfully used in NHs to reduce physical restraint use, enhance management of urinary incontinence, identify and

Table 8-1 Comparison between clinical quality assurance (QA) techniques in the nursing home and the total quality management (TQM) approach

	Classical QA	TQM
Time of data collection	Retrospective	Real time and continuous
Data collection	Quality assurance staff	Workers
Work sampling goals	Achieve predetermined outcomes	Control variability in outcomes
Statistical analysis	Minimal	Sophisticated, searches for most common cause(s) of problem
Staff (customer) feedback	Irregular and mainly to managers	Regular and to all staff
Employee training	Classroom	On the job
Employee involvement	Low	High–includes employees' suggestions for corrections
Employee motivation	Reprimands, merit awards, facility citations, facility fines	Motivation comes predominantly from involvement in process and achieving improved outcomes

correct nutritional problems, to improve overall care in individual NHs and to improve quality in large numbers of facilities on a state-wide basis. In many cases, increased regulatory requirements have driven the development of innovative quality improvement programs in NHs.

The St Louis University Geriatric Group has examined the areas in NH care considered most amenable to quality improvement by practicing geriatricians and an expert panel (**Table 8-2**). The expert panel rated TQM, clinical care guidelines and clinical care outcomes as the quality improvement processes most likely to have a positive effect on NH care. The expert panel was poorly supportive of the role of State License Review and Minimum Data Set.

The first clearly defined TQM system for a NH was developed by Jacob Dimant, a medical director in New York. His approach demonstrated that major improvements can be achieved in a facility by identifying problem areas and developing and implementing systems that result in continuous improvement in multiple processes of care. One of us (JM) has reported marked alterations in physician behavior in responses to a nurse practitioner-driven continuous quality improvement program. Feedback to physicians concerning possible deviations from modern geriatric practices proved to be a powerful tool in producing positive alternations in physician behavior.

In the next section specific monitoring techniques that have proven useful in identifying problematic outcomes and their causes. Specific examples of quality improvement programs that have improved outcomes will also be discussed.

Table 8-2 Areas in nursing home care considered most amenable to quality improvement by practicing geriatricians and an expert panel[a]

Priority ranking	Geriatricians	Expert panel
1	Undernutrition (85)	Depression
2	Incontinence (70)	Polypharmacy
3	Decubiti (70)	Decubiti
4	Falls (54)	Undernutrition
5	Polypharmacy/Compl. (49)	Falls
6	Depression (38)	UTI
7	Behavior Problems (36)	Behavior Problems
8	Dementia (34)	Incontinence
9	Heart disease (25)	Dementia
10	UTI (22)	Heart Disease

[a]From data in Miller et al: *J Am Geriatr Soc* 41:60, 1994.

MONITORING SYSTEMS

All NHs should utilize at least two ongoing monitoring systems. The first is to monitor changes in clinical outcomes in the facility on a monthly basis. The second is to compare the performance of their own facility to the performances of other facilities. When a facility shows a statistically meaningful deviation from its own norm of from the average of other facilities, further investigations of the cause(s) of the variation are warranted. Data collection concerning specific causes of the variation is then pursued. The findings of this study are then subjected to a Pareto analysis to pinpoint the major causes of the identified problem. The Pareto analysis is based on the principle that a small number of causes will be responsible for the majority of cases. An example of a Pareto analysis is illustrated in the next paragraph.

Facility B was having a problem with an increase in falls. The data on falls were abstracted and analyzed according to the wing and shift time at which they occurred (**Fig. 8-1**). As might be expected, a few individuals accounted for the majority of the falls. No specific cause could be identified. However, there was an excessive number of falls on the 3 pm to 11 pm shift and the majority occurred on wing B. Further investigation identified two aides who were abusing some of the residents on Wing B.

Statistical quality control charts can be utilized to monitor monthly fluctuations in quality of care. The data are presented as a percentage to allow for monthly variations in the census. These graphs need to include lines setting the upper and lower limits of acceptable levels for the item being measured. An example of this monitoring approach is shown in **Fig. 8-2**. An example of the monthly quality assurance data collection form is given in the Appendix.

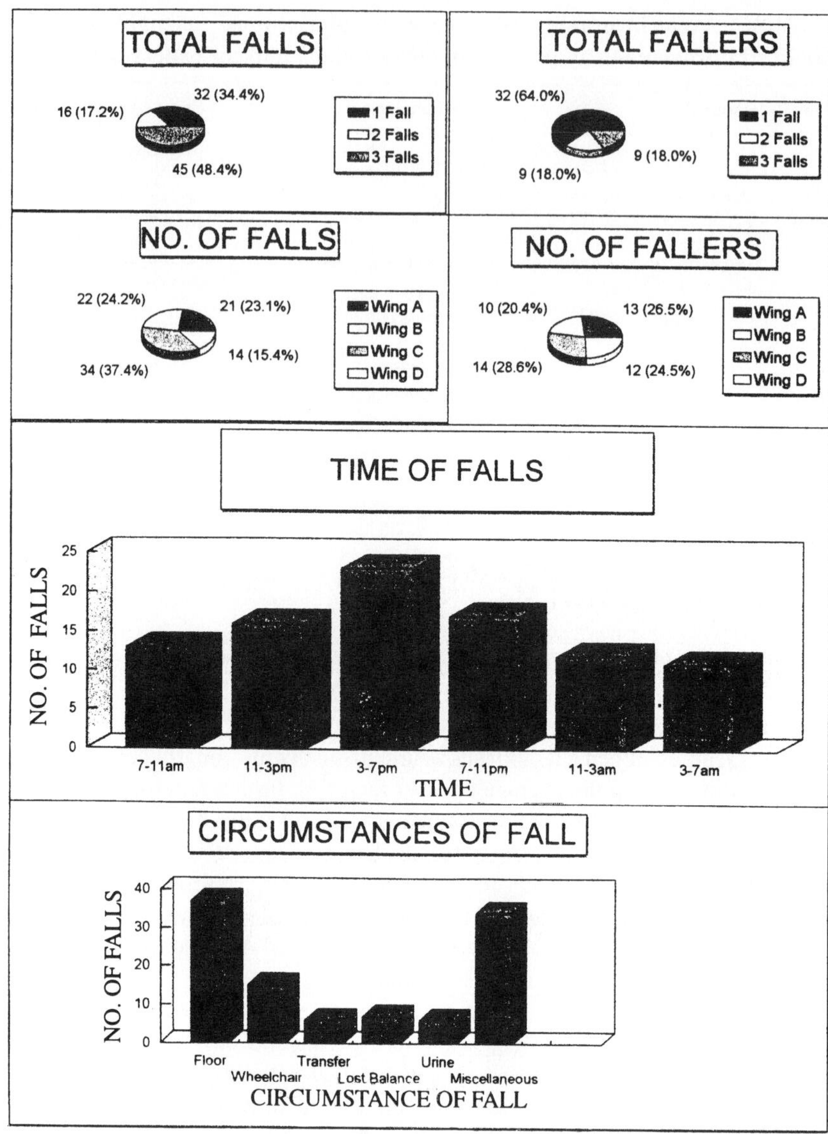

Figure 8-1 Quality improvement data collected on falls in a nursing home.

A key to quality care is the appropriate monitoring of drug utilization. Most major pharmacies can provide comparisons to other facilities they serve in the same are a (**Table 8-3**). Components of appropriate drug utilization monitoring include scheduled medications per resident, as needed medications per resident, number of drugs passed per shift (this highlights if too many

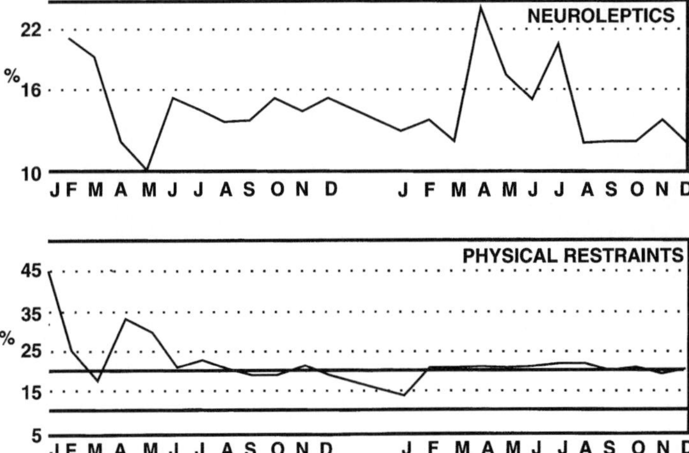

Figure 8-2 Example of a statistical control (p) chart being utilized to monitor alterations in restraint use and neuroleptics in a nursing home.

Table 8-3 Example of a monthly pharmacy report to a nursing home comparing the home's performance to others in the area

Item	General medical information Current period	 Previous period	 IPS average
Average number of scheduled medications per resident	5.27	5.00	5.59
Average number of PRN medications per resident	1.94	1.86	2.94
Average number of scheduled treatments per resident	1.18	1.13	1.66
Average number of PRN treatments per resident	0.29	0.27	0.72
Number of medications passed on the day shift	11175	1134	N/A
Average number of medications per resident passed on the shift	5.88	5.53	6.43
Number of medications passed on the evening shift	760	744	N/A
Average number of medications per resident passed on the evening shift	3.80	3.63	3.85
Number of medications passed on the night shift	288	236	N/A
Average number of medications per resident passed on the night shift	1.14	1.15	1.32

Table 8-4 Abstraction of some of the key data available on the OSCAR reports[a]

	Percentage of residents			
	Facility	Region	State	Nation
Catheters	3.1	6.7	6.7	7.4
Pressure sores	3.7	6.8	6.3	6.0
Physical restraints	6.7	13.1	11.8	22.0
Rehabilitation	31.3	16.9	16.7	16.7

[a]OSCAR reports are based on Minimum Data Set (MDS) reporting.

medications are not being used in their long-acting forms), percent of residents receiving neuroleptics, percent of residents receiving anxiolytics and cost per medication.

The availability of Online Survey on Certification and Reporting system (OSCAR) reports of each facility and its comparisons to other facilities on a regional, state and nationwide basis revolutionizes the ability to compare the performance one facility to another. The OSCARs are based on reporting to the state through the Minimum Data Set (MDS) forms. Thus, they are only as accurate as the MDS reporting. However, as state surveyors utilize these forms to carry out their inspections, reporting quality should improve. An example of abstracted data from the OSCAR is given in **Table 8-4**.

A variety of quality indicators derived from MDS data have been developed by Zimmerman under contract with the Health Care Financing Administration (HCFA) (**Table 8-5**). Other countries are using different strategies based on MDS data. Geronte (**Fig. 8-3**) is the French equivalent of the MDS. This simple drawing of a person divided into multiple parts representing each potential functional problem allows all the staff and the physician to recognize resident problems after briefly viewing a single sheet. Areas that are impaired are colored in. This diagram has been adapted to the computer. It can be rapidly filled in during the interdisciplinary team meeting at which the MDS is being completed. Staff can then rapidly update the figure when new functional problems occur.

Another source of between facility comparisons comes from commercial chains. These chains commonly collect a variety of data comparing the performances of their facilities. An example of comparing weight loss between different facilities in one region of a commercial chain is given in **Table 8-6**.

Physicians are often unaware of the large amount of outcomes data that are available in NHs. Distribution of these data to physicians represents an important quality assurance strategy as there is a major need for conformation towards the norm among many NHs and health professionals.

Table 8-5 Quality indicators derived from MDS data[a]

Domain	Quality indicator
Accidents	Prevalence of any injury Prevalence of falls
Behavioral and emotional patterns	Prevalence of problem behavior toward others Prevalence of symptoms of depression Prevalence of symptoms of depression with no treatment
Clinical management	Use of 9 or more scheduled medications
Cognitive patterns	Incidence of cognitive impairment
Elimination and continence	Prevalence of bladder or bowel incontinence Prevalence of occasional bladder or bowel incontinence without a toileting plan Prevalence of indwelling catheters Prevalence of fecal impaction
Infection control	Prevalence of urinary tract infections Prevalence of antibiotic or anti-infective use
Nutrition and eating	Prevalence of weight loss Prevalence of tube feeding Prevalence of dehydration
Physical functioning	Prevalence of bedfast residents Incidence of decline in late-loss activities of daily living Incidence of contractures Lack of training or skill practice or range of motion
Psychotropic drug use	Prevalence of antipsychotic use in the absence of psychotic and related conditions Prevalence of antipsychotic daily dose in excess of surveyor guidelines Prevalence of hypnotic drug use on a scheduled or as-needed basis greater than twice in last week Prevalence of use of any long-acting benzodiazepine
Quality of life	Prevalence of daily physical restraints Prevalence of little or no activity
Sensory functional and communication	Lack of corrective action for sensory or communication problems
Skin care	Prevalence of stage 1–4 pressure ulcers Insulin-dependent diabetes with no foot care

[a]Based on the work of Zimmerman and colleagues (see "Suggested Readings")

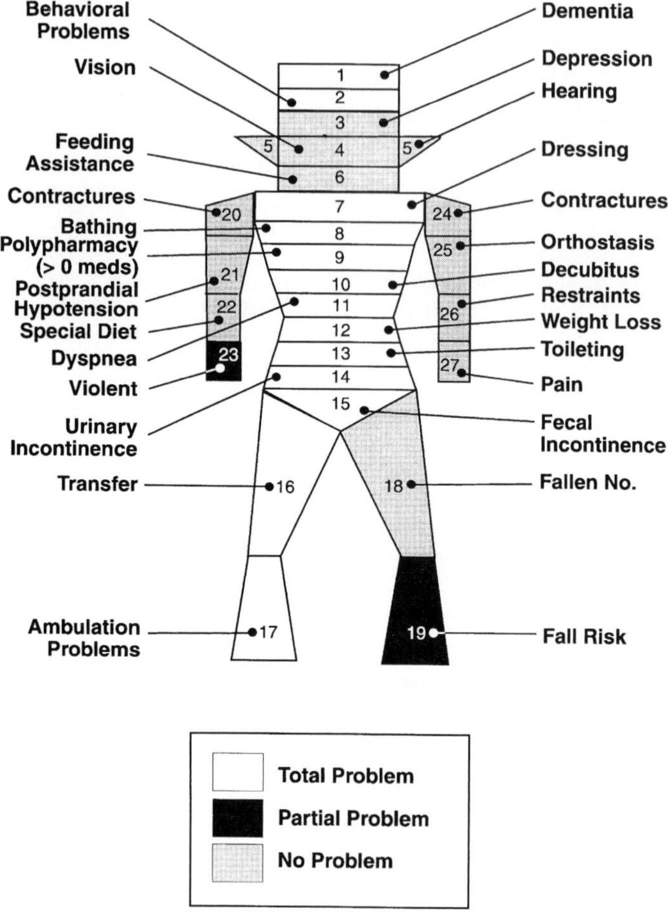

Figure 8-3 Figure used as a basis of the French equivalent of the Minimum Data Set ("Geronte", see text).

AN EXAMPLE OF THE MEDICAL DIRECTOR'S ROLE: REVIEW OF NEUROLEPTIC AND ANXIOLYTIC USE

In a number of facilities one of us (JM) has developed a yearly medical director's review of all residents on neuroleptics and/or anxiolytics. The medical record of each resident who is on psychoactive drugs is reviewed and the resident is interviewed and examined to determine the appropriateness of the psychoactive drug use. A medical director's note, such as the one illustrated in **Table 8-7**, record summarizes the typical findings of a review at one facility. The medical director's note represents a powerful tool to alter physician behavior. **Table 8-8**

Table 8-6 Comparison of weight loss greater than 10 percent between different facilities in one region of a commercial chain

	Percentage of Residents		
Facility	**June**	**July**	**August**
A	7	3	7
B	12	8	12
C	5	4	2
D	6	3	10
E	10	12	8
F	4	3	6
G	2	1	7
H	0	2	0
Own Home	2	2	4

illustrates an example of a monthly review of psychotropic medication use in an entire facility.

EXAMPLES OF INTERDISCIPLINARY QUALITY IMPROVEMENT

Reduction of physical restraint use is a major need in many facilities. A highly successful approach has been to form a team of a nurse practitioner, nurse supervisor, unit coordinator and physical therapist to do monthly rounds to identify residents who may be inappropriately restrained. Discussion of the

Table 8-7 Medical director's psychotropic drug review

This resident is on Haldol 0.5 mg daily; lorazepam 0.5 mg q 6 hours p.r.n.

Findings

1. No diagnosis is given for the use of the haldol
2. The resident has dementia and may have been agitated in the past
3. The resident does not have hallucinations or paranoia
4. The nurses' notes make no mention of agitation and lorazepam has not been given for the last three months
5. The resident is mildly dysphoric with a Geriatric Depression Scale of 14/30
6. The resident has early Parkinsonism
7. There is no tardivedyskinea

Recommendations

1. Discontinue both the haloperidol and lorazepam
2. Add trazodone 50 to 100 mg at night. This will help treat the dysphoria and also decrease agitation

Table 8-8 Example of a facility review of psychotropic medication use

	This Month	Last Month	Pharmacy Average
Number of residents receiving antipsychotic medications	20	20	N/A
% of resident population receiving antipsychotics	10%	10%	14.43%
Number of residents receiving sedative/hypnotic/anxiolytic medications	19	20	N/A
% of resident population receiving sedative/hypnotic/anxiolytic medications	9.5%	10%	23.14%
Number of residents receiving antidepressant medications	79	76	N/A
% of resident population receiving antidepressants	39.5%	37%	29%
Total number of residents receiving psychotropics	95	100	N/A
% of resident population receiving psychotropics	47.5%	49%	49.53%
Total number of resident receiving chemical restraints (not including antidepressants)	36	37	N/A
Percent of resident population receiving chemical restraints (not including antidepressants)	18%	18%	N/A
Average cost per Rx	$32.79	$35.23	N/A

N/A = Data not available.

problem with the nurses aides looking after the resident enhances outcomes. Physician support is often needed when dealing with families who are apposed to restraint reduction. An example of an assessment for the need for restraint use is discussed in Chapter 16.

A high prevalence of orthostatic hypotension was recognized in a 200–bed NH. A review of the medical records demonstrated that many of the residents with orthostasis were on a low salt diet **Table 8-9**. The data were presented in an interdisciplinary quality improvement meeting during which the food manager stated that in view of the large number of residents on a low salt diet she had decided to only cook low salt food and allow the residents not on the diet to add salt to taste. Unfortunately, many of the demented residents failed to add sufficient salt to their diet. The medical director and administrator agreed to only

Table 8-9 Effects of low salt diets in a nursing home[a]

	Low-salt diet	Regular diet	*P*
Orthostatic hypotension	79%	46%	<0.05
Albumin <3.5 g/dl	66%	33%	<0.05
Weight loss	53%	43%	Not significant

[a]From Morley et al: *Nurs Home Med* 2:11–17, 1994.

allow low salt diets after consultation with the medical director. All diets were then cooked with salt. Full interdisciplinary discussion of the problem and physician agreement to limit the use of low salt diets were keys to success of the program.

In a facility in Rolla, Missouri, there was an increase in skin tears. An interdisciplinary meeting identified the cause as the sharp edges of wheelchairs. The maintenance engineer solved the problem by placing old tire strips over the sharp edges of the wheelchairs.

Schnelle and colleagues have described in detail the use of principles of TQM and statistical quality control to improve the interdisciplinary management of urinary incontinence. In their system wetness rates are measured periodically by nursing supervisors. These wetness rates are then plotted on a quality control chart such as the one illustrated in **Fig. 8-4**. The key to the

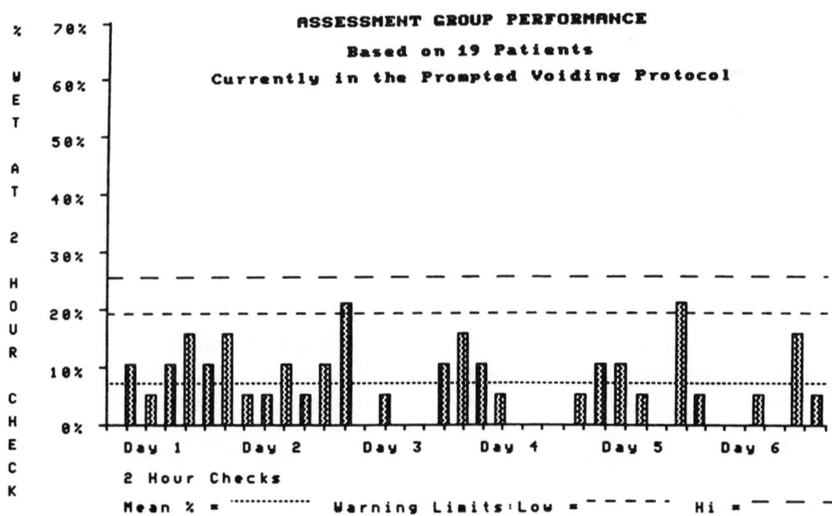

Figure 8-4 Example of a statistical quality control chart used to monitor wetness rates and maintain effectiveness of a prompted voiding program for urinary incontinence.

system, however, is the targeting of the intervention (in this case prompted voiding) to residents who are responsive to the intervention (as identified in a 3-day trial period of the intervention) so that an expected performance level (wetness rate) without extreme variability, and associated warning limits can be established.

CUSTOMER SATISFACTION: THE KEY TO QUALITY MANAGEMENT

Monitoring of customer satisfaction is an important component of quality management. It needs to be recognized that quality of care is often poorly related to resident and/or family satisfaction. When resident satisfaction is very low, consideration needs to be given to the possibility that depression is being undertreated. Reliable and valid measurement tools are currently being developed and tested to assess resident and family satisfaction with care. The high prevalence of dementia among NH residents makes the accurate measurement of satisfaction particularly difficult and challenging.

In addition to residents and families, the NH staff represent a third set of customers. Positive physician interactions with the staff can greatly enhance quality of care for the residents. It is particularly important to be respectful to the staff and enforce the importance of the job they are doing.

CONCLUSION

TQM techniques have an important role to play in improving quality of life of NH residents. **Table 8-10** provides examples of topics and outcomes that can be used for improving quality improvement in the NHs. Other chapters in this text elaborate in detail on the clinical guidelines that can be utilized to improve the process, outcomes and overall quality of care.

Table 8-10 Examples of selected areas in which data collection can be targeted for quality improvement in nursing homes

Falls	Infections
Incontinence	Chronic indwelling bladder, catheter use
Weight loss	Pressure ulcers
Psychotropic drug prescriptions	Skin tears
Medications in general	Hospital transfers
Contractures	Depression

SUGGESTED READINGS

Dimant J: From quality assurance to quality management in long term care. *QRB* 207–215, 1991.

Schnelle JF, Ouslander JG, Osterweil D, and Blumenthal S: Total quality management: Administrative and clinical applications in nursing homes. *J Am Geriatr Soc* 41:1259–1266, 1993.

Miller DK, Coe RM, Morley JE, and Romeis JC: *Total Quality Improvement in Geriatric Care*. New York, Springer, 1995.

Miller DK, Coe RM, Romeis JC, and Morley JE: Improving quality of geriatric health care in four sites: Suggestions from practitioners and experts. *J Am Geriatr Soc* 41:60–65, 1994.

Morley JE, Kraenzle D, Jensen JM, Gettman J, and Tetter L: The role of a nurse practitioner in quality improvement in nursing homes. *Nurs Home Med* 2:11–17, 1994.

Vetel JM: Geronte: A low-cost tool to increase the quality of care of elderly persons. *Danish Medical Bulletin Suppl* 5:93–95, 1987.

Zimmerman DR, Karon SL, Arling G, Clark BR, Collins T, et al: Development and testing of nursing home quality indicators. *Health Care Financing Review* 16:107–127, 1995.

CHAPTER

NINE

THE ROLE OF THE NURSE PRACTITIONER AND PHYSICIAN'S ASSISTANT

Nurse practitioners (NPs) and physician's assistants (PAs) can play an important role in nursing home (NH) care. NPs are (as of 1991) master's prepared registered nurses who are educated to perform advanced physical assessment, order and interpret laboratory tests, provide health promotion and disease prevention, manage and monitor acute simple health problems and chronic health problems. Nurse practitioners practice under their own licensure and certification and enter into collaborative practice agreements with physicians to provide the patient care which falls beyond the NP's scope of practice. PAs have multiple levels of entrance into practice; from associates degree to masters level preparation. The majority of PAs have bachelor's degrees. PA's are educated to provide health care services with the direction and responsible supervision of a doctor of medicine or osteopathy. The functions include performing diagnostic therapeutic preventive and health maintenance services in any setting in which a physician renders care. Medicare reimbursement can be obtained for both types of providers for services they provide in the NH and, importantly, and services can be provided without on-site physician supervision. State regulations regarding the involvement of NPs and PAs vary, and providers should be knowledgeable of relevant legislation. Although clinical service, especially the initial assessment of acute conditions, will be a predominant activity, NPs and PAs can potentially play a number of roles in the NH setting that will lead to improvements in medical care as well as interdisciplinary communication. Several studies have documented that NPs can play an important role in improving the outcomes of NH residents.

No studies have specially examined the impact of PAs in the NH, but their clinical training is clearly compatible with the role of a clinician in the NH setting. NPs have one important advantage: their background in nursing. Many of the day-to-day issues that arise in the care of NH residents are nursing-oriented, and much of the care depends on effective communication between the nursing staff and primary-care physicians. In our experience, the NPs' nursing background has been critical in their roles in the NH and has enabled them to act as effective liaisons between the nursing and medical staffs. Whether NPs or PAs are employed, their success is critically dependent on their ability to interact in a nonthreatening manner with the nursing staff and other members of the interdisciplinary team and on clearly defined roles, responsibilities, clinical privileges, and place within the organizational structure of the facility.

ROLES AND RESPONSIBILITIES

NPs and PAs can participate in a number of different clinical, administrative, educational, and research activities (**Table 9-1**). The extent of their participation will depend on a number of factors, including their qualifications and experience, who hires them, how they fit into the organizational structure of the facility, and the policies and extent of activities (e.g., educational, research) within the facility.

Clinical activities will be the basis of the NP's or PA's role and responsibilities in the vast majority of settings. These responsibilities can range from serving as a primary care provider in conjunction with the physician, to the assessment and management of acute and subacute conditions, to serving as a consultant to the interdisciplinary team and family members. With respect to primary care, the NP or PA can assist with readmission assessments in stable residents after hospitalizations, carefully documenting baseline findings, problems, and goals. He or she can also perform some of the required periodic visits as well as annual reassessments in conjunction with the primary-care physician. Federal regulations relevant to the primary care role of NPs and PAs are summarized in **Table 9-2**. With respect to consultant activities, the NP or PA can play an integral role in the evaluation of specific geriatric conditions which might be identified by the Minimum Data Set (MDS) assessment and trigger the relevant resident assessment protocol (RAP) (such as dementia, incontinence, and recurrent falls) or common chronic problems, such as diabetes and hypertension. The NP or PA can also serve as a valuable consultant to the interdisciplinary team and family members, especially since most primary care physicians spend limited time at the facility. The NP or PA can explain the medical regimen and the rationale for it; discuss the results of diagnostic tests and their implications; and assist the team, the resident, and the

Table 9-1 Potential roles and responsibilities for nurse practitioners and physician's assistants

A. Clinical
   1. Primary care (in conjunction with primary physician)
   2. Assist with re-admission assessments (after hospitalization in stable residents)
   3. Periodic (e.g., annual) medical and functional assessments
   4. Assessment of acute changes in status
   5. Management of subacute illness
   6. Participation in discharge planning at acute hospital
   7. Consultant
      (a) Serve as a resource to implement the Resident Assessment Protocols (RAPs) for specific conditions identified on the Minimum Data Set (MDS)
         (1) Dementia
         (2) Incontinence
         (3) Falls
         (4) Functional decline
         (5) Others
      (b) Serve as consultant to interdisciplinary team and family members
         (1) Explain medical care regimens and diagnostic test results
         (2) Discuss ethical issues and advance directives
         (3) Assist in the development of mutually acceptable, realistic expectations and goals of care

B. Administrative
   1. Participate in interdisciplinary team meetings
   2. Participate in medical and nursing committees and meetings
   3. Assist in the development of policies, procedures and protocols
   4. Assist the medical director in administering an employee health program
   5. Participate in quality assurance activities
      (a) Review and ensure appropriate documentation in progress notes and problem lists
      (b) Assist in the implementation and completion of screening, health maintenance and preventive protocols (see Chapter 4)
      (c) Perform selected quality assurance audits
      (d) Serve on institutional committees (e.g., infection control, pharmacy, ethics)

C. Educational
   1. Participate in the in-service education program for nursing staff
   2. Make presentations to residents and families
   3. Participate in undergraduate education programs for medical and nursing students
   4. Participate in graduate education programs for medical residents, geriatric medicine fellows, master's nursing students and nurse practitioner trainees
   5. Represent the facility at community educational programs

D. Research
   1. Consult with investigators on the design of protocols to be implemented in the facility
   2. Facilitate the implementation of approved studies
   3. Assist with data collection (time should be supported by research funds if appropriate)
   4. Design and conduct independent clinical research projects

Table 9-2 Summary of federal guidelines relevant to the primary care role of nurse practitioners and physician assistants in nursing homes[a]

Regulation	Guidance to surveyors
At the option of the physician, required visits to SNFs after the initial visit (once every 30 days for the first 90 days, and at least once every 60 days), may alternate between personal visits by the physician and visits by a physician assistant, nurse practitioner or clinical nurse specialist (in States allowing their use)	Visits performed by these other providers do not relieve the physician of the obligation to visit a resident when the resident's medical condition makes that visit necessary. When one of these providers determines that the resident's condition warrants direct contact between the physician and the resident, the physician must follow-up promptly with a personal visit.
A physician may delegate tasks to a physician assistant, nurse practitioner or clinical nurse specialist who: (1) Meets the applicable definition; (2) Is acting within the scope of practice as defined by State law; and (3) Is under the supervision of the physician A physician may not delegate a task when the regulations specify that the physician must perform it personally, or when the delegation is prohibited under State law or by the facility's own policies. At the option of the State, any required physician task in a NF (including tasks which the regulations specify must be performed personally by the physician) may also be satisfied when performed by a nurse practitioner, clinical nurse specialist or physician assistant who is not an employee of the facility but who is working in collaboration with a physician.	"Nurse practitioner" is a registered professional nurse now licensed to practice in the State and who meets the State's requirements governing the qualifications of nurse practitioners. "Clinical nurse specialist" is a registered professional nurse currently in practice in the State and who meets the State's requirements governing the qualifications of clinical nurse specialist. "Physician assistant" is a person who meets the applicable State requirements governing the qualifications for assistants to physicians. When *personal* performance of a particular task by a physician is specified in the regulations, performance of that task cannot be delegated to anyone else. The tasks of examining the residents, reviewing the resident's total program of care, writing progress notes, and signing orders may be delegated according to state law. The extent to which physician services are delegated to physician extenders in SNFs will continue to be determined by Federal provisions, while the extent to which these services are performed by physician extenders in NFs will be determined by the individual States. NP/clinical nurse specialist/PA progress notes and orders must follow the scope of practice allowed by State law. There must be evidence of physician supervision of NPs or PAs (for example, do physicians countersign NP/PA orders, if required by State law).

[a]Table based on HCFA State Operations Manual, June 1995.
SNF, state nursing facility.

family in developing realistic expectations and goals of care. The NP or PA can therefore play a critical role in enhancing communication and establishing the medical care plan.

Perhaps the most important clinical role and responsibility of the NP or PA is to assess acute changes in status and oversee the management of subacute problems in the NH. In the absence of NPs and PAs, the vast majority of acute problems are evaluated over the telephone, frequently result in an emergency room visit, and too often lead to a costly and unnecessary hospitalization. Although many factors influence decisions as to whether or not to hospitalize a NH resident (see Chapter 5), the availability of an on-site NP or PA will decrease the likelihood of unnecessary and expensive emergency room visits. Many acute and subacute conditions can be assessed and managed in a typical community NH by a NP or PA. Protocols are available and others can be developed that are mutually acceptable to the medical director, medical staff, nursing staff, and NH administration. These protocols are discussed further under "Clinical Privileges and Protocols," below.

NPs and PAs can also play an important role in a variety of administrative activities (**Table 9-1**). They may be especially valuable in working with nursing staff to develop and implement policies and procedures related to medical and nursing care, such as "Immediate versus Nonimmediate Physician Notification" (see Appendix). The NP and PA staff can also play a critical role in the employee health program by performing on-site initial assessments of illness and injury within the facility's guidelines regarding workers compensation issues. This may save the facility a considerable amount of money by reducing the number of emergency room and physician visits made by employees. Adult and family NPs (as opposed to geriatric NPs) are especially well prepared to participate in facilities' employee health programs. The NPs and PAs can also play an important role in a variety of medical quality assurance activities (**Table 9-1**).

In facilities with active educational and research programs, appropriately qualified and experienced NPs and PAs can be active participants in enhancing these programs. All facilities have in-service programs for staff, and the NP or PA can assist in the development of curricula and in making selected presentations. The NP and PA can also make valuable contributions to the undergraduate and graduate education of physicians and nurses in facilities with university affiliations. Many NPs and PAs may qualify for appointments at the university's nursing or medical school. If the facility serves as a site for clinical research, the NP or PA can assist investigators in the development of appropriate protocols for the NH setting and facilitate the implementation of the research, especially by serving as a liaison between the investigators and the medical and nursing staff. Some NPs and PAs may want to design and conduct their own research projects or participate actively in projects being implemented at the facility. Whenever appropriate, time spent by NPs and PAs on funded research projects should be supported by research funds.

CLINICAL PRIVILEGES AND PROTOCOLS

No matter what the precise roles and responsibilities of the NP or PA in a particular NH may be, a specific set of clinical privileges and protocols should be developed, in addition to a complete job description to serve as a clean delineation of the role for NH staff.

Whether or not state laws require the NP or PA to have an explicit written agreement with a supervising physician, a list of clinical privileges should be developed and agreed upon by the NP or PA, the medical director, members of the medical staff who work collaboratively with the NP or PA, the director of nursing, and the facility administrator. This list of privileges serves to clarify for everyone involved what the NP or PA is qualified to do independently and what activities require consultation with the medical director or supervising physician. An example of a list of clinical privileges is included in the Appendix.

Clinical protocols are also a valuable tool in clearly defining the general approach that NPs or PAs will take toward their clinical care activities. As discussed in Chapter 4, the medical director and primary medical staff should develop standardized approaches to admission, readmission, and periodic (e.g., monthly, annual) assessments, which the NP or PA can use as guidelines in carrying out these activities. Examples of such databases are illustrated in Chapter 4, for the monthly progress note and in the Appendix for admission and annual assessments. Examples of clinical protocols for the evaluation of five common acute conditions—fever, change in mental status, dyspnea, abdominal pain, and gastrointestinal bleeding are illustrated in **Figs. 9-1 through 9-5**.

PLACE WITHIN THE FACILITY'S ORGANIZATIONAL STRUCTURE

In order for NPs or PAs to function effectively in a NH setting, their place within the facility's organizational structure must be clearly defined. There are a number of different possibilities, but some general principles should be adhered to. First, irrespective of who the employer is, NPs or PAs should have a written job description that clearly defines their roles and responsibilities and refers to the clinical privileges and protocols discussed above. Second, the job description should be reviewed and approved by the medical director, director of nursing, and administrator of the facility. Third, the clinical supervision and performance evaluations must be done by an appropriately qualified individual; administrators and directors of nursing should be responsible for supervision and performance evaluation only if they themselves are qualified and experienced NPs, PAs, or MDs. It is also important to clearly separate the role and responsibilities of the NP or PA from those of the licensed nursing staff. Finally, state and federal regulations need to be considered in arranging employment agreements, as they may affect the role of NPs and PAs.

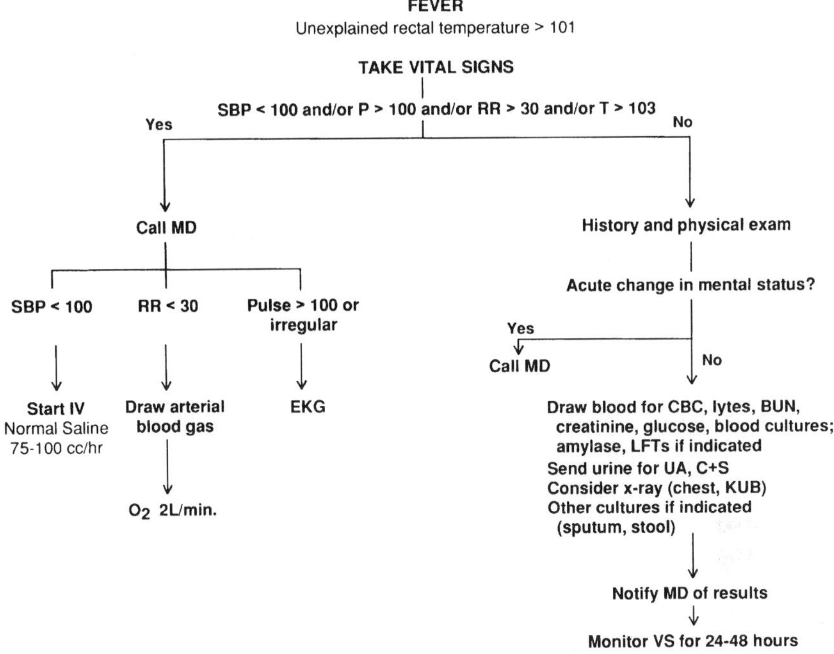

Figure 9-1 Example of clinical protocol for use by NPs or PAs in the assessment and management of fever in the NH.

In our experience, NPs have functioned most effectively when they are basically considered active members of the primary medical staff, limited only by their clinical privilege statement. **Fig. 9-6** illustrates the way in which the NP or PA fits into the facility's organizational structure under two different employment conditions: employed by the facility or employed by a physician or group of physicians. Other models exist as well. For example, an NP may have direct reporting responsibilities to the medical director for resident care activities and to the director of nursing for nursing education, consultations with nursing staff, and nursing research.

EMPLOYMENT AND REIMBURSEMENT CONSIDERATIONS

The employer of the NP or PA is generally a facility, a physician, or a group of physicians. Joint employment by the facility and a physician or physician group is possible but would probably make things unnecessarily complicated. Some health maintenance organizations (HMOs) have hired NPs and PAs to participate in the care of members of their plan who reside in NHs. NPs are able to bill Medicare directly for services they provide in NHs at 85 percent

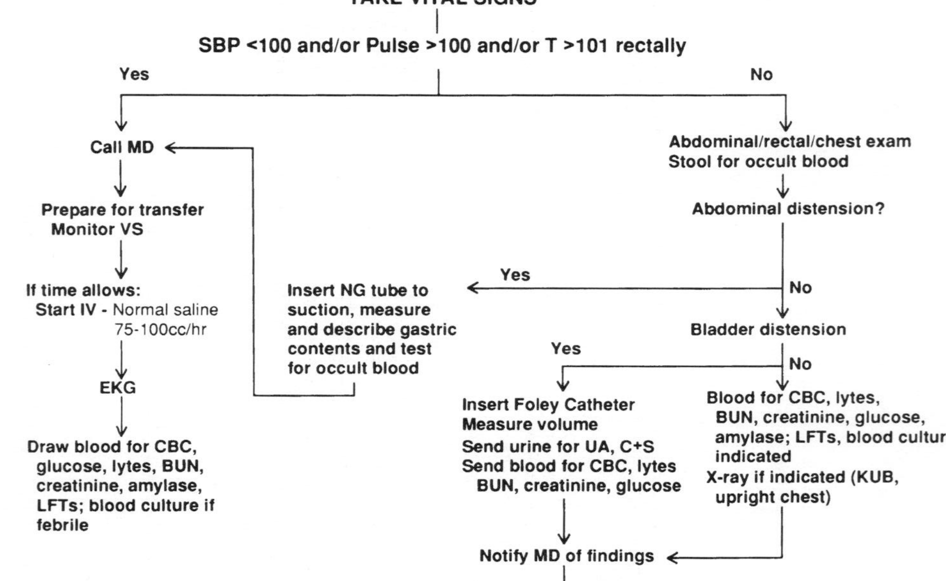

Figure 9-2 Example of clinical protocol for use by NPs or PAs in the assessment and management of acute abdominal pain in the NH.

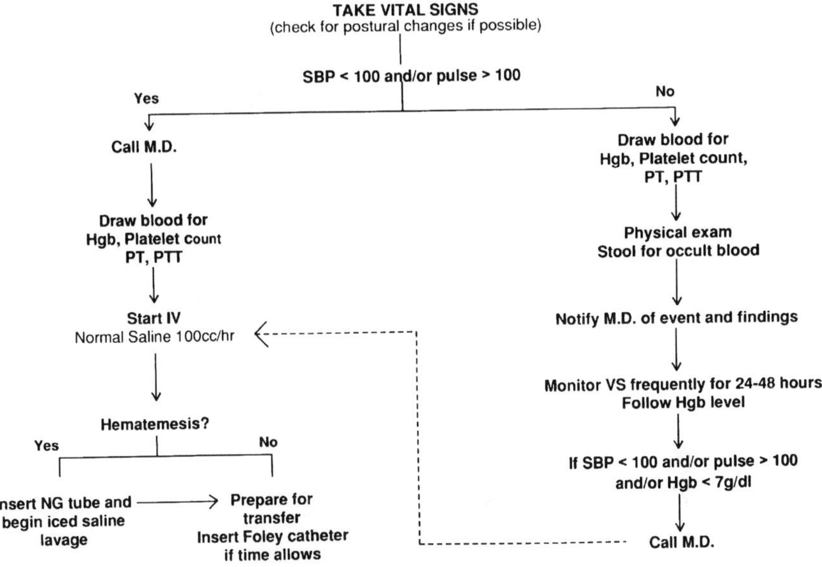
GASTROINTESTINAL BLEEDING
Symptoms: Resident or staff report hematemesis, tarry stool and/or red blood per rectum
TAKE VITAL SIGNS
(check for postural changes if possible)
SBP < 100 and/or pulse > 100
Yes
No
Call M.D.
Draw blood for
Hgb, Platelet count
PT, PTT
Start IV
Normal Saline 100cc/hr
Hematemesis?
Yes
No
Insert NG tube and
begin iced saline
lavage
Prepare for
transfer
Insert Foley catheter
if time allows
Draw blood for
Hgb, Platelet count,
PT, PTT
Physical exam
Stool for occult blood
Notify M.D. of event and findings
Monitor VS frequently for 24-48 hours
Follow Hgb level
If SBP < 100 and/or pulse > 100
and/or Hgb < 7g/dl
Call M.D.

Figure 9-3 Example of clinical protocol for use by NPs or PAs in the assessment and management of gastrointestinal bleeding in the NH.

of the rate for physicians. PAs can bill indirectly for their services in the NH through the physician's provider number with a modifier, or through the NH; in either case it is billed at 85 percent of the physician's rate. When NPs or PAs bill, however, the physician cannot also request reimbursement for the same activity. The current *Medicare Carrier Manual* allows physician reimbursement for one visit per calendar month, with further visits reimbursable only in situations where the physician has adequately substantiated the need for more frequent reimbursement. However, for nursing home residents who receive visits from a member of a physician/PA/NP team, 1.5 routine visits per month (averaged over a 4–6 month period) are allowed (in addition to nonroutine visits for acute illnesses which are adequately substantiated). A "team" is defined as a physician and PA working under the physician's supervision, and/or a NP working in collaboration with the physician. "Team" cannot be used to describe a medical group that does not employ either PAs or NPs. Whether NPs or PAs bill Medicare directly or their services are billed for by the facility or a physician or physician group, net clinical revenues are unlikely to support their entire salary and benefits. In the Los Angeles area, the median salary for an NP in 1996 is approximately $60,000, with salaries for PAs being slightly lower. Thus, creative methods of supplementing clinical revenues must be developed. In some cases, the NH will support part of the

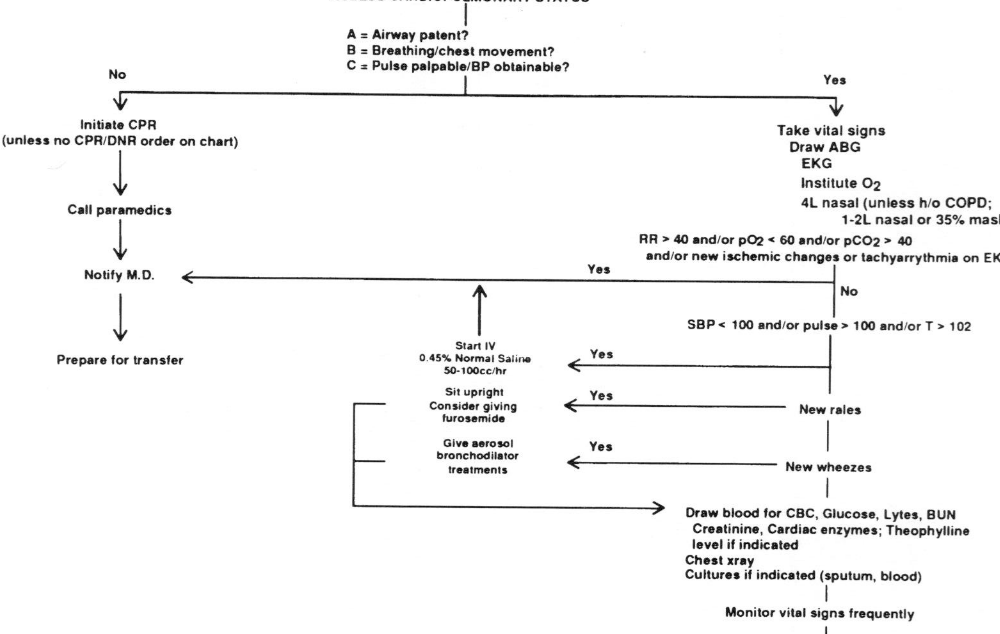
ACUTE DYSPNEA
Symptoms: Sudden onset of shortness of breath, with or without cough/wheezing
ASSESS CARDIOPULMONARY STATUS
A = Airway patent?
B = Breathing/chest movement?
C = Pulse palpable/BP obtainable?
No
Yes
Initiate CPR
(unless no CPR/DNR order on chart)
Call paramedics
Notify M.D.
Prepare for transfer
Take vital signs
Draw ABG
EKG
Institute O2
4L nasal (unless h/o COPD;
1-2L nasal or 35% mask)
RR > 40 and/or pO2 < 60 and/or pCO2 > 40
and/or new ischemic changes or tachyarrythmia on EKG
Yes
No
SBP < 100 and/or pulse > 100 and/or T > 102
Start IV
0.45% Normal Saline
50-100cc/hr
Yes
Sit upright
Consider giving
furosemide
Yes
New rales
Give aerosol
bronchodilator
treatments
Yes
New wheezes
Draw blood for CBC, Glucose, Lytes, BUN
Creatinine, Cardiac enzymes; Theophylline
level if indicated
Chest xray
Cultures if indicated (sputum, blood)
Monitor vital signs frequently
Notify M.D. of results

Figure 9-4 Example of clinical protocol for use by NPs or PAs in the assessment and management of acute dyspnea in the NH.

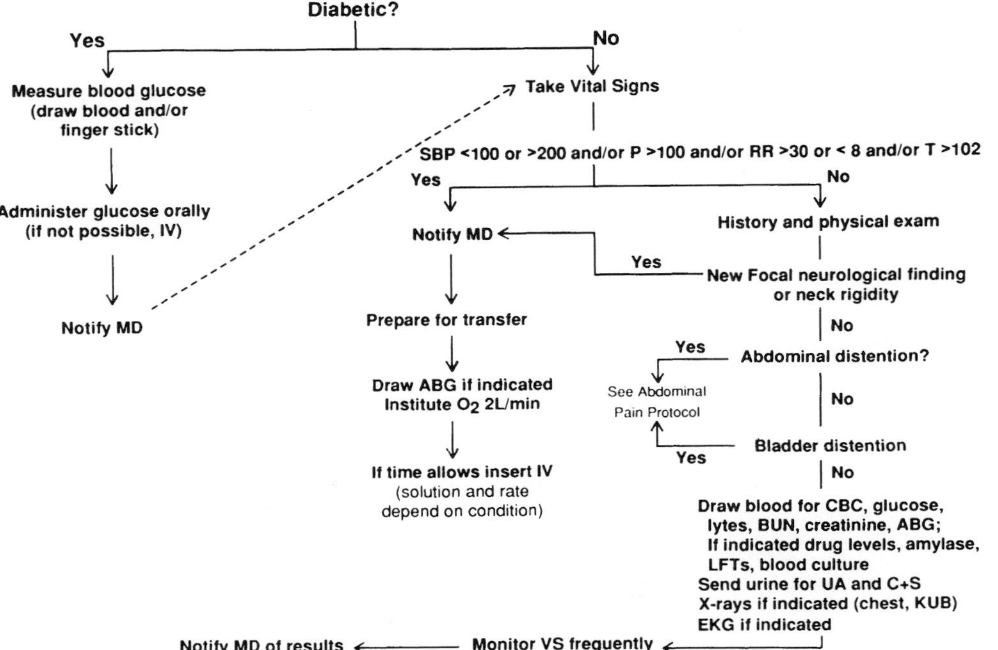

Figure 9-5 Example of clinical protocol for use by NPs or PAs in the assessment and management of an acute change in mental status in the NH.

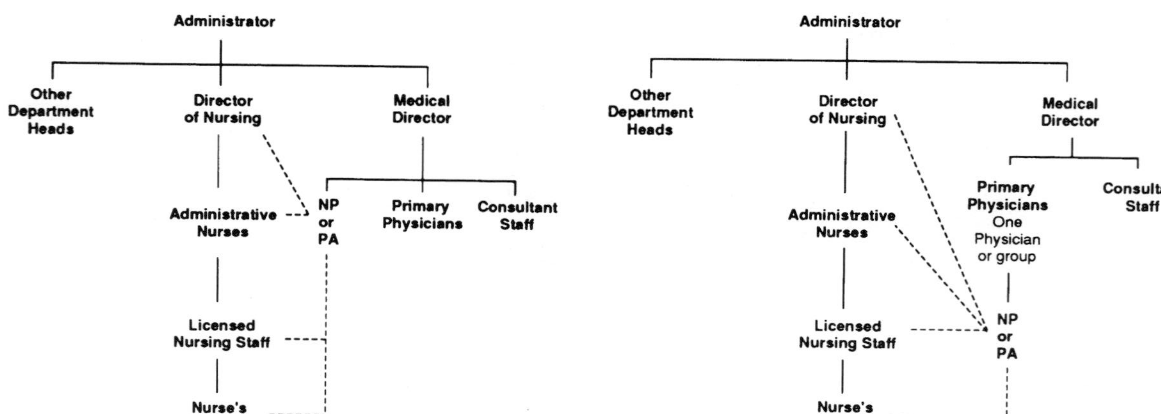

Figure 9-6 The place of the NP or PA in the organizational structure of an NH. Solid lines imply direct supervision and lines of reporting. Dotted lines refer to frequent interaction on clinical and administrative issues. In the diagram on the left, the NP or PA is employed by the facility; in the diagram on the right, she/he is employed by a physician or group of physicians who provide primary care at the facility.

salary through its nursing and/or administrative budget. Similarly, a physician or physician group may support part of the salary from other income. If NPs or PAs do not spend full time at the NH, they may engage in other revenue-generating activities (e.g., clinical practice in a geriatric clinic or other geriatric program). Other possibilities are partial support from an affiliated acute care hospital for participating in discharge planning and quality assurance activities related to geriatric care or from a funded research project.

SUGGESTED READINGS

American College of Physicians: Physician Assistants and Nurse Practitioners. *Ann Intern Med* 121:714–716, 1994.

Jones EP, Cawley JF: Physician assistants and health system reform: Cliincal capabilities, practice activities and potential roles. *JAMA* 271:1266–1272, 1994.

Garrard J, Kane RL, Radosevich DM, et al: Impact of geriatric nurse practitioners on nursing-home residents' functional status, satisfaction, and discharge outcomes. *Med Care* 28:271–283, 1990.

Kane RL, Garrard J, Skay CL, et al: Effects of a geriatric nurse practitioner on process and outcome of nursing home care. *Am J Pub Health* 79:1271, 1989.

Kane RL, Garrard J, Buchanan J, et al: The geriatric nurse practitioner as a nursing home employee: Conceptual and methodological issues in assessing quality of care and cost effectiveness, in Mezey MD, Lynaugh JE, and Cartier MM (eds): *Nursing Homes and Nursing Care: Lessons from the Teaching Nursing Homes*. New York, Springer, 1989.

Kane RA, Kane RL, Arnold S, et al: Geriatric nurse practitioners as nursing home employees: Implementing the role. *Gerontologist* 28:469–477, 1988.

Martin SE, Turner CL, Mendelsohn SE, et al: Assessment and initial management of acute medical problems in a nursing home, in Bosker G (ed): *Principles and Practice of Acute Geriatric Medicine*, 2nd ed. St Louis, Missouri, Mosby, 1990.

Mezey MD, McGivern, DO: *Nurses, Nurse Practitioners Evolution to Advanced Practice*. New York, Springer Publishing Company, 1993.

Wieland D, Rubenstein LZ, Ouslander JG, et al: Organizing an academic nursing home. *JAMA* 255:2622–2627, 1986.

CHAPTER
TEN

INTERDISCIPLINARY TEAMS

The use of the team approach has become part of the essence of geriatrics. Interdisciplinary teams were originally developed in missionary hospitals in the 1920s and were academized by the team developed by physiatrists at Montefiore Hospital in New York in the 1940s. Interdisciplinary teams represent a coordinated effort by a number of health professionals to develop a shared treatment plan for a given patient. They differ from the classical multidisciplinary approach of health care delivery where a physician makes all decisions for the patient, utilizing the services of others as consultants. Central to the interdisciplinary team approach is the concept that the sharing of information by all the health professionals caring for the patient will lead to better management decisions.

When interdisciplinary teams originally developed in missionary hospitals, there was a shortage of available physician time, forcing other members of the health care team to shoulder more responsibilities. Similarly, in America, the greatest cohesiveness and success of interdisciplinary teams have been in situations where there is less physician availability, such as in the nursing home (NH). Recently, interdisciplinary teams in the NH have been demonstrated to decrease emergency department visits, decrease drugs prescribed and decrease mortality.

POTENTIAL FUNCTIONS OF INTERDISCIPLINARY TEAMS

Interdisciplinary teams serve several purposes and can have multiple functions (**Table 10-1**). The first purpose of the interdisciplinary team is to allow the

Table 10-1 Functions of interdisciplinary teams

1. Sharing of specialized knowledge between team members from different backgrounds
2. Obtaining a composite view of the resident
3. Development of a unified approach to residents with behavioral problems
4. Evaluation of rehabilitation potential
5. Evaluation of the potential for the resident to return to noninstitutional living
6. Resolution of interpersonal conflicts
7. Formal and mutual education
8. Discussion of administrative issues
9. Acting as part of the facility's quality assurance program
10. Alleviation of caregiver stress
11. Development of a comprehensive individualized plan of care (**see Tables 10-2 and 10-3**)
12. Restraint reduction

sharing of specialized information between health professionals of differing backgrounds. Thus, for example, the team allows the physical therapist to communicate the importance of the nursing staff's active involvement in ongoing physical therapy programs. The dietician may be able to highlight the severity of malnutrition in a resident and stress the need for encouraging her or him to complete all meals. The occupational therapist can work with the nursing staff to develop a program designed to assess and improve activities of daily living. The physician or pharmacist may share with other members of the team information about the specific potential side effects of a drug.

The second purpose of the interdisciplinary team is the sharing of different viewpoints of the resident experienced by different members of the team. This can be particularly useful in assessing the resident's motivation. It can also help to ensure that a quiet resident is not ignored.

The third purpose of the interdisciplinary team is to facilitate a unified approach to residents with behavioral problems. It is essential that team members agree to not allow a resident to play one team member against another. In these cases it is also important that all team members impart the same information to the resident on key issues, such as an impending discharge, setting limits on behavioral disorders, and the prognosis and management of a specific clinical condition.

A fourth purpose of the interdisciplinary team is to evaluate the rehabilitation potential of the resident. Coupled with this is the fifth purpose, which is to evaluate the discharge potential and make discharge plans for residents when appropriate. Clearly, multiple inputs including the social workers' assessment of the resident's social situation, the knowledge derived from a home visit by the occupational therapist, and the input of those who see the resident's functioning throughout the 24-hour period are all essential in order to determine whether the resident is capable of returning home.

The sixth purpose of the interdisciplinary team is to give the team members an opportunity to resolve interpersonal conflicts. This is an extremely important part of teamwork, and time should always be allocated to explore perceived and potential conflicts at team meetings.

The seventh purpose of the interdisciplinary team is to provide an opportunity for formal education for the group as a whole. The team meeting is a time when new information about management of nursing home (NH) residents with interdisciplinary implications can be shared by the group. An example might be data indicating that blood pressure can drop after meals and cause falls. The team meeting is also an excellent time to share articles or recent data on specific management problems with the group as a whole.

The eighth purpose of the interdisciplinary team is to share thoughts on administrative policies and procedures and also to help enforce old ones. The team meeting can also be a time when problems with administration can be fully explored.

The ninth purpose of the interdisciplinary team is to provide a part of the quality assurance program of the facility. For this reason, careful and accurate recording of both the team's plans and also the outcome of these plans is essential.

The final purpose of the team is to help alleviate caregiver stress. If the team is carrying out the first nine functions adequately, this goes a long way toward alleviating caregiver stress. In some cases the expertise of a psychologist may be necessary to diffuse stress among the members of the team.

In summary, the major functions of an interdisciplinary team involve improved communication and development of specific management plans as well as mutual education and a method of alleviating caregiver stress. An example of an individualized plan of care developed by an interdisciplinary team is given in **Table 10-2**.

COMPOSITION OF INTERDISCIPLINARY TEAMS

The development of the appropriate composition of the interdisciplinary team depends on the needs of the resident population to be served and the goals the team wishes to achieve. The core team always includes members of the nursing staff. Beyond this, there is no agreement on the optimal composition of the interdisciplinary team. A review of 200 health care teams suggests that almost as many disciplines can be involved as there are teams. While most texts include the physician as part of the core team, the physician is not an essential member of all interdisciplinary teams in the NH setting. The major focus of an interdisciplinary team should be on the functional, social, dietary, and psychological needs of the resident. In this case, the nurse, or—ideally, if available—the nurse practitioner or physician's assistant can substitute for the physician. This often results in an appropriately less medicalized care plan. It is essential, however, that the physician review this care plan. A number of other professionals such as pharmacists, medical specialists, and dentists can act as consultants to the team.

Table 10-2 Example of an interdesciplinary care plan

Original date	Problem	Goals	Target date	Approaches	Discipline[a]
8/20/90	Incontinent of urine	Resident will be continent during the day	9/20/90	Toilet every 2–4 h	NSG
				Place resident on bedpan every 4 h at night or place bedpan in bed with resident	NSG
				Rearrange room to provide access to bathroom	Hskp NSG NP
				Assess urine for infection	MD NSG
				Catheterize for residual to rule out urinary retention	MD NP
8/20/90	Inability to dress and groom self	Resident will have clothing on correctly with snaps, buttons, etc., in place	9/20/90	Refer to therapies	MD NP
				Assess ADL skills	OT
				Provide easy access to toilet articles	
				Teach resident techniques for self-help	NSG
				Provide resident with assistive devices as necessary	OT PT
					OT PT NSG
8/15/90	Edema, both feet	Edema will decrease in one month Resident will not develop venous stasis ulcers	9/20/90	Elevate feet while sitting	NSG
				Limit intake of high sodium foods	MD RD
				Monitor weekly weights	
				Diuretics if indicated	NSG
				ROM exercises, every shift	

8/1/90	Does not attend recreational group programs	Resident will attend two programs every month	Ongoing	Investigate possibility of volunteer to visit once a week Staff visitation once a week to develop hobbies, interests Encourage family visitation	ACT ACT NP ACT NSG SW
8/1/90	Poor hygiene	Resident will have showers twice a week and bed bath three times a week	Ongoing	Assess ability to perform independently Maintain privacy Assist resident as necessary with bath using mild soap and warm water	NSG NSG NSG
8/1/90	Tendency toward constipation	Resident will have normal bowel movements at least four times a week	Ongoing	Provide high fiber diet, include prune juice, bran cereal, wheat breads, and fresh vegetables daily 1 tablespoon bran in orange juice or applesauce daily Promote exercise if feasible Encourage fluids Meds as ordered	RD NP NP NSG OT PT MD NSG MD
8/1/91	Inability to transfer	Resident will be able to transfer self and be independent in wheelchair mobility	10/30/90	Exercises three times a week for balance and muscle strengthening Passive and active ROM all extremities every shift Assist with transfers and use of wheelchair twice daily	PT MD NSG PT NSG

[a]NSG = nursing; Hskp = housekeeping; NP = nurse practitioner; MD = physician; OT = occupational therapy; PT = physical therapy; RD = dietition; ACT = activities director; SW = social worker.

In the nursing home the key members of the interdisciplinary team are the nurses and/or nurse's aides, dietician, physical and occupational therapists, social worker, and recreation therapist. The physician can act as a consultant to this team. The golden rule of teams should be remembered: the smaller the team, the more functional it is likely to be. Larger teams often have increased interpersonal conflicts.

A team meeting that we have found particularly useful for handling the medical problems of residents includes the physician, registered nurse, nurse specialist (e.g., mental health nurse) and nurse practitioner and/or physician assistant. In a large NH (150 or more beds), a weekly meeting of this team can rapidly review medical problems of residents and make appropriate management decisions. This team format is also an excellent educational vehicle. Another advantage of utilizing this team is it separates the discussions of medical problems from the recreational, rehabilitation, and psychological needs of the resident. This prevents the medicalization of the regular NH interdisciplinary team meeting.

Specialized interdisciplinary teams can be developed to handle specific problems. One example of this is the restraint reduction team which includes nurses, physical therapists and occupational therapists. This team reviews the appropriateness of residents in restraints monthly. Our experience and that of others is that this is an excellent approach to restraint reduction.

Team leadership is often a problem. In traditional teams, the physician uses the authority of his or her position to be the leader. However, many teams function much better when another member of the team assumes the leadership role. The concept of allowing all team members equal opportunity for participation and thus to spread responsibility for decisions to all team members can lead to a healthy work situation. Leadership can be shifted depending on which team member has the most knowledge in a particular situation. In all team meetings, a team recorder should be designated; he or she should be responsible for maintaining a record of all team decisions. The recorder should not be the team leader, as this can result in incomplete and in some cases biased recording.

RESIDENTS, FAMILY MEMBERS, AND THE TEAM

It can be very useful for a NH resident (or a designated family member if the resident is not capable) to be invited to be part of the nonmedical interdisciplinary team meeting. To prevent this becoming a situation of "misplaced hospitality," the resident and/or family member needs to be aware of and adhere to certain rules, such as the following: (1) the discussion will be time-limited; (2) negative comments may be made about the resident, which may be upsetting; (3) the resident and/or family member is a guest and will act predominantly as an observer; and (4) explanations of the discussion will be given to the resident and/or family member by individual team members after the meeting and should not be expected to be provided during the meeting. Some feel strongly that residents and family members should not be included in team meetings. Many staff members find the inclusion of residents or relatives threatening and find it difficult to have a frank discussion under these circumstances. Careful education, which is sensitive to the staff's feelings, can often overcome this problem. Teams that include the resident and family may, in fact, fail to reduce caregiver stress because they do not allow the staff to vent their feelings fully.

TEAM DEVELOPMENT AND MAINTENANCE

The first task of an interdisciplinary team is to develop rules of procedure and define the areas over which the team has authority. It is important to realize that decisions can be made unanimously, by consensus, through majority vote, by unilateral decision of the person with the authority (e.g., administrator, director of nursing, or medical director), or through failure of the group to form an adequate response. In certain circumstances each of these processes may be appropriate.

When conflict occurs in the team, it must be recognized and openly discussed. The team should not take sides but rather attempt to find an acceptable compromise. When this is not possible, there should at least be a full discussion of the confrontation, with a review of both the facts and feelings involved. It is important that conflicts be resolved without compromising the major functions of the team.

Table 10-3 lists the major dynamic techniques involved in allowing an interdisciplinary team to complete its functions. Numerous different behaviors can help to facilitate these roles. When team functions are being completed, minor disagreements should be ignored. It is important to see that one member

Table 10-3 Dynamic techniques necessary for successful functioning of interdisciplinary teams

1. Informative questions and reports
2. Opinions solicited and opinions given
3. Elaborations on 1 and 2
4. Coordination to see that all are given an opportunity to participate in 1 through 3
5. Enumeration of all problems
6. Evaluation and criticism of information and problems
7. Development of solutions to problems
8. Encouragement of team members
9. Maintenance of time schedule
10. Recognition and solution of conflict
11. Distribution of specific tasks
12. Recording of problems and team decisions

of the team is not isolated from the rest of the team because of personality conflicts. When teams become truly dysfunctional, it may be helpful to obtain consultation from a team facilitator. Such a consultant can assess the dynamics of the team and attempt to solve problems by meeting with both individual team members and the whole team. When caregiver stress is particularly high, the services of a psychologist to provide group therapy may be extremely useful.

SUGGESTED READINGS

Cavalieri TA, Chopra A, Gray-Miceli D, Shreve S, Waxman M, and Forman LJ: Geriatric assessment teams in the nursing home: Do they work? *J Am Osteopath Assoc* 1993;12:1247–1248.

Cole KD, Jones FA: Interdisciplinary teams for the solution of nutritional problems, in Morley JE, Glick Z, Rubenstein LZ (eds): *Geriatric Nutrition: A Comprehensive Review.* New York, Raven Press, 1990, pp 457–470.

Evans MK: Multidisciplinary teams in geriatric wards: Myth or reality. *J Adv Nurs* 6:205, 1981.

Foley CJ, Libow LS, Charatan FB: The team approach to geriatric care, in Hazzard WR, Andres R, Bierman EL, Blass JP (eds): *Principles of Geriatric Medicine and Gerontology.* New York, McGraw-Hill, 1990, pp 184–191.

Sandel M, Garrett RM, and Horn RD: Restraint reduction in the nursing home and its impact on employee attitudes. *J Am Geriatr Soc* 42:381–387, 1994.

Tsukuda RA: Interdisciplinary collaboration: Teamwork in geriatrics, in Cassel CK, Riesenberg DE, Sorensen LB, Walsh JR (eds): *Geriatric Medicine* 2d ed, New York, Springer-Verlag, 1990, pp 668–676.

Wright BA: Behavior diagnoses by a multidisciplinary team to create a plan of care of an elderly patient in a nursing home, members of multidisciplinary teams must lend a common language. *Ger Nurs* 16:30–35, 1993.

PART TWO

CLINICAL CONDITIONS

What Do You See?

What do you see nurses. What do you see.
Are you thinking. When you are looking at me?
A crabbit old woman, not very wise,
Uncertain of habit, faraway eyes,
Who dribbles her food, and makes no reply,
When you say in a loud voice, "I do wish you'd try."
Who seems not to notice, the things that you do,
And forever is losing, a stocking or shoe.
Who unresisting or not lets you do as you will,
When bathing and feeding, the long day to fill.
Is that what you are thinking, is that what you see?
Then open your eyes nurse, you are not looking at me.

I'll tell you who I am, as I sit here so still.
As I use at your bidding, as I eat at your will.
I'm a small child of ten, with a father and mother,
Brothers and sisters, who love one another.
A young girl of sixteen, with wings on her feet,

Dreaming that soon now a lover she'll meet.
A bride soon at twenty, my heart gives a leap,
Remembering the vows, that I promised to keep.
At twenty-five now, I have young of my own.
Who need me to build a secure happy home.
A woman of thirty, my young now grow fast.
Bound to each other, with ties that should last.
At forty my young sons now grow and will be gone,
But my man stays beside me to see, I don't mourn.
At fifty, once more babies play round my knee,
Again we know children, my loved ones and me.

Dark days are upon me, my husband is dead.
I look at the future I shudder with dread.
For my young are all busy, rearing young of their own.
And I think of the years, and the Love that I've known.
I'm an old woman now, and nature is cruel.
It's her jest, to make old age look like a fool.
The body it crumbles, grace and vigor depart,
There is now a stone, where I once had a heart.
But inside this old carcass, a young girl still dwells,
And now and again, my battered heart swells,
I remember the joys, I remember the pain,
And I'm loving and living, life all over again.
I think of the years, all too few—gone too fast,
And accept the stark fact, that nothing can last.
So open your eyes, nurses, open and see,
Not a crabbit old woman. Look closer—see me.

Anonymous

protocols (RAP) for delirium and/or dementia (see following sections). The 30–point Mini Mental State Examination (MMSE) is a popular scale used to assess and follow cognitive function in geriatric patients. Scores less than 17 (very common among NH residents) are considered "severe" cognitive impairment. Thus the MMSE may not be helpful in discriminating the severity of cognitive impairment at the lower end of the scale. Scores on the MMSE may fluctuate by a few points over the course of a short period of time (even within a day), but changes of 3–4 points or more probably represent a clinically significant change in cognitive function.

The MDS items (**Fig. 11-1**) can be used to generate a cognitive performance scale (CPS) (**Fig. 11-2**). When the MDS items are completed by trained observers using specific definitions, the CPS correlates well with the MMSE and is more discriminating at the lower end of the scale. The stability of the CPS and its sensitivity to changes in cognitive function over time have not as yet been well studied. Other brief screening tests, such as clock drawing, may be helpful in identifying cognitive impairment in visuospatial skills and other areas.

DELIRIUM

Delirium is an acute confusional state involving a global disorder of cognition and attention associated with a decreased level of consciousness. **Table 11-2** outlines the diagnostic criteria for delirium. Individuals with delirium usually have sleep disturbances, with wakefulness at night and drowsiness during the day. The onset is generally acute or subacute, with mental status changes occurring over hours to a few days. Symptoms tend to fluctuate and are often worse at night. Delirium may be either of the agitated or apathetic type. Delirium may be subtle with the sign being a lack of attention by the resident. A resident with new onset of falls should be screened for delirium, as falls are one of the subtle presentations of delirium. Almost any medical disorder and a variety of drugs can precipitate delirium in a NH resident (**Table 11-3**). The common causes can be reimbursed by the acronym "DELIRIUMS":

D = drugs
E = emotional (agitated depression, mania)
L = low oxygenation (myocardial infarction, exacerbation of chronic pulmonary disease or congestive heart failure, pulmonary embolus)
I = infection
R = retention of urine and/or feces
I = ictal states
U = undernutrition, dehydration
M = metabolic (organ failure, thyroid disorder)
S = stroke, subdural hematoma

Table 11-2 Diagnostic criteria for delirium[a]

1. Disturbance of consciousness (that is, reduced clarity of awareness of the environment) in conjunction with reduced ability to focus, sustain, or shift attention
2. A change in cognition (e.g., impaired memory, orientation, or language) or the development of a perceptual disturbance that is not explained by preexisting dementia
3. Mental status changes develop over a brief period (usually hours to days) and tend to fluctuate during the course of the day
4. Evidence from the history, physical examination, or laboratory findings that the disturbance is caused by:
   (a) A general medical condition
   (b) A substance intoxication or side effect
   (c) A substance withdrawal
   (d) Multiple factors

[a]Based on *Diagnostic and Statistical Manual of Mental Disorders*, 4th ed.

Table 11-3 Common causes of delirium in the nursing home

Metabolic disorders
- Hypoglycemia
- Hyperglycemia
- Hypoxia
- Hyponatremia
- Hypercarbia
- Hypercalcemia
- Azotemia

Infections

Decreased cardiac output
- Dehydration
- Acute blood loss
- Acute myocardial infarction
- Congestive heart failure

Central nervous system disorders
- Stroke
- Subdural hematoma

Drugs
- Anticholinergics
- Narcotics
- Psychotropics

Acute psychosis

Transfer to unfamiliar surroundings (especially when sensory input is diminished)

Other
- Fecal impaction
- Urinary retention

The cornerstone of treating delirium is the identification and treatment of the underlying cause. This basically requires a thorough physical and laboratory evaluation. **Table 11-4** outlines the key aspects of the delirium RAP. In NHs, the most common cause of delirium is infection. Thus, acutely altered mental status should initially be treated as an infection until other potential causes are excluded. Among diabetic residents who are on hypoglycemic agents, a change in mental status should immediately precipitate a blood glucose determination by finger stick if available. The medication list of any NH resident who becomes delirious should be reviewed and, where possible, any medications that may be responsible for the delirium should be discontinued. Silent myocardial infarction can also cause acute delirium in older persons; therefore, if the cause of the delirium is unclear, an electrocardiogram should be done.

Residents with mental status changes and a change in heart and/or respiratory rate should have a blood gas or pulse oximetry performed. A delirious

Table 11-4 Key aspects of the delirium resident assessment protocol (RAP)

1. Evaluation
   - (a) Staff should become familiar with resident's cognitive function so that subtle but important changes can be recognized
2. Diagnoses and conditions
   - (a) Most common causes: circulatory, respiratory, infectious and metabolic disorders
   - (b) Drug side effects and dehydration are common contributing factors
3. Medications
   - (a) Review medication orders carefully
   - (b) Look for new medications corresponding to the onset of mental status changes
   - (c) Commonly prescribed drugs that can cause delirium
     - (1) Psychotropics
     - (2) Narcotic analgesics
     - (3) Other (less common causes of mental status changes) e.g., cardiac drugs, H_2 antagonists, anti-inflammatory agents
4. After serious illness and drug toxicity ruled out, consider psychosocial factors
   - (a) Isolation
   - (b) Recent loss of family or friend
   - (c) Depression, anxiety
   - (d) Restraints
   - (e) Recent relocation
5. Sensory loss may contribute
   - (a) Hearing loss
   - (b) Vision impairment
6. Clarifying information
   - (a) Assess for sleep disturbance, previous diagnosis of dementia syndrome, timing of onset of new mental status changes
7. Environment conducive to reducing symptoms
   - (a) Quiet, well-lit, calm environment with familiar objects

resident should be kept in a well-lit environment with minimal disturbances. Physical restraints are contraindicated, as they can make the symptoms of delirium worse. If the delirious resident is severely agitated or assaultive, the use of low-dose haloperidol (0.5 to 1 mg one or two times per day) may be helpful until the delirium clears. This drug should be discontinued as rapidly as possible to avoid side effects. Occasionally residents will have a reaction to haloperidol and become more, rather than less agitated. When this occurs, the drug should be discontinued immediately. More sedating drugs should be avoided if possible because they can cause disturbances of consciousness that can mask recovery from the underlying delirium.

DEMENTIA

Definition

Dementia is defined as a loss of intellectual abilities of sufficient severity to interfere with an individual's ability to function. Dementia is a syndrome that can involve several distinct types of impaired intellectual functioning. Demented individuals generally have impaired memory and orientation; they may also

Table 11-5 DSM-IV diagnostic criteria for alzheimer's dementia[a]

A. The development of multiple cognitive deficits manifested by both
   1. Memory impairment (impaired ability to learn new information or to recall previously learned information)
   2. One (or more) of the following cognitive disturbances:
      (a) Aphasia (language disturbances)
      (b) Apraxia (impaired ability to perform motor activities despite intact motor function)
      (c) Agnosia (failure to recognize or identify objects despite intact sensory function)
      (d) Disturbance in executive functioning (that is, planning, organizing, sequencing, abstracting)

B. The cognitive deficits in criteria A1 and A2 each cause severe impairment in social or occupational functioning and represent a major decline from a previous level of functioning

C. The course is characterized by gradual onset and continuing cognitive decline

D. The cognitive deficits in criteria A1 and A2 are not due to any of the following:
   1. Other central nervous system conditions that cause progressive deficits in memory and cognition (for example, cerebrovascular disease, Parkinson's disease, Huntington's disease, subdural hematoma, normal-pressure hydrocephalus, brain tumor)
   2. Systemic conditions known to cause dementia (for example, hypothyroidism, vitamin B_{12} and folic acid deficiency, niacin deficiency, hypercalcemia, neurosyphilis, HIV infection)

E. The deficits do not occur exclusively during the course of a delirium

F. The disturbance is not better accounted for by other axis I disorder (for example, major depressive disorder, schizophrenia)

[a]Based on the *Diagnostic and Statistical Manual of Mental Disorders* (DSM-IV), 4th ed.

Table 11-6 Key features differentiating delirium from dementia

Feature	Delirium	Dementia
Onset	Acute, often at night	Insidious
Course	Fluctuating, with lucid intervals, during day; worse at night	Generally stable over course of day
Duration	Hours to weeks	Months to years
Awareness	Reduced	Clear
Alertness	Abnormally low or high	Usually normal
Attention	Hypoalert or hyperalert, distractible; fluctuates over course of day	Usually normal
Orientation	Usually impaired for time, tendency to mistake unfamiliar place and persons	Often impaired
Memory	Immediate and recent impaired	Recent and remote impaired
Thinking	Disorganized	Impoverished
Perception	Illusions and hallucinations (usually visual) relatively common	Usually normal
Speech	Incoherent, hesitant, slow, or rapid	Difficulty in finding words
Sleep-wake cycle	Always disrupted	Often fragmented sleep
Physical illness or drug toxicity	Either or both present	Often absent, especially in Alzheimer's disease

After Lipkowski: *JAMA* 258:1789–1792, 1987.

exhibit impaired abstract thinking and judgment, apraxia (inability to carry out motor activities), agnosia (inability to recognize common objects), visuospatial disturbances, and alterations in personality. An underlying delirium must be ruled out before dementia can be diagnosed. **Table 11-5** summarizes the diagnostic criteria for Alzheimer type dementia. **Table 11-6** lists features that help distinguish delirium from dementia.

Causes

The most common cause of dementia is Alzheimer's disease, and the next most common is multiple infarcts within the brain (vascular dementia). Many NH residents may have both. There are a number of less common causes of nonreversible dementia such as frontal lobe dementia, dementia associated with Parkinson's disease, Pick's disease, Creutzfeld–Jakob disease, AIDS, Huntington's disease, and cerebellar degeneration. Creutzfeld–Jakob disease is one of the slow virus diseases which is associated with an abnormality in the prior gene. Persons who received growth hormone in their youth are particulary prone to develop this disease and recently, it has been associated with mad cow disease. Persons with AIDS dementia need to have unusual injections of the central nervous system (CNS) excluded. In the NH it is important to distinguish these predominantly untreatable dementias from those that are treatable. Although completely reversible dementias are rare, the causes of such dementias should be kept in mind. **Table 11-7** lists the causes of reversible dementia. Among these, depression and medications are the most common. Withdrawal of suspect medications and/or a trial of antidepressant therapy for possible depression should always be attempted before labeling a demented NH resident as untreatable, because depression and Alzheimer's disease often coexist. A careful assessment should be undertaken to identify a potentially treatable depression. Clinical clues to depression in a NH resident with dementia include: (1) the abrupt onset and rapid progression of cognitive deficits; (2) recognition of the deficits by the resident; (3) a tendency to answer questions with "I don't know" or to make no attempt to answer; and (4) an apathetic or agitated affect. If depression is suspected, a therapeutic trial should be undertaken (see Chapter 12). The dementia may not reverse completely, but the resident's functioning and quality of life may improve.

Table 11-7 Causes of treatable or potentially reversible dementias[a]

D	– Drugs
E	– Emotional (depression)
M	– Metabolic (e.g., hypothyroidism, vitamin B_{12} deficiency)
E	– Ear and eye impairment (sensory deprivation)
N	– Normal-pressure hydrocephalus
T	– Tumors and masses (e.g., subdural hematoma)
I	– Infection
A	– Anemia

After Lamy PP: *Prescribing for the Elderly.* Littleton, Massachusetts, PSG Publishing, 1980.

[a]Completely reversible dementias are rare in the NH population. Management of these conditions may, however, improve or delay progression of cognitive function, and improve the quality of life of the resident.

Other causes of reversible dementia are much less common. Normal-pressure hydrocephalus is distinguished by dementia coexisting with acute-onset incontinence and an ataxic gait disturbance. Residents with normal-pressure hydrocephalus who will respond to treatment usually show an improved gait after the removal of substantial amounts of cerebrospinal fluid. Vitamin B_{12} deficiency may be a cause of dementia. However, it is now recognized that individuals with dementia may develop low vitamin B_{12} levels, perhaps related to coexistent malnutrition. It is possible that dementia in these individuals may be improved by treatment with vitamin B_{12} as well as by adequate nutritional intake.

Diagnostic Evaluation

The goals of assessing cognitive dysfunction in a NH resident are to: (1) define the nature and extent of the cognitive deficits; (2) rule out delirium and potentially reversible causes of dementia; (3) determine the etiology of the dementia; and (4) identify behavioral disturbances that require management. The assessment is generally multidisciplinary, involving input from the physician, nursing staff, and social worker. When appropriate, an evaluation by occupa-

Table 11-8 Key aspects of the resident assessment protocol for cognitive loss/dementia

1. Neurological disorder
   (a) Consider coexisting delirium
   (b) Assess recent changes in cognitive and functional limitations to develop reasonable expectations and care plans that enhance quality of life
   (c) Be aware of the increasing numbers of mentally retarded older adults being admitted to NHs
2. Mood/behavior
   (a) Some behavior problems will not be reversible
   (b) For residents with declining cognitive function and behavioral problems consider:
      (1) Is the decline due to psychotropic drug toxicity and/or a reaction to physical restraints?
      (2) Have cognitive skills improved subsequent to initiating a behavioral management program?
      (3) Has staff assistance enhanced resident self-performance?
3. Concurrent medical problems
   (a) Identify and treat major medical problems
   (b) Comfort (pain avoidance) should be a paramount goal
4. Failure to thrive
   (a) As residents become more disabled the risk of complications (e.g., pressure sores) increases. Staff should review
      (1) Emotional, social and environmental factors which might need to be intervened upon
      (2) Interventions to decrease complications such as fecal impaction, fever, pain, pressure sores
5. Functional limitations
   (a) Can the resident be more independent?
   (b) Is the resident going downhill?
6. Sensory Impairments
   (a) Visual problems may contribute and may be difficult to diagnose
   (b) Individualized approaches may be helpful to enhance meaningful communication
7. Medications
   (a) Psychoactive and other medications can be a factor in cognitive decline
8. Involvement factors
   (a) Staff can encourage residents to participate in self-care and activities
   (a) Decline in one functional area should not be interpreted as an indication of inevitable decline in other areas

tional therapists may assist in objectively assessing functional capabilities, and an evaluation by an experienced psychiatrist or psychologist may provide very valuable input on the nature of cognitive deficits and behavioral disturbances.

Table 11-8 outlines the key aspects of the resident assessment protocol (RAP) for cognitive loss/dementia. The basic evaluation should include a history, physical examination, careful mental status examination, and selected laboratory studies. A careful history obtained by an experienced social worker can be extremely valuable in providing essential background information. The medical evaluation should include a thorough physical examination (to identify treatable conditions) and selected laboratory studies. **Table 11-9** lists studies that may be

Table 11-9 Evaluating dementia: diagnostic studies[a]

Blood studies
- Complete blood count
- Glucose
- Urea nitrogen
- Electrolytes
- Calcium and phosphorus
- Liver function tests
- Vitamin B_{12} level
- Human immunodeficiency antibodies*
- VDRL*

Radiographic studies
- Chest X-ray
- Computerized axial tomography or magnetic resonance imaging of the head (see Table 11–11)*

Other studies
- Electrocardiogram (Holter monitor if indicated)
- Urinalysis
- Electroencephalogram*
- Neuropsychological testing*
- Lumbar puncture*

[a]There is not consensus on the required studies. The studies marked by an asterisk (*) are not recommended for routine screening, but may be helpful in some instances (see text).

helpful in evaluating NH residents with dementia. There is no consensus on what studies are required. The diagnostic evaluation should be tailored to the individual based on their history and other findings. The routine use of neuroimaging techniques remains controversial. We recommend that all NH residents with cognitive impairment of unclear etiology or who have had a rapid and clinically significant decline in cognitive function (in the absence of delirium) have either a computed tomography (CT) or magnetic resonance imaging (MRI) scan to rule out tumors and subdural hematomas. Although these conditions are unusual, it is impossible to exclude them on the basis of clinical

Table 11-10 Imaging techniques in the diagnosis of dementia

	Common findings
Computerized tomography (CT)	Shows cortical atrophy with enlargement of the ventricula and sulci. Not very different from findings in many cognitively intact individuals.
Magnetic resonance imaging (MRI)	In Alzheimer's disease will show same as above. Some will show high intensity signals in the white matter which are also seen in nonimpaired elderly. More sensitive than CT in detecting multiple infarcts.
Position emission tomography (PET)	Not widely available. Involves injecting radioactively labeled dioxy-glucose which is metabolized and enables visualization of active parts of the brain. Scans of patients with Alzheimer's are dark, indicating less activity than the bright images shown by active brains in normal individuals. Early in the disease the temporal and parietal cortex show the most prominent deficits.
Single photon emission computerized tomography (SPECT)	Shows the blood flow through the brain, rather than the rate of brain metabolism. Not yet widely available.

examination alone, and they are treatable. **Table 11-10** describes selected neuroimaging techniques.

The cornerstone of the assessment of cognitive impairment is the mental status examination. This should include several components (**Table 11-1** and **Figures 11-1, 11-2**). For some residents with dementia and psychiatric symptoms, an assessment by an experienced psychiatrist or psychologist, when available, can be valuable. Because of the high prevalence of behavioral disturbances in NH residents with dementia, an assessment of behavior should be carried out by nursing and/or social work staff. Such assessments are discussed in Chapter 12.

The vast majority of demented NH residents have either Alzheimer's disease, multi-infarct dementia, or a combination of both. Features that suggest a vascular multi-infarct dementia include: (1) history of hypertension, stroke or transient ischemic attack; (2) focal neurological symptoms or signs; (3) an abrupt onset with stepwise deterioration; and (4) emotional lability. In the NH, from a practical standpoint, the management of Alzheimer's disease and multi-infarct dementia is the same. Control of risk factors for multi-infarct dementia is important in both Alzheimer's and vascular (as well as other) dementias, since vascular disease may worsen cognitive deficits in any type of dementia syndrome. As more effective targeted therapies (e.g., drug treatment) become available, the diagnostic distinction between Alzheimer's and vascular dementias will become increasingly important.

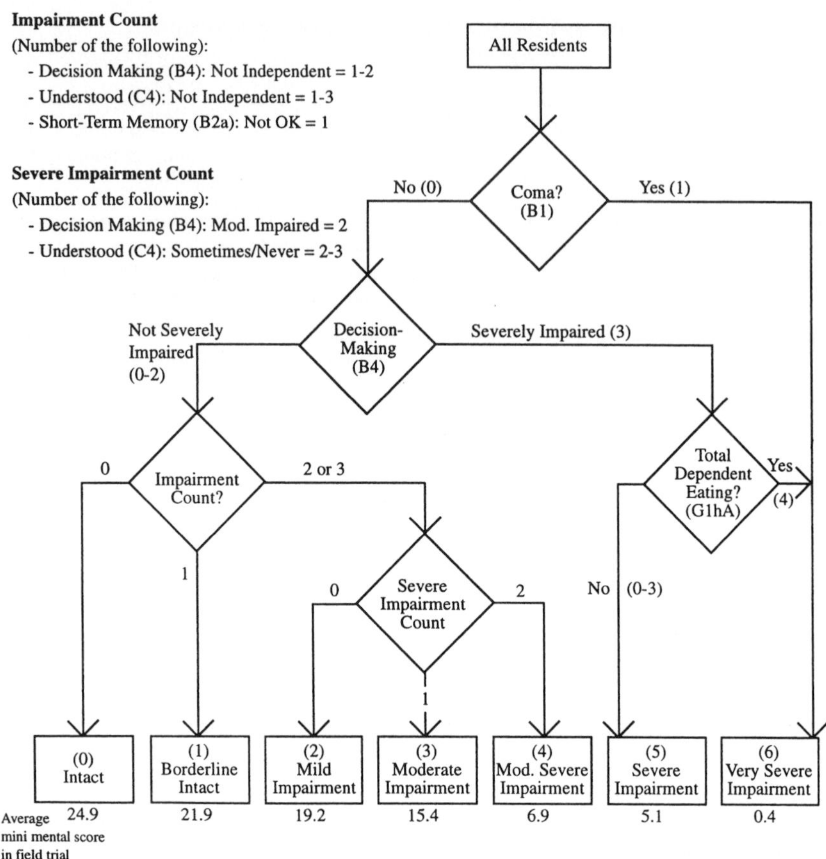

Figure 11-2 Scoring rules for the MDS cognitive performance scale. Original reference: Morris JH, Fries BF, et al: MDS Performance Scale. *J Gerontology* 1994; 49, m174–m182. Figure taken from: US Department of Health and Human Services State Operation Manual: Resident Assessment Instrument; MDS Version 2.0.

Management of Residents with Dementia

The basic principles of managing residents with dementia are not different from those that govern the management of other NH residents described throughout this text. The focus is on providing a safe environment that will compensate for cognitive impairments and appropriate management of behavioral disturbances, such as wandering and agitation, while minimizing the use of physical or chemical restraints. Findings from the MDS and other multidisciplinary assessments should be incorporated into the resident's care plan. The care plan should address issues such as wandering and other behavioral disturbances, sleep disorders, nutrition, potential for falling, and functional capabilities. The treatment of underlying medical conditions should be optimized. Because small infarcts may worsen cognitive function, significant hypertension (i.e., systolic above 160; diastolic above 95) should be controlled to the extent possible without causing side effects. Tacrine (tetrahydroaminocrine) is a Food and Drug Administration (FDA) approved drug for treating persons with Alzheimer's disease. It has not proved extremely useful as its use is limited by side effects (liver dysfunction) and it appears to be marginally efficacious. Newer agents are currently being developed. Many residents with dementia gradually develop malnutrition, which should be managed aggressively to prevent complications (see Chapter 13). Residents with dementia who are capable of carrying out their activities of daily living (ADL) but who tend to require cuing for eating and toileting and/or who tend to get lost require a structured environment with appropriate staffing to supervise them. It is usually not until a resident reaches an advanced stage of dementia that he or she loses the ability to perform all basic ADL. Other significant management problems include behavioral disturbances and feeding problems, which are discussed in Chapters 12 and 13. At present drugs available to treat the cognitive impairment of Alzheimer's disease (such as tetrahydroaminocrine (Tacrine)) have questionable efficacy. The "Suggested Readings" includes sources that also provide more detailed discussions of managing dementia.

Caregivers

Caring for a demented loved one, even if he or she is in a NH, is associated with tremendous emotional strain and disruption of normal personal, household, and work activities. These stresses place family caregivers at high risk for developing health problems of their own. The process that families undergo when they turn care over to others is painful and may have significant consequences, including depression, guilt, anger, and other psychological problems. Assisting and supporting a caregiver through this process should be part of NH admission and ongoing care. Many family caregivers continue to engage in caregiving by managing their relative's finances and legal matters, and they must cope with a range of social and psychological problems after NH admission. In addition, family caregivers play an important role in medical decision making for demented NH residents who are no longer capable of making their own decisions (see Chapter 27). Family caregivers may be helpful by participating in some aspects of care (feeding, for example) in conjunction with NH staff. Many family caregivers benefit from this participation and learn how to interpret the eating behaviors of their relative. Such participation may help family members develop a more positive attitude to their relative as well as a better appreciation of the care their relative is receiving. Family members should also be encouraged to contact the local Alzheimer's Association. This association provides much useful information on dementia at a level aimed at the lay public; it also offers a variety of support groups. In the US, the Association is headquartered in Chicago ((800) 272–3900).

Special Care Units for Residents with Dementia

Special care units (SCUs) for NH residents with dementia have become increasingly popular. SCUs are intended to provide a safe, therapeutic environment that will compensate for cognitive deficits and resultant disabilities. **Table 11-11** describes some of the characteristics of SCUs. SCUs should be preferably limited in size and have stable, well-trained staff who take pride in this unique working environment. A well-organized unit should provide effective staff and family support so as to reduce "burnout." Preventing burnout is critical in maintaining stable, competent staff- critical in the management of residents with dementia. A support group for staff, as well as staff involvement in continuous quality improvement activities, may be helpful in this regard.

Although the concept of the SCU may be sound, there has been little data documenting a significant impact on the course of dementia or on secondary complications. Most studies suffer from methodological limitations that limit generalization of their findings. Many SCUs simply segregate demented residents rather than offer alternative approaches to their care. One of the primary reasons for placement in a SCU is, in fact, to prevent demented residents from wandering and injuring themselves. This objective is likely to be met if the

Table 11-11 Characteristics of special care units (SCU) for demented nursing home residents

Staffing

- Staff ratios on SCUs are often higher than other units
- Staff are specially trained in the causes and manifestation of dementia
- Team approach is used involving social worker, nurse, medical and psychiatry/psychology input
- Meetings held regularly to review and modify programs

Programs

- More emphasis on reality orientation
- More emphasis on music programs (may facilitate reminiscence more than other activities)
- More textural materials are used in enriched arts and crafts programs
- Special feeding programs
- Finger foods are provided to encourage independent eating
- Frequent snacks are available

Environmental

- Special exit doors with alarms for wandering residents
- Furniture has rounded edges
- More space for recreational activity
- Quiet rooms provided for small gatherings or behaviorally disturbed residents
- The dining room is set up for optimal feeding of residents (some have single seat size serving tables)
- The nursing station is located near elevators or exits to facilitate monitoring of wandering residents
- Pets are sometimes permanent "residents" of the unit
- Pictures and other designs are used to cue residents to finding the proper locations of their room, etc.

environment is designed appropriately. Whether health status and/or longevity are affected is still to be determined. We believe that well run SCUs may have a measurable impact on caregivers (staff and families) and possibly on the quality of life of demented NH residents. It may be possible to create SCUs at a lower level of care, such as assisted living, and still maintain a safe, effective level of care at a lower cost. The potential benefits may include improved quality of life, minimization of the use of chemical and physical restraints, improved nutrition, and a reduction in the frequency of falls and other accidents. It is important that SCUs have special programs (e.g., music therapy, exercise programs); otherwise there is a marked possibility that they will become areas that segregate the unwanted resident and provide below-average care.

SCUs can certainly provide an appropriate milieu for education and research. SCUs with specific admission criteria may become teaching sites for nurses' aides, nursing staff, medical and other health professional students. Units that accept residents with particular diagnoses may be an excellent place in which to study the natural course of institutionalized demented persons. These units can also serve as sites for controlled trials of interventions, such as a restraint reduction, the effectiveness of exercise in improving sleep patterns, reality orientation and feeding programs, and the effects of certain drugs on behaviors and cognition. Observation of noncommunicative residents during interactions with staff or in response to environmental stimuli such as music, light/darkness, and food may provide insight into the complex issue of quality of life in the demented elderly, so that better units can be designed in the future.

SUGGESTED READINGS

American Psychiatric Association: *Diagnostic and Statistical Manual of Mental Disorders* (4th ed). Washington DC, American Psychiatric Association, 1994.

Calkins MP: *Design for Dementia: Planning Environments for the Elderly and the Confused.* Baltimore, National Health Publishing, 1988.

Carlson DL, Fleming KC, Smith GE, Evans JM: Management of dementia-related behavioral disturbances: A nonpharmacologic approach. *Mayo Clin Proc* 70:1108–1115, 1995.

Cohen U, Kay K: *Contemporary environments for people with dementia.* Baltimore, Maryland: Johns Hopkins University Press, 1993.

Cummings JL, Miller BL (eds): *Alzheimer's Disease: Treatment and Long Term Management.* New York, Marcel Dekker, Inc, 1990.

Fleming KC, Adams AC, and Petersen RC: Dementia: Diagnosis and evaluation. *Mayo Clin Proc* 70:1093–1107, 1995.

Fleming KC, and Evans JM: Pharmacologic therapies in dementia. *Mayo Clin Proc* 70:1116–1123, 1995.

Hartmaier SL, Sloane PD, Guess HA, Koch GG, et al: Validation of the minimum data set cognitive performance scale: Agreement with the mini-mental state examination. *J Gerontol Med Sci* 50AM128–M133, 1995.

Joint Commission for the Accreditation of Healthcare Organizations: *1996 Accreditation Manual for Long Term Care—Including Scoring Guidelines for Dementia Special Care Units.* Chicago, Illinois, JCAHO, 1996.

Lipkowski ZJ: Delirium (acute confusional states). *JAMA* 258:1789–1792, 1987.

Mace NL (ed): *Dementia Care: Patient, Family, and Community.* Baltimore, Maryland, Johns Hopkins University Press, 1990.

Moletta G (ed): *Treatment considerations for Alzheimer's disease and related dementing illnesses. Clinics in Geriatric Medicine, vol 4.* Philadelphia, Pennsylvania, WB Saunders Co, 1988.

Morris JN, Fries BE, Mehr DR, et al: MDS cognitive performance scale. *J Gerontol Med Sci* 49:M174–M182, 1994.

NIH Consensus Conference: Differential diagnosis of dementing diseases. *JAMA* 258:3411–3416, 1987.

Office of Technology Assessment: *Special care units for people with Alzheimer's and other dementias: Consumer education, research, regulatory, and reimbursement issues.* Washington, DC, US Government Printing Office, 1992.

Rovner BW, Steele CD, Shmuely Y, Folstein MF: A randomized trial of dementia care in nursing homes. *J Am Geriatr Soc* 44:7–13, 1996.

Rummans TA, Evans JM, Krahn LE, Fleming KC: Delirium in elderly patients: Evaluation and Management. *Mayo Clin Proc* 70:989–998, 1995.

Sloane PD, Mathew LJ, (eds): *Dementia Units in Long-Term Care.* Baltimore, Maryland, Johns Hopkins University Press, 1991.

Sloane PD, Mathew L, Scarborough M, et al: Physical and chemical restraint of dementia patients in nursing homes: Impact of specialized units. *JAMA* 265:1278–1282, 1991.

Sloane PD, Lindeman DA, Phillips C, Moritz DJ, Koch G: Evaluating Alzheimer's special care units: Reviewing the evidence and identifying potential sources of study bias. *Gerontologist* 35:103–111, 1995.

Winograd CH, Jarvik LF: Physician management of the dementia patient. *J Am Geriatr Soc* 34:285–308, 1986.

CHAPTER
TWELVE

PSYCHIATRIC AND BEHAVIORAL DISORDERS

A hallmark of a good nursing home (NH) is adequate attention to the identification and appropriate management of psychiatric and behavioral disorders. The prevalence of psychiatric and behavioral disorders among NH residents has been estimated to be between 68 and 94 percent. Psychological problems in the NH include depression, cognitive disorders, late-life paranoia, anxiety and panic disorders, and behavioral disorders. In addition, NH personnel need to be aware of psychopathology among relatives of residents; they must also be able to deal with psychological reactions among staff caregivers. This chapter reviews the diagnosis and management of common psychiatric and behavioral disorders seen in the NH. The diagnosis and management of dementia and delirium are discussed in Chapter 9.

DEPRESSION

The prevalence of major depression among NH residents has been reported to range from 9 to 38 percent. In addition, dysphoria, particularly at the time of admission to the NH, is common. In one well-designed study 16 percent of persons displayed major depression and 17 percent minor depression. Major depression is an independent risk factor for death in NH residents, increasing the risk by 59 percent. The diagnosis of depression in older individuals involves the same diagnostic criteria as those utilized in younger persons (**Table 12-1**). To be considered depressed, the resident must have had at least a 2-week period of dysphoria or loss of interest or enjoyment in activities. In addition, at least two

Table 12-1 Criteria for major depressive episode—DSM IV

A. Five (or more) of the following symptoms have been present during the same 2-week period and represent a change from previous functioning; at least one of the symptoms is either (1) depressed mood or (2) loss of interest or pleasure.

Note: Do not include symptoms that are clearly due to a general medical condition, or mood-incongruent delusions or hallucinations.

(1) depressed mood most of the day, nearly every day, as indicated by either subjective report (e.g., feels sad or empty) or observation made by others (e.g., appears tearful)
(2) markedly diminished interest or pleasure in all, or almost all, activities most of the day, nearly every day (as indicated by either subjective account or observation made by others)
(3) significant weight loss when not dieting or weight gain (e.g., a change of more than 5 percent of body weight in a month), or decrease or increase in appetite nearly every day
(4) insomnia or hypersomnia nearly every day
(5) psychomotor agitation or retardation nearly every day (observable by others, not merely subjective feelings of restlessness or being slowed down)
(6) fatigue or loss of energy nearly every day
(7) feelings of worthlessness or excessive or inappropriate guilt (which may be delusional) nearly every day (not merely self-reproach or guilt about being sick)
(8) diminished ability to think or concentrate, or indecisiveness, nearly every day (either by subjective account or as observed by others)
(9) recurrent thoughts of death (not just fear of dying), recurrent suicidal ideation without a specific plan, or a suicide attempt or a specific plan for committing suicide

B. The symptoms cause clinically significant distress or impairment in social, occupational, or other important areas of functioning.

C. The symptoms are not due to the direct physiological effects of a substance (e.g., a drug of abuse, a medication) or a general medical condition (e.g., hypothyroidism).

D. The symptoms are not better accounted for by bereavement, i.e., after the loss of a loved one, the symptoms persist for longer than 2 months or are characterized by marked functional impairment, morbid preoccupation with worthlessness, suicidal ideation, psychotic symptoms, or psychomotor retardation.

of the following symptoms must be present: appetite disturbance or weight loss, fatigue or decreased energy, psychomotor agitation or retardation, guilt, sleep disturbance, altered cognition or concentration, and suicidal ideas. Older persons with depression are more likely to have weight loss and less likely to express suicidal ideation. Nursing home residents with depression often have atypical presentations (**Table 12-2**). Depressed NH residents are more likely to have pain than nondepressed residents.

Delusions and agitated behavior may be particularly common presentations of depression in the NH. Pain syndromes such as jaw, abdominal or musculoskeletal pains for which there is no obvious explanation may also constitute the presentation of depression. Malnutrition is another very common presentation of depression in NH residents.

On admission to the NH, all residents should be screened with an objective test such as the Yesavage Geriatric Depression Scale (YGDS) (**Table 12-3**) in

Table 12-2 Atypical presentation of depression in the nursing home

Anxiety/agitation
Delusions
Depressive dementia ("pseudodementia")
Malnutrition
Atypical pain syndromes
Passive suicide

Table 12-3 Yesavage Geriatric Depression Scale (YHDS)

Choose the best answer for how you felt the past week:		
1. Are you basically satisfied with your life?	Yes	No[a]
2. Have you dropped many of your activities and interests?	Yes	No
3. Do you feel that your life is empty?	Yes	No
4. Do you often get bored?	Yes	No
5. Are you hopeful about the future?	Yes	No[a]
6. Are you bothered by thoughts you can't get out of your head?	Yes	No
7. Are you in good spirits most of the time?	Yes	No[a]
8. Are you afraid that something bad is going to happen to you?	Yes	No
9. Do you feel happy most of the time?	Yes	No[a]
10. Do you often feel helpless?	Yes	No
11. Do you often get restless and fidgety?	Yes	No
12. Do you prefer to stay at home, rather than going out and doing new things?	Yes	No
13. Do you frequently worry about the future?	Yes	No
14. Do you feel you have more problems with memory than most?	Yes	No
15. Do you think it is wonderful to be alive now?	Yes	No[a]
16. Do you often feel downhearted and blue?	Yes	No
17. Do you feel pretty worthless the way you are now?	Yes	No
18. Do you worry a lot about the past?	Yes	No
19. Do you find life very exciting?	Yes	No[a]
20. Is it hard for you to get started on new projects?	Yes	No
21. Do you feel full of energy?	Yes	No[a]
22. Do you feel that your situation is hopeless?	Yes	No
23. Do you think that most people are better off than you are?	Yes	No
24. Do you frequently get upset over little things?	Yes	No
25. Do you frequently feel like crying?	Yes	No
26. Do you have trouble concentrating?	Yes	No
27. Do you enjoy getting up in the morning?	Yes	No[a]
28. Do you prefer to avoid social gatherings?	Yes	No
29. Is it easy for you to make decisions?	Yes	No[a]
30. Is your mind as clear as it used to be?	Yes	No

[a]These questions are scored 1 point for a "no" answer; other questions are scored 1 point for a "yes" answer. Mean scores are as follows: normal (not depressed), 5; mildly depressed, 15; very depressed, 23. Scores of 15 and above generally indicate depression (see text and Fig. 10-1).

SECTION E. MOOD AND BEHAVIOR PATTERNS

1.	INDICATORS OF DEPRESSION, ANXIETY, SAD MOOD	***(Code for indicators observed in last 30 days, irrespective of the assumed cause)*** 0. Indicator not exhibited in last 30 days 1. Indicator of this type exhibited up to five days a week 2. Indicator of this type exhibited daily or almost daily (6, 7 days a week) **VERBAL EXPRESSIONS OF DISTRESS** **a.** Resident made negative statements—e.g., "*Nothing matters; Would rather be dead; What's the use; Regrets having lived so long; Let me die*" **b.** Repetitive questions—e.g., "*Where do I go; What do I do?*" **c.** Repetitive verbalizations—e.g., calling out for help, ("*God help me*") **d.** Persistent anger with self or others—e.g., easily annoyed, anger at placement in nursing home; anger at care received **e.** Self deprecation—e.g., "*I am nothing; I am of no use to anyone*" **f.** Expressions of what appear to be unrealistic fears—e.g., fear of being abandoned, left alone, being with others **g.** Recurrent statements that something terrible is about to happen—e.g., believes he or she is about to die, have a heart attack **h.** Repetitive health complaints—e.g., persistently seeks medical attention, obsessive concern with body functions **i.** Repetitive anxious complaints/concerns (non-health related) e.g., persistently seeks attention/reassurance regarding schedules, meals, laundry, clothing, relationship issues **SLEEP-CYCLE ISSUES** **j.** Unpleasant mood in morning **k.** Insomnia/change in usual sleep pattern **SAD, APATHETIC, ANXIOUS APPEARANCE** **l.** Sad, pained, worried facial expressions—e.g., furrowed brows **m.** Crying, tearfulness **n.** Repetitive physical movements—e.g., pacing, hand wringing, restlessness, fidgeting, picking **LOSS OF INTEREST** **o.** Withdrawal from activities of interest—e.g., no interest in long standing activities or being with family/friends **p.** Reduced social interaction	
2.	MOOD PERSISTENCE	**One or more indicators** of depressed, sad or anxious mood **were not easily altered by attempts to "cheer up", console, or reassure the resident over last 7 days** 0. No mood indicators 1. Indicators present, easily altered 2. Indicators present, not easily altered	
3.	CHANGE IN MOOD	Resident's mood status has changed as compared to status of **90 days ago** (or since last assessment if less then 90 days) 0. No change 1. Improved 2. Deteriorated	
4.	BEHAVIORAL SYMPTOMS	**(A) *Behavioral* symptom *frequency in last 7 days*** 0. Behavior not exhibited in last 7 days 1. Behavior of this type occurred 1 to 3 days in last 7 days 2. Behavior of this type occurred 4 to 6 days, but less than daily 3. Behavior of this type occurred daily **(B) *Behavioral* symptom *alterability in last 7 days*** 0. Behavior not present OR behavior was easily altered 1. Behavior was not easily altered **a.** WANDERING (moved with no rational purpose, seemingly oblivious to needs or safety) **b.** VERBALLY ABUSIVE BEHAVIORAL SYMPTOMS (others were threatened, screamed at, cursed at) **c.** PHYSICALLY ABUSIVE BEHAVIORAL SYMPTOMS (others were hit, shoved, scratched, sexually abused) **d.** SOCIALLY INAPPROPRIATE/DISRUPTIVE BEHAVIORAL SYMPTOMS (made disruptive sounds, noisiness, screaming, self-abusive acts, sexual behavior or disrobing in public, smeared/threw food/feces, hoarding, rummaged through others' belongings) **e.** RESISTS CARE (resisted taking medications/ injections, ADL assistance, or eating)	(A) (B)
5.	CHANGE IN BEHAVIORAL SYMPTOMS	Resident's behavior status has changed as compared to **status of 90 days ago** (or since last assessment if less than 90 days) 0. No change 1. Improved 2. Deteriorated	

SECTION F. PSYCHOSOCIAL WELL-BEING

1.	SENSE OF INITIATIVE/ INVOLVE-MENT	At ease interacting with others	a.
		At ease doing planned or structured activities	b.
		At ease doing self-initiated activities	c.
		Establishes own goals	d.
		Pursues involvement in life of facility (e.g., makes/keeps friends; involved in group activities; responds positively to new activities; assists at religious services)	e.
		Accepts invitations into most group activities	f.
		NONE OF ABOVE	g.
2.	UNSETTLED RELATION-SHIPS	Covert/open conflict with or repeated criticism of staff	a.
		Unhappy with roommate	b.
		Unhappy with residents other than roommate	c.
		Openly expresses conflict/anger with family/friends	d.
		Absence of personal contact with family/friends	e.
		Recent loss of close family member/friend	f.
		Does not adjust easily to change in routines	g.
		NONE OF ABOVE	h.
3.	PAST ROLES	Strong identification with past roles and life status	a.
		Expresses sadness/anger/empty feeling over lost roles/status	b.
		Resident perceives that daily routine (customary routine, activities) is very different from prior pattern in the community	c.
		NONE OF ABOVE	d.

Figure 12-1 Mood and behavior and psychosocial well-being items from the Minimum Data Set.

addition to the Minimum Data Set (MDS). The MDS items on mood and behavior are illustrated in **Fig. 12-1**. Residents with a score of 15 or greater should be considered for treatment of depression. Residents with scores between 10 and 14 often revert to nondepressed levels within 4 to 6 weeks without pharmacological therapy. For this reason, we recommend repeating the YGDS 6 weeks after admission for residents with scores in this range. The utility of the YGDS is limited among residents with moderate to marked dementia. In these residents careful behavioral observation by the nursing staff is necessary to make the diagnosis. Also if the resident makes little attempt to answer mental status questions this may suggest an underlying depression.

When the diagnosis of depression is made, it is important to exclude any treatable medical causes (**Table 12-4**). In addition, physicians need to be aware that following a stroke, 1 in 3 NH residents will develop depression within the next 2 years. Thus, these NH residents should be screened for depression every 3 months for 2 years following a stroke. A careful review of all medications must be conducted for any depressed resident, because many medications may contribute to depression (**Table 12-4**).

The mood state resident assessment protocol is outlined in **Table 12-5**, and an approach to the treatment of depression among NH residents is illustrated in **Fig. 12-2**. When the diagnosis of depression is made and the resident is not agitated and has no major sleep disturbance, treatment is initiated with desipramine 25 mg in the evening for 3 days. It is then increased to 50 mg. Postural vital signs should be monitored at least once or twice per week during this time, and other potentially bothersome side effects should be identified (see

Table 12-4 Treatable medical causes of depression

Endocrine
Thyroid disease
Hyperparathyroidism
Chronic infections
Malnutrition
Tumors
Central nervous system
Pancreatic carcinoma
Other
Electrolyte imbalances and dehydration
Medications
Antihypertensives
Propranolol
Reserpine
Psychotropics
Neuroleptics
Benzodiazopines
Hormones
Corticosteroids
Analgesics
Indomethacin
Other
Narcotics
Digoxin
Amantadine

below). Residents with prolonged PR intervals or QRS durations on electrocardiogram should have a repeat electrocardiogram to identify any progression of heart block. After 2 weeks, the YGDS is repeated. If the score is still greater than 15, the dose of desipramine is increased to 75 mg daily for 1 week and then to 100 mg daily. The depression scale is repeated 8 weeks later. If the resident is still depressed, she/he is given a trial of a selective serotonin uptake inhibitor (SSRI), and if this fails psychiatric consultation should be obtained. At the start of therapy, nursing staff are informed that the resident is depressed. They are asked to increase positive verbal interactions with the resident and to consistently encourage her or him to become involved in group activities.

If the resident is agitated or has severe sleep disturbances, then trazodone (which has mild to moderate sedative effects) is used instead of desipramine, starting at a dose of 50 mg in the evening for 1 week and increasing the dose by 25 mg every week to a maximum dose of 150 mg a day. If this fails to normalize the YGDS, trial of an SSRI or referral to a psychiatrist is appropriate. Although

Table 12-5 Summary of the mood state resident assessment protocol (RAP)[a]

Trigger	Guidelines	Care plan

A mood problem suggested if one or more of following is present:
• Resident made negative statements
• Repetitive questions
• Repetitive verbalizations
• Persistent anger with self or others
• Self deprecation
• Expressions of what appear to be unrealistic fears
• Recurrent statements that something terrible is about to happen
• Repetitive health complaints
• Repetitive anxious complaints/concerns
• Unpleasant mood in morning
• Insomnia/change in usual sleep pattern
• Sad, pained, worried facial expressions
• Crying, tearfulness
• Repetitive physical movements
• Withdrawal from activities of interest
• Reduced social interaction
• Mood persistence
	Indicators of the need to consider a new/altered care strategy:
	• Mood decline
	• Mood unimproved and reversible conditions present
	  • Recent move int/within facility
	  • Delirium, cognitive decline, delusions, hallucinations
	  • Communication decline
	  • Grief due to loss
	  • ADL decline
	  • Use of meds know to cause mood shifts (e.g., antihypertensives, cimeidine, clonidine, cytoxic agents, digitalis, guanethidine, immunosuppressive, methyldopa, nitrates, propranolol, reserpine, steroids, stimulants)
	• Mood unimproved and indication of problem with cognitive ability/ memory, decision-making ability, and ability to understand and any of following:
	  • Little or no initiative shown
	  • Little or no involvement in activities
	  • No psychotropic medications
	  • No psychological therapy
	• Behavioral or relationship problems present
		• Confirm presence of depression with Geriatric Depression Scale or DSM IV criteria[a]
		• Increase psychosocial activities
		• Have social worker evaluate for possible response to psychotherapy
		• Consider pet therapy (bird)
		• Consider use of antidepressants
		• Consider psychiatric consult if no improvement in 3 months or severe weight loss, etc., may be appropriate
		• Consider stopping anxiolytics or neuroleptics that may cause depressed mood
		• Educate family and caregivers concerning approach to depressed person

	Confounding issues to be considered: • Communication skills • Diseases: Thyroid disease, cardiac disease, neurological disease, anxiety, depression, schizophrenia, cancer, other psychosis, hypercalcemia, Cushing's, Addison's, hypoglycemia, hypokalemia, porphyria	

[a]In our experience the MDS correctly identifies depressed patients less than half the time.

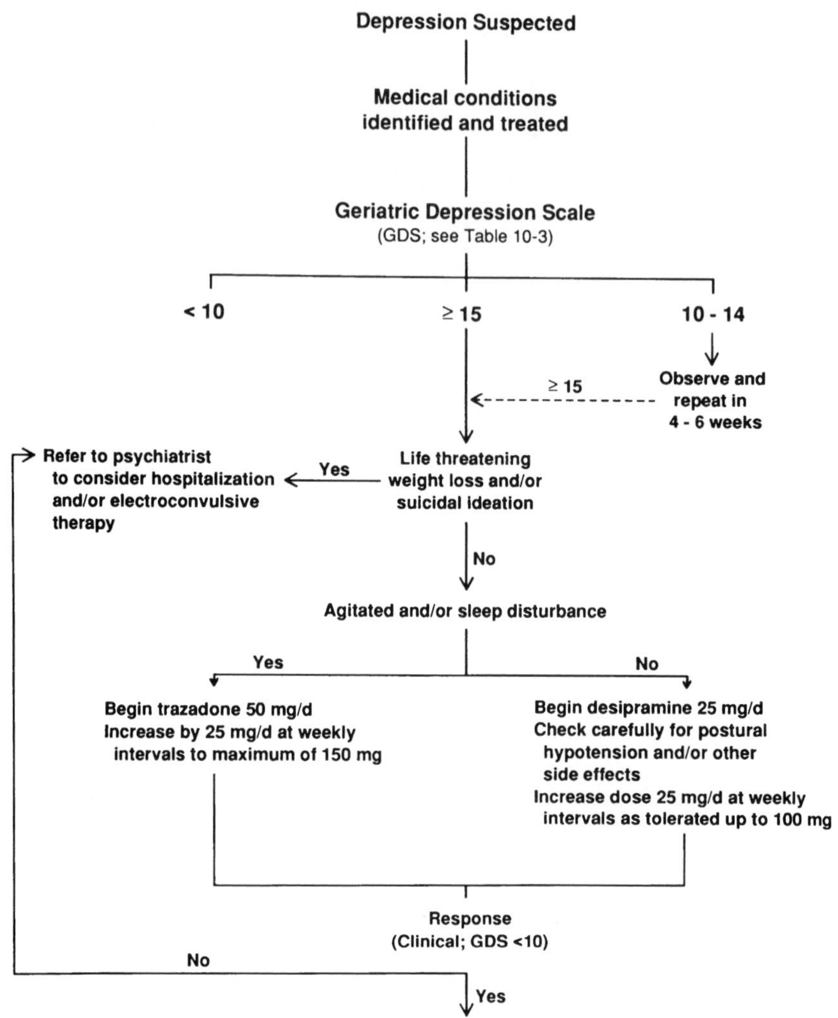

Figure 12-2 Approach to depression in the nursing home. If the resident fails to respond to this approach or develops intolerable side effects, trials of serotonin reuptake inhibitors or other agents may be appropriate.

many physicians now use SSRIs as first line drugs others feel they should be reserved for primary treatment in residents with orthostasis or those who develop symptomatic postural hypotension during treatment with tricyclic antidepressants and those who fail to respond to tricyclics (**Fig. 12-3**). Most experience has been obtained with sertraline and paroxetin, though a number of other agents are now available. The major side effect is weight loss and weight needs to be carefully

PHARMACOTHERAPEUTIC

Geriatric Depression Scale (GDS) ≥15

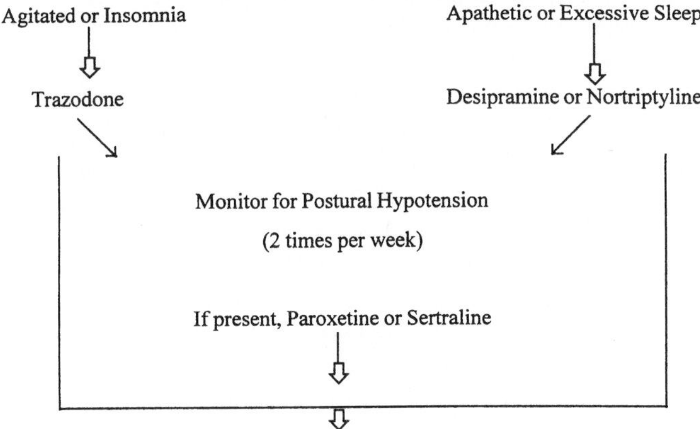

Repeat GDS 2-3 Months. If ≥ 15, refer to Psychiatrist

Medication	Start Dose	Increase by (change interval)	Maximum Dose	Main Side Effects	Costs[1]
Trazodone[2]	25-50mg[3]	25-50mg (every 3-7 days)	150mg	Orthostatic hypotension Drowsiness	$15
Desipramine[4]	25-50mg	25-50mg (every 3-7 days)	100mg	Orthostatic hypotension	$15
Nortriptyline[4]	10-30mg	10-20mg (every 3-7 days)	50mg	Orthostatic hypotension	$60
Paroxetine	10-20mg[5]	10mg (every 7-14 days)	40mg	Somnolence <u>or</u> insomnia Agitation/anxiety GI upset/nausea	$60
Sertraline	25-50mg[5]	25mg (every 7-14 days)	100mg		$60

1 Estimated average for one month supply in 1994

2 Trade Brand (DESYREL) approximately 4 times the cost

3 Usually given in one dose at bedtime. Can be given in divided dose if agitation during day

4 Usually given in a.m., but if medication causes drowsiness, can be given at bedtime. Higher doses given in divided doses

5 For older patients with renal or hepatic impairment, use lower dose

Note: Fluoxetine (PROZAC) relatively contraindicated in older persons because of long-half life (36 hours) and risk of anorexia

Figure 12-3 Pharmacotherapeutic algorithm for treating depression among nursing home residents (Adapted with permission from Morley JE: Clinical guidelines: depression. *Nursing Home Medicine* 2(3):44, 1994).

monitored during treatment. The SSRIs are much more expensive, have almost the same occurrence of side effects (although the profile is different) and may be less effective than tricyclics in older persons.

Desipramine is preferred to nortriptyline because it has slightly less anticholinergic side effects. The major anticholinergic side effects of these secondary amines are urinary retention in residents with prostatic enlargement, decreased visual acuity, constipation, and dry mouth. A major potential side effect is orthostatic hypotension, which can result in falls. Orthostatic blood pressure measurements should be done at regular intervals (at least twice per week) while a NH resident is being stabilized on an appropriate dose of desipramine. Trazodone produces a greater degree of sedation and less anticholinergic side effects than desipramine. Occasional residents may benefit from the addition of small doses of lithium to the antidepressant. If lithium is prescribed, blood levels should be monitored carefully. The use of methylphenidate (Ritalin) is sometimes effective, but it should be limited to prescription and oversight by psychiatrists. Fluoxetine should generally not be used in NH residents, because it can precipitate agitated behavior and also cause life-threatening weight loss. The extremely long half-life of fluoxetine makes it less suitable than the other SSRIs in the NH. Side effects of monoamine oxidase inhibitors usually limit their use in the NH population, but they may occasionally stimulate appetite in malnourished residents. Venaflaxine modulates both norepinephrine and serotonin. Its use should be limited to those residents resistant to other forms of treatment.

In severely depressed residents with significant weight loss, malnutrition, or high suicide potential, electroconvulsive therapy (ECT) is the treatment of choice. It should also be considered for residents who fail an adequate trial of antidepressant therapy. Serum levels of antidepressants should be obtained to demonstrate that a sufficiently high dosage was given before treatment was considered unsuccessful. ECT is an excellent therapy for residents who scream continuously, presumably as screaming in demented residents is a depression variant.

Severely depressed residents should be given a room near the nursing station to permit regular observation. These residents should be carefully monitored to identify any suicidal ideation. As a first step, residents should be asked directly if they have any suicidal thoughts or wish to die. If they respond positively, they should be asked if they have made any specific plans. Residents who have specific plans (e.g., hoarding pills, suffocation) should be taken seriously and hospitalized for more intensive management. In most NHs, staffing is inadequate to monitor these residents for suicide attempts. Severely depressed residents should be checked regularly, especially after being outside the NH or in the hospital, to ensure that they are not hiding medications that could be used to commit suicide. The early phase of recovery from depression is also a time of higher risk for suicide.

LATE-LIFE PARANOIA

Isolated late-life paranoia is a relatively unusual condition, but residents who develop it can be very disruptive. They may become suspicious and develop delusions that caregivers or other residents are trying to poison them or steal from them. The affected resident may focus on a single fellow resident or staff member and attempt to enlist the help of other staff and residents to prove the guilt of the person who has been singled out. As stealing and other unacceptable behaviors can occur among staff, the resident's paranoid complaints should be evaluated carefully. When paranoid delusions are present and disruptive, the resident may respond well to low doses of haloperidol or resperidol (the latter is more expensive) (see Chapter 23).

ANXIETY AND PANIC DISORDERS

Anxiety is a common problem in NH residents. Approximately 20 percent of NH residents exhibit some degree of anxiety. Common signs and symptoms of anxiety include palpitations, tremors, hyperventilation, insomnia, confusion, hypochondriasis, generalized fears, and feelings of hopelessness and helplessness. When a NH resident develops these symptoms, a careful assessment should be undertaken to exclude treatable medical conditions that might underlie the symptoms. Anxiety may also be based on a legitimate concern, such as the fear of falling, that is then blown out of proportion.

Whenever possible, anxiety should be treated nonpharmacologically. Acute adjustment reactions to NH admission are best treated by supportive psychotherapy. Biofeedback and relaxation techniques and participation in activity programs may be useful for some residents with anxiety. Buspirone or short-acting benzodiazepines without active metabolites may be useful (see Chapter 23). Buspirone has minimal side effects but takes 4 to 6 weeks before its effects are seen. Once symptoms are under control, an attempt should be made to wean anxious residents from drug therapy, and nonpharmacologic interventions should be provided.

Late-life onset of panic disorders is being more commonly recognized. Buspirone, a nonbenzodiazepine anxiolytic, may be particularly useful in treating NH residents with panic disorders. Late-life onset of mania must also be recognized, as the treatment of choice for this disorder is lithium. When supportive measures and drug treatment fail, residents with severe anxiety or panic disorders should be evaluated by a psychiatrist.

SLEEP DISTURBANCES

With advancing age there is a tendency for older individuals to spend more time in bed, sleep less, take longer to fall asleep, have decreased sleep efficiency, and have increased episodes of wakefulness after falling asleep. For this reason, complaints about sleep tend to increase with advancing age, and it is important to distinguish pathological sleep disturbances from the normal age-related changes.

Table 12-6 Causes of chronic insomnia in the nursing home

Excessive daytime naps
Resident being awakened after falling asleep at night (e.g., for medication dosage)
Psychological disturbances
Depression
Dementia
Anxiety
Late-life panic disorder
Mania
Medical conditions
Heart failure (orthopnea, nocturia)
Esophageal reflux
Hyperthyroidism
Head injury
Venous insufficiency (nocturia)
Insufficient light during day (midwinter insomnia/indoor insomnia)
Chronic pain
Sleep apnea
Nightmares/night fears
Nocturnal myoclonus
Drugs
Withdrawal from alcohol or sedative/hypnotics
Caffeine
Theophylline

Insomnia can be transient, such as the sleeplessness that may occur on first being admitted to a NH or when a resident's room is changed. Reassurance that normal sleep patterns will return is usually sufficient in these cases. Insomnia lasting for more than 3 weeks requires a careful diagnostic workup. The major causes of chronic insomnia are listed in **Table 12-6**.

The treatment of insomnia involves explaining to the resident the normal, age-related changes in sleep patterns as well as the appropriate management of the treatable causes, listed in **Table 12-6**. A list of simple techniques for promoting improved sleep for residents with insomnia is given in **Table 12-7**. Some residents may benefit from administration of a bright light (2500 lux) for an hour in the morning. Nocturnal myoclonus may respond to treatment with a muscle relaxant (e.g., baclofen or a short-acting benzodiazepine). Daytime exercises and the planning of meals and social activities so as to keep the resident awake later at night may also be useful. Use of hot milk before sleep remains an excellent placebo. Melatonin which is available in health food stores promotes sleep in older persons. Sedatives and hypnotics are discussed in Chapter 23. The long-term use of hypnotics should be avoided whenever possible. At the St Louis Veteran's Administration Nursing Home Care Unit, a majority of residents have

Table 12-7 Sleep improvement program in the nursing home

1. Avoid daytime naps
2. Do not awaken resident after he/she has fallen asleep
3. Implement consistent times for sleep and awakening
4. Do not allow resident to rest frequently in bed or to be on the bed to watch television or read
5. See that resident exercises in the afternoon
6. Reduce resident's caffeine intake
7. Do not allow resident to fall asleep immediately after evening meal
8. Provide hot milk and a snack at bedtime (trytophan loading)
9. Do not restrain resident in bed, so that normal sleep movements can occur
10. If the resident is not asleep within 30 min, have him or her get up for at least 30 min before making another attempt to go to sleep
11. Use muted night light if resident has anxiety or night fears
12. Keep disturbing noises and lights to a minimum
13. Restrict fluids for 3 h before bedtime in order to decrease nocturia when necessary

been successfully weaned from sleeping medications without any appreciable difference in complaints concerning sleep.

Hypersomnolence during the daytime hours is also not a rare phenomenon in the NH. The most common causes are obstructive sleep apnea and nocturnal myoclonus. Narcolepsy is a rare condition. Fatigue following infection and other acute illnesses and day–night reversal among residents with dementia may both result in excessive sleep during the day. Drugs are probably the major cause of excessive sleepiness during the day. Carryover sleepiness from benzodiazepines given the previous evening is very common. Ambien, a nonbenzodiazepine hypnotic, causes less carryover sleepiness and as such appears to be the hypnotic of choice for older persons. Antihistamines, trazodone and other antidepressants, methyldopa, and antipsychotic drugs can all cause hypersomnolence and should be discontinued if this becomes a problem.

BEHAVIORAL DISORDERS—GENERAL

Behavioral disorders are common among NH residents. They may be expressed as overtly aggressive antisocial behaviors or as passive aggression. In some cases, the behavioral disorder is a symptom of an underlying psychiatric disorder. When this is the case, therapy should be directed toward the underlying disorder. In other cases, behavioral disorders represent the expression of a lifelong personality disorder. Inappropriate methods that the resident may have used to cope with stressors in the past may become accentuated in his or her later years. These individuals often show marked dependency and require constant reassurance and direction. Other individuals may have outbursts of anger when frustrated. Phobias concerning potential injury may discourage the resident from leaving his or her chair or cause inappropriate screams for help.

A major reason for the onset of new behavioral disturbances is related to the loss of locus of control that many residents experience on entry to the NH. These residents may respond by attempting to regain their locus of control by using manipulative behaviors. Refusal to eat is one such behavior. Others will constantly demand attention. In some cases, residents will be verbally abusive toward staff in an attempt to prove that they can still be in charge. This can lead to a vicious cycle in which the abused staff member retaliates, potentially creating a situation of resident abuse. Early recognition of this problem and the provision of support groups for staff are important steps in preventing resident abuse.

An outline of behavioral disorders commonly observed in the NH is given in **Table 12-8**. Management of these disorders begins by recognizing their existence. The first approach should be to provide residents with reassurance that their needs will be met. An approach of rewarding appropriate behaviors and not rewarding inappropriate behaviors is often successful. When behaviorally difficult residents are recognized, the staff should receive support and recognition of the difficulties involved in handling such residents. Staff should be encouraged to express their anger to other staff and should be made aware of the fact that anger and dislike resulting from problematic resident behaviors are appropriate

Table 12-8 Behavioral problems commonly seen among nursing home residents

Disruptive
- Shouting
- Breaching privacy of others
- Deliberately attempting to interfere with staff when they are busy

Demanding
- Attention seeking
- Food refusal
- Continuous seeking of reassurance
- Inappropriately summoning staff
- Dependency behaviors

Distressful
- Hitting
- Biting
- Crying
- Other forms of agitation (see Table 12-9)
- Paranoia
- Emotional liability

Offensive
- Verbal abuse
- Sexually inappropriate behavior
- Undressing in public
- Abnormal feeding behaviors (e.g., sloppiness, pica)

Table 12-9 Causes of nocturnal agitation

A. New onset
  1. Environmental change
  2. Delirium
  3. Bereavement (including death of another resident)

B. Recurrent

  Diseases:

  1. Dementia
  2. Depression
  3. Late-life mania
  4. Late-life panic disorder
  5. Anxiety disorder
  6. Sleep apnea
  7. Medications
  8. Medication withdrawal

  Precipitating factors:

  1. Environmental—lighting, illusionogenic objects, physical restraints
  2. Sensory isolation syndrome—visual, auditory, immobility, social
  3. Nocturnal enuresis
  4. Chronic pain syndromes
  5. Altered circadian rhythm
  6. Frequent awakenings for medical treatment
  7. Social fear of the dark
  8. Night hunger
  9. Staff or family burnout

Table 12-10 Key aspects of the behavioral symptoms resident assessment protocol (RAP)

Trigger	Guidelines

• Wandering
• Verbally abusive
• Physically abusive
• Socially inappropriate
• Resists care
• Behavior improved
	• Review and evaluate the seriousness and stability or change in behavioral symptoms
	• Review potential causes that could be addressed or resolved:
	  • Cognitive status problems, delirium, dementia, stroke
	  • Mood or relationship problems especially depression
	  • Environmental changes
	  • Acute illness or worsening of chronic illnesses
	  • Communication deficits
	  • Sensory impairments
	  • Drugs: antipsychotics, antianxiety, antidepressants, hypnotics
	  • Behavior management program
	  • Physical restraints

feelings. However, the staff must be aware that it is inappropriate to express such feelings to the resident or to allow them to interfere with the care plan. Recognition and elimination of environmental and staff problems that trigger behavioral disorders represent an important part of the management. Short-acting benzodiazepine anxiolytics or buspirone may be useful in allowing the resident to adapt to the environment and benefit from appropriate attempts by staff at behavior modification. All residents who are excessively demanding should have a contract drawn up with the staff, setting forth clearly defined limits. It is important that all staff work together in this regard, not allowing the resident to manipulate one staff member against another. The establishment of a monthly support group for staff, where they can discuss their problems with behaviorally disruptive residents in a supportive environment, often dissipates latent anxiety among the staff and may decrease unplanned leave. **Table 12-9** lists the common causes of nocturnal agitation. **Table 12-10** summarizes the resident assessment protocol (RAP) for behavioral symptoms.

BEHAVIORAL DISORDERS ASSOCIATED WITH DEMENTIA

In the NH, the major need in the management of residents with dementia is to control the secondary symptoms (**Table 12-8**). **Table 12-11** illustrates an agitation inventory developed by Dr Jiska Cohen-Mansfield that may be helpful to NH staff in identifying the nature and frequency of specific behaviors, and for monitoring the response of these behaviors to the various management approaches. Agitated behavior may be worse at night ("sundowning"). Sundowning that occurs after the evening meal may be due to glucose fluctuations and may be improved by the use of frequent small snacks. Factors that may precipitate the sundown syndrome are given in **Table 12-12**. Sometimes residents with dementia who become agitated at night respond to frequent reorientation. Night lights should be kept on in the rooms of residents with sundowning. Residents who frequently pace at night should be placed in exercise programs. Residents who are agitated at night should be carefully observed for precipitating causes of their agitation; where possible, these causes should be removed. Only when behavior modification fails should the use of low-dose neuroleptics (such as haloperidol) or short-acting benzodiazepines be tried. In some cases trazodone (50 to 100 mg) at night will prove to be useful. High doses of a beta blocker may decrease agitation in some residents for whom there are no contraindications to these agents.

Aggressive behavior can be either physical or verbal. Verbally aggressive behavior may sometimes be controlled by ignoring the resident during the outbursts and increasing attention at other times. Verbal aggression may be precipitated by the inability of the resident to hear or understand complex instructions or answers to questions. Thus, simplification of dialog with the resident may result in improved behavior. Verbal aggression should never be

Table 12-11 The Cohen-Mansfield Agitation Inventory[a]

Frequency of the following behaviors are rated by nursing staff for the previous 2 weeks on a 7-point scale:

1 = Never
2 = Less than once/week
3 = Once or twice/week
4 = Several times/week
5 = Once or twice/day
6 = Several times/day
7 = Several times/h

Pacing, aimless wandering
Inappropriate dress or disrobing
Spitting (include at meals)
Cursing or verbal aggression
Constant unwarranted requests for attention or help
Repetitive sentences or questions
Hitting (including self)
Kicking
Grabbing onto people
Pushing
Throwing things
Strange noises (weird laughter or crying)
Screaming
Biting
Scratching
Trying to get to a different place (e.g., out of the building)
Intentional falling
Complaining
Negativism
Eating/drinking inappropriate susbstances
Hurting self or other (cigarette, hot water, etc.)
Handling things inappropriately
Hiding things
Hoarding things
Tearing things or destroying property
Performing repetitious mannersims
Making verbal sexual advances
Making physical sexual advances
General restlessness

[a]Copyright Cohen-Mansfied, 1986. Reprinted with permission.

Source: Cohen-Mansfield J, Marx MS, Rostenthal AS: A description of agitation in a nursing home. *J Gerontol* 44(3):M77–M84, 1989.

treated with psychotropic drugs. Physical aggression is best treated by giving residents sufficient space of their own. Many staff, wittingly or unwittingly, taunt residents and precipitate physical outbursts. Residents with Alzheimer's disease may have visual defects which cause them to startle easily when rapidly approached, especially from behind. This can give the appearance of violent

Table 12-12 Postulated factors that may precipitate the sundown syndrome

A. Phase shift in circadian rhythm of activity peak to later in the afternoon
B. Postprandial hypotension
C. Glucose fluctuations
D. Oxygen desaturation following feeding in persons with chronic obstructive pulmonary disease
E. Environmental and endogenous sensory isolation
F. Hunger "pangs"
G. Societal factors related to a meal:
  - interaction with other residents
  - anger at delay in being served
  - reminiscence of previous positive meal-related behaviors
H. Inadequate lighting

behavior. If physical aggression is unresponsive to behavior modification, isolation of the resident in his or her own room may be appropriate. Low doses of an antipsychotic may also be necessary in some cases and would be acceptable under Omnibus Budget Reconciliation Act (OBRA) regulations, provided that the need is documented (see Chapter 23). Valproic acid has come into vogue as a treatment to decrease agitation. It is not on the OBRA '87 list of restricted drugs. Trazodone is also an excellent drug to calm the agitated resident.

Approximately 10 percent of NH residents are wanderers. Positive effects of wandering include exercise and decreased tension. Negative effects of wandering include the risk of being lost or sustaining injury, the problem of invading the privacy of others, and the creation of staff stress and an increase in time necessary to observe the resident. The wanderer costs a NH approximately $2500 per year extra in staff time in order to monitor the wandering behavior.

The management of wandering requires both staff and environmental modifications (**Table 12-13**). Restraints (physical or chemical) should never be used to manage the wandering resident. Exercise programs and other organized group activities represent a cost-effective response to monitoring groups of wanderers. Elimination of stressors that may trigger wandering is an important part of the overall approach. A lounge or garden specifically designed for wandering can be particularly useful. Adequate signposting to help residents to find their own rooms, the bathroom, and the dining room is very important. The placement of a picture of the resident at the entrance to his or her room may be most useful in this regard. A strip of masking tape on the floor may be a sufficient barrier for some residents. For others, the use of "Dutch doors" (half doors) or door-locking devices that work on a code known only to the staff may be appropriate.

The advent of high technology in the NH has led to the development of a number of sophisticated systems to monitor wandering residents. Door monitoring systems can be activated to sound an alarm when residents wearing

Table 12-13 Approaches to managing wandering behavior

Staff intervention
Adequate and repeated resident orientation
Exercise
Planned group activities
Distraction techniques
Elimination of stressors that trigger wandering
Placing pictures and items from home in resident's room
Behavior modification
Placing picture of resident outside room
Using bracelets to indentify residents
Environmental modifications
Clear sign posting
Dutch doors
Wandering garden/lounge
Door-monitoring systems
Perimeter monitoring systems
Door-locking devices
Electronic locator systems
Administrative modifications
Environmental design and space allocation
Staff training
Staff support

bracelet activators pass though them. Other units allow the wanderer to wear a transmitter which activates an alarm in a receiver when a preselected perimeter distance is exceeded. One company has developed a locator system that displays the locations of individuals on a microcomputer screen.

Inappropriate sexual behavior is most often represented by public masturbation and verbal and sexual overtures to staff and other residents. Residents who masturbate should be encouraged to do this in private, and staff should be counseled that this is a normal behavior. Residents who make verbal or physical sexual overtures should be counseled and firmly told that such behavior is unacceptable. The need of some residents to touch and hug other people should be distinguished from true sexual overtures. When two demented or demented and nondemented residents form romantic attachments, a number of ethical questions arise. Overall, the major criteria for allowing such relationships should be the ability of both residents to understand the implications of their behavior. It should not be automatically assumed that mildly demented residents cannot carry on normal relationships. Finally, all NHs should provide a quiet room where residents can be assured privacy to entertain a spouse or partner when so desired. In-service programs for staff should include discussions of normal and acceptable sexual behavior in the NH. Staff should also be encouraged to express their feelings about these matters.

Screaming is a particularly disturbing problem in some residents. Frequent orientation and keeping the resident near the nurses' station may decrease the frequency of screaming. High-dose beta blockers and/or trazodone may also be useful for some of these residents. Good results may be obtained with some chronic screamers through the use of electroconvulsive therapy.

Social isolation and withdrawal are common problems in demented residents. This behavior may lead to depression and deterioration in self-care skills. Care must be taken to see that attempts to increase socialization result in meaningful experiences for the residents. Social interaction can be increased by, for example, arranging chairs in small groupings and having refreshment areas throughout the NH. Spirituality groups which emphasize touching and overt religious expression may be especially useful for some residents. Tai chi (Chinese exercise) done to music may also increase participation in social activities. Television and radio may play a role in keeping residents in touch with society. However, some demented residents may incorporate events seen on television or heard on the radio into their versions of reality. Hallucinations or delusions may, in fact, be the reality of a television program.

Self-care skills can sometimes be improved by retraining, even among residents with dementia. Rewarding the performance of self-care tasks by tokens redeemable for small luxuries or treats has been reported to increase some NH residents' self-care skills. Such a reward system may slow the development of disability.

Many demented residents respond to reality orientation. This involves constant reminders about real events that are going on in the NH and the community. Correction of mistaken ideas is undertaken. Residents are continuously reminded of where they are and oriented to time and place. Staff are instructed to work with the residents to establish positive attitudes. Such approaches can greatly improve both resident and staff morale. Finally, reminiscing may be very helpful for some residents and can be carried out in a group setting.

PHYSICAL RESTRAINTS

A common response to agitated behaviors, wandering, or a fear of falling has been to restrain NH residents physically. Restraint usage has been increasing in the United States. Up to 50 percent of NH residents are in some type of physical restraint for some portion of the day. This is in stark contrast to the extremely rare use of restraints in Europe. The most common types of restraints are wrist, chest, and jacket restraints. Sheet restraints confining agitated residents to their beds are not rare. Bed rails are virtually universal.

The major reasons for the use of restraints are listed in **Table 12-14**. However, a majority of these have no scientific basis. In one Canadian nursing home, reduction in the use of physical restraints resulted in no significant

Table 12-14 Rationale given for the application of physical restraints in nursing homes

Rationale	Evidence that restraints are useful for this purpose
To prevent falls	No
To prevent wandering	Yes, but at expense of resident freedom
To reduce agitated behavior	No, actually increases such behavior
To avoid litigation	No
For posture improvement	In some cases
To substitute for insufficient staffing	May utilize more staff if properly monitored
To satisfy staff and administration	Yes
As a punitive measure in cognitively impaired residents for "misbehaving"	Certainly punitive but no evidence that it produces appropriate behavior modification
Protection of staff and residents from violent behavior	In most cases confinement to a room is better
To allow medical treatment, such as feeding tubes and intravenous lines, to be administered without interference	In some cases necessary, but alternatives should be tried first

increase in falls. At the St Louis Veterans Administration Medical Center's 150-bed Nursing Home Care Unit, reduction of physical restraints from 38 to 9 percent resulted in a significant decrease in falls. Other studies have suggested that the application of restraints increases agitated behavior. Recent court cases in the United States have found liability for the NH when residents injure themselves while they are being restrained. The rationale in these cases has been that the application of physical restraints to an individual implies that the resident is in danger and requires 24-hour-a-day observation. On the other hand, courts have failed to assign culpability to the institution in most cases when a nonrestrained resident falls.

The application of physical restraints has been associated with a number of adverse effects (**Table 12-15**). **Table 12-16** lists examples of management decisions that result in restraint reduction. The single most important decision is for managers not to demand restraints to prevent injury. Restraint programs work better when the nurses' aides and licensed nurses are asked to come up with strategies allowing the removal of restraints. An example of an assessment that addresses safety and the potential need for restraints is discussed in Chapter 16. Such an assessment may be helpful for NH staff in making decisions about restraints. Monthly feedback on number of restraints in the facility and number of falls also reinforces a restraint-reduction program and is an excellent proactive quality-assurance measure. In some cases, the use of seat belts like those on airplanes (manufactured by J. T. Posey Co., Arcadia, California 91006) will remind the resident not to rise from the chair while still allowing her or him freedom to remove the belt.

Table 12-15 Potential adverse effects of physical restraints

Deconditioning
Falls and injuries
Death
Strangulation
Overall increased mortality
Abrasions, sheet burns
Incontinence
Contractors
Increased agitation
Depression
Anxiety (e.g., inability to get out in case of fire)
Anorexia and protein-energy malnutrition
Dehydration
Decreased functional status
Loss of locus of control
Osteopenia
Regressive behavior
Pressure sores

Table 12-16 Approaches to restraint reduction

1. Administration should mandate restraint reduction and remove pressures from staff when residents wander or fall
2. Staff education concerning problems associated with restraints
3. Emotional appeal to staff: "How would you like to be tied down?"
4. Licensed nurses and nurses' aides should be asked for their suggestions for restraint reduction and rewarded for good suggestions
5. Measure restraints and falls on a monthly basis, graph results, and share with staff
6. Consider use of seat belts like those on airplanes (Posey)
7. Identify high-risk fallers and place them near nursing station
8. Document resident feelings about restraints and their comments after removal
9. Institute conditioning program for deconditioned residents
10. Increase awareness that many falls occur in bathrooms
11. Develop contractual arrangements with residents not to leave chairs without help
12. Continual reinforcement and praise

SUMMARY

The management of psychiatric and behavioral disorders among NH residents is a difficult and challenging task. The precise nature and frequency of these disorders must be carefully defined, and treatable medical conditions that can cause or exacerbate these disorders should be identified and treated. Optimal management requires an interdisciplinary team approach. Psychiatrists and psychologists as well as clinical social workers should work together with

Table 12-17 Sample care plan for complex, behaviorally disturbed residents

Behaviors

Yelling and screaming on frequent basis
Insomnia
Uncooperativeness
Demandingness
Attention seeking
Restlessness
Abusive language
Potential assaultiveness to staff
Disruption of unit and staff with noise (i.e., crying out and shouting at mealtime—demanding immediate service)
Unsteady gait with need at present for restraints
Request for bathroom after every few minutes

Goals

To resolve pain sustained from fall
To decrease agitation precipitated by fall and the use of restraints
To achieve safe ambulation as soon as possible
Reevaluation of behavioral changes and mobility every 2 weeks

Interventions

Follow-up psychiatric consultation
Toilet resident every hour *only* at appointed hour and explain procedure to resident. With each toileting, have resident ambulate as much as possible. At night, toilet when resident awakes and asks to be toileted.
May use geri-chair *only* for mealtime. If resident becomes disruptive to the rest of the residents, move resident out of the dining hall to finish meal.
If resident is agitated, try
- Walking with resident in the halls
- Moving resident to another area
- Sitting and talking calmly with resident. Find a topic of interest (e.g., resident's relatives, past life experiences)
- Sitting quietly with resident, holding his/her hand and offering reassurance

If behavior becomes disruptive, noisy, and out of control, use unit manager's office as a quiet room until resident calms down. Do not leave resident alone.
Under no circumstances allow a resident who is shouting and asking for assistance to be ignored
When resident is quiet and cooperative, give praise and reward resident's good/appropriate behavior. Rewards are
- Praise
- Attention
- Sweets (candy bars)
- Popcorn

Medicate freely as needed for hip and thigh pain
Give resident sleep medication at night as needed
Give haloperidol prn as ordered for agitation that is not resolved by other measures
Protect resident from injury: Use Posey seat belt if necessary for safety
Set limits firmly but with kindness and tell resident when behavior is *not* appropriate
Do *not* reward resident for inappropriate behavior
Rotate staff to work with resident throughout the shift to prevent exhaustion and burnout

medical and nursing staff to identify and treat these disorders. An example of an interdisciplinary care plan for a complex resident with severe behavioral disturbances is outlined in **Table 12-17**. Physical restraints and psychotropic medications should be avoided in the management of behavioral disturbances. When they are used, the reasons should be clearly documented and the behavioral responses closely monitored. Attempts should be made to reduce or eliminate the use of these interventions as soon as feasible.

SUGGESTED READINGS

Carlson DL, Fleming KC, Smith GE, Evans JM: Management of dementia-related behavioral disturbances: A nonpharmacologic approach. *Mayo Clin Proc* 70:1108–1115, 1995.

Cohen-Mansfield J, Marx MS, Rosenthal AS: A description of agitation in a nursing home. *J Gerontol* 44(3):M77–M84, 1989.

Cohen-Mansfield J, Werner P, Marx MS: Screaming in nursing home residents. *J Am Geriatr Soc* 38:785–792, 1990.

Cohen-Mansfield J: Assessment of disruptive behavior/agitation in the elderly: function, methods, and difficulties. *J Geriatr Psy & Neurol* 8:52–60, 1995.

Cohen-Mansfield J, Marx MS: Pain and depression in the nursing home: Corroborating results. *J Gerontol* 48:6–7, 1993.

Evan LK, Stumpf NE: Tying down the elderly: A review of the literature on physical restraints. *J Am Geriatr Soc* 37:67–74, 1989.

Fitten LJ, Morley JE, Gross PL, et al: Depression. *J Am Geriatr Soc* 37:459–472, 1989.

Gillin JC, Byerly WF: The diagnosis and management of insomnia. *N Engl J Med* 322:239–247, 1990.

Grossberg G, Massan R, Szwabo P, et al: Psychiatric problems in the nursing home. *J Am Geriatr Soc* 38:907–917, 1990.

Katz IR, Parmelee PA, Beaston-Wimmer P, and Smith BD: Association of antidepressants and other medications with mortality in the residential-care elderly. *J Geriatr Psy & Neurol* 7:221–226, 1994.

Morley JE: Nocturnal agitation in sleep disorders and insomnia in the elderly, in Albarede JL, Morley JE, Roth T, Vellas BJ (eds). Serdi, Paris, pp 109–117, 1993.

Parmelee PA, Katz IR, and Lawton MP: Incidence of depression in long-term care settings. *J Gerontol* 47:M189–M196, 1992.

Powell C, Mitchell-Pedersen L, Fingerote E, Edmund L: Freedom from restraint: Consequences of reducing physical restraints in the management of the elderly. *Can Med Assoc J* 141:561–564, 1989.

Rovner BW: Depression and increased risk of mortality in the nursing home patient. *Am J Med* 94:19S–22S, 1993.

Rovner BW, Edelman BA, Cox MP, Shmuely Y: The impact of antipsychotic drug regulations on psychotropic prescribing practices in nursing homes. *Am J Psy* 149:1390–1392, 1992.

Tinetti M, Liu WL, Marottoli RA, and Ginter SF: Mechanical restraint use among residents of SNF. *JAMA* 265(4):468–447, 1991.

Werner P, Cohen-Mansfield J, Braun J, Marx MS: Physical restraints and agitation in nursing home residents. *J Am Geriatr Soc* 37:1122–1126, 1989.

Winograd CH, Jarvik LF: Physician management of the demented patient. *J Am Geriatr Soc* 34:295–308, 1986.

CHAPTER
THIRTEEN

NUTRITION

Malnutrition is very common in the nursing home (NH). The prevalence varies based on the case mix and socioeconomic status of the resident population in different institutions. The most common form of malnutrition among NH residents is protein–energy malnutrition, which occurs in up to 66 percent. Insufficient caloric intake has been documented in 5 percent to 18 percent of NH residents. In addition, a recent study has demonstrated a tendency of nursing staff to overestimate the amount the amount of food eaten by residents. Along with malnutrition, vitamin and trace mineral deficiencies occur in a substantial proportion of NH residents. This chapter highlights the specific nutritional problems often seen in NH residents and gives a practical approach to their management.

PROTEIN-ENERGY MALNUTRITION

Diagnosis

Elements of the Minimum Data Set (MDS) for oral and nutritional status are shown in **Fig. 13-1**. Protein–energy malnutrition can present either with weight loss alone with maintenance of serum albumin levels (marasmus) or with low serum albumin levels (kwashiorkor). A marasmus-like picture is a more common presentation, as most older individuals in institutions are ingesting at least 800 to 1000 calories, which is sufficient to maintain serum albumin at the expense of muscle protein. In patients with marasmus, the onset of infection leads to release

SECTION K. ORAL/NUTRITIONAL STATUS

1.	ORAL PROBLEMS	Chewing problem	a.
		Swallowing problem	b.
		Mouth pain	c.
		NONE OF ABOVE	d.
2.	HEIGHT AND WEIGHT	*Record (**a.**) **height in inches** and (b.) **weight in pounds**. Base weight on most recent measure in **last 30 days**; measure weight consistently in accord with standard facility practice—e.g., in a.m. after voiding, before meal, with shoes off, and in nightclothes*	
		a. HT (in.) **b.** WT (lb.)	
3.	WEIGHT CHANGE	**a. Weight loss**—5 % or more in **last 30 days**; or 10 % or more in **last 180 days** 0. No 1. Yes	
		b. Weight gain—5 % or more in **last 30 days**; or 10 % or more in **last 180 days** 0. No 1. Yes	
4.	NUTRITIONAL PROBLEMS	Complains about the taste of many foods — a. Regular or repetitive complaints of hunger — b.	Leaves 25% or more of food uneaten at most meals — c. *NONE OF ABOVE* — d.
5.	NUTRITIONAL APPROACHES	***(Check all that apply in last 7 days)*** Parenteral/IV — a. Feeding tube — b. Mechanically altered diet — c. Syringe (oral feeding) — d. Therapeutic diet — e.	Dietary supplement between meals — f. Plate guard, stabilized built-up utensil, etc. — g. On a planned weight change program — h. *NONE OF ABOVE* — i.
6.	PARENTERAL OR ENTERAL INTAKE	***(Skip to Section L if neither 5a nor 5b is checked)***	
		a. Code the proportion of **total calories** the resident received through parenteral or tube feedings in the **last 7 days** 0. None 1. 1% to 25% 2. 26% to 50% 3. 51% to 75% 4. 76% to 100%	
		b. Code the average **fluid intake** per day by IV or tube in **last 7 days** 0. None 1. 1 to 500 cc/day 2. 501 to 1000 cc/day 3. 1001 to 1500 cc/day 4. 1501 to 2000 cc/day 5. 2001 or more cc/day	

SECTION L. ORAL/DENTAL STATUS

1.	ORAL STATUS AND DISEASE PREVENTION	Debris (soft, easily movable substances) present in mouth prior to going to bed at night	a.
		Has dentures or removable bridge	b.
		Some/all natural teeth lost—does not have or does not use dentures (or partial plates)	c.
		Broken, loose, or carious teeth	d.
		Inflamed gums (gingiva); swollen or bleeding gums; oral abcesses; ulcers or rashes	e.
		Daily cleaning of teeth/dentures or daily mouth care—by resident or staff	f.
		NONE OF ABOVE	g.

Figure 13-1 Minimum Data Set (MDS) assessment of oral/nutritional status.

Table 13-1 Indicators of protein-energy malnutrition

Indicator	Critical Level
Weight loss	5 lb in 6 months or less
Low body weight	Less than 10 percent of average weight
Mid-arm circumference	Less than 10.4 in.
Albumin	Less than 4.0 g/dl in ambulatory and less than 3.5 g/dl in recumbent
Cholesterol	Less than 150 mg/dl

of interleukins and tumor necrosis factor, which results in a decrease in serum albumin levels.

The best indicators of protein–energy malnutrition in a NH resident are weight loss, low body weight, low mid-arm muscle circumference, low cholesterol levels and low albumin levels (**Table 13-1**). Low cholesterol and low albumin levels usually represent a combination of protein–energy malnutrition and cytokine release secondary to a variety of disease processes. Cytokines cause muscle wasting and anorexia. The single best predictor of death in a malnourished NH resident is a cholesterol below 150 mg/dl. Other predictors of death are recent weight loss, low mid-arm muscle circumference, albumin below 4 g/dl, and hematocrit below 41 percent. The use of regular monthly weights is recommended for monitoring NH residents. It is essential that the scales be checked regularly, and standard procedures for weighing should be used (e.g., no shoes, no jackets, no sweaters, and empty pockets). There must be regular in-service training on procedures for weighing, and a random sample (e.g., 5 percent) of residents should have their weights checked by a registered nurse (RN) supervisor on a monthly basis. In residents who have fluid shifts—such as those with congestive heart failure, renal failure, or dehydration—measurement of mid-arm circumference should replace weighing. Use of skin-fold thickness generally shows too high an interindividual variation to be useful as a routine method of assessing nutritional status. **Table 13-2** lists average body weights and normal mid-arm circumference values.

Causes

The major causes of protein–energy malnutrition are outlined in **Table 13-3** and as an easy to remember mnemonic in **Table 13-4**. Every effort should be made to separate the less impaired from the more impaired residents at mealtimes. This allows residents to enjoy their meals and, where possible, promotes social interaction. Room dividers can be very useful in this regard. Eating habits of different residents need to be carefully observed and table pairings made on this basis. Ethnic food preferences also need to be determined.

Table 13-2 Limits for standard body weight per inch of height (± 10 percent)

Height, inches	65–69	70–74	Age, years 75–79	80–84	85–89	90–94
			Men			
61.........	156–128	153–125	151–123			
62.........	158–130	155–127	153–125	148–122		
63.........	161–131	157–129	155–127	150–122	146–120	
64.........	164–134	161–131	157–129	152–124	148–122	
65.........	166–136	164–134	160–130	155–127	153–126	143–117
66.........	169–139	167–137	163–133	158–130	156–128	146–120
67.........	172–140	170–140	166–136	162–132	160–130	150–122
68.........	175–143	174–142	169–139	165–135	163–133	154–126
69.........	179–147	178–146	174–142	169–139	167–137	158–130
70.........	184–150	182–148	178–146	175–143	172–140	164–134
71.........	189–155	186–152	183–149	180–148	176–144	169–139
72.........	195–159	190–156	188–154	187–153	182–148	
73.........	200–164	196–160	192–158			
			Women			
58.........	146–120	138–112	135–111			
59.........	147–121	140–114	136–112	122–100	121–99	
60.........	148–122	142–116	139–113	130–106	124–102	
61.........	151–123	144–118	141–115	133–109	128–104	
62.........	153–125	147–121	144–118	136–112	132–108	131–107
63.........	155–127	151–123	147–121	141–115	136–112	131–107
64.........	158–130	154–126	151–123	145–119	141–115	132–108
65.........	162–132	158–130	154–126	150–122	146–120	136–112
66.........	166–136	162–132	157–128	154–126	152–124	142–116
67.........	170–140	166–136	161–131	158–130	156–128	
68.........	175–143	170–140				
69.........	180–148	176–144				

Source: After Master A, Lasser R: *JAMA* 172:658, 1960.

Restrictive diets in NHs are more likely to cause protein–energy malnutrition than they are likely to improve the status of other diseases. For example, the prescription of severely sodium-restricted diets in NHs has been questioned. In one study, switching NH residents from a 3 g to a 4 g sodium diet resulted in no significant changes in control of heart failure. Studies in NHs have clearly implicated low salt diets as a major cause of malnutrition. Similarly, there is little evidence that American Diabetic Association (ADA) diabetic diets have a major role in NH residents. A "no free sugar" diet may be equally effective and allow residents more variety. There is also no evidence that low-cholesterol diets benefit NH residents. An optimal cholesterol level for a NH resident is 240 to 280 mg/dl. In addition to a routine diet order, bedtime nourishment should be offered to all NH residents.

Table 13-3 Causes of protein–energy malnutrition in the nursing home

Social
- Monotonous institutional meals
- "Disgust" with surroundings and/or behaviorally disturbed residents
- Lack of ethnic foods
- Unnecessary dietary restrictions (e.g., low salt, low cholesterol, ADA diabetic)

Psychological
- Depression
- Dementia
- Anorexia nervosa
- Anorexia (tardive)
- Sociopathy–loss of locus of control
- Mania
- Overwhelming burden of life (passive suicide)

Medical
- Increased metabolism
  - Hyperthyroidism
  - Pheochromocytoma
- Anorexia
  - Drugs
    - Digoxin
    - Psychotropics
    - Fluoxetine
  - Esophageal candidiasis
  - Hyperparathyroidism
  - Intestinal ischemia
  - Zinc deficiency
  - Altered taste and smell
- Malabsorption
- Cancer
- Chronic obstructive pulmonary disease (increased metabolism and anorexia)
- Dysphagia

Table 13-4 "Meals-on-wheels" mnemonic for treatable causes of malnutrition in nursing home residents

Medications (e.g., digoxin, cimetidine, fluoxetine
Emotional problems (depression)
Anorexia tardive (nervosa)
Late-life paranoia
Swallowing disorders (dysphagia)

Oral factors
No money (insufficient funds in Medicaid facilities for palatable, individualized diets and consultant dietician)

Wandering and other dementia-related behavior (e.g., forget to eat, apraxia)
Hyperthyroidism, hyperparathyroidism, hypoadrenalism
Enteric problems (malabsorption)
Eating problems (inability to feed oneself)
Low-salt, low-cholesterol diets
Social problems (ethnic food preferences, isolation, "disgusting" food habits of other residents)

Table 13-5 Techniques for oral feeding

Proper positioning to maximize ability to swallow
Nondistracting environment
Food preparation
Palatably warm—not hot
Gelatinous consistency
Avoid rice and applesauce
Try macaroni and cheese, meatloaf and gravy
If there is excessive mucus, exclude milk products and chocolate

Depression is a common, treatable cause of weight loss. One study in a NH where there was little polypharmacy and the nursing staff placed a premium on feeding residents found that depression was the most common cause of malnutrition, accounting for a third of all cases. Adequate treatment of depression resulted in return to normal weight in nearly 70 percent of these cases. Two other studies using different methodologies have similarly highlighted the prominent role depression can plays in the pathogenies of malnutrition. All NH residents with weight loss should therefore be screened for depression. The multiple other causes of weight loss in NH residents with dementia are outlined in **Table 13-5**. One study demonstrated that 18 minutes per day was spent feeding demented NH residents, compared with 99 minutes per day when the same individuals were managed at home. The use of a semicircular table where one aide can feed four or five residents at a time is one innovative solution to this problem. To overcome the apraxia of swallowing, nurse's aides need to be taught to instruct the residents to swallow. Residents with loss of locus of control often attempt to use food to regain this control. Thus, food refusal may represent a manipulative behavior. Other residents notice that residents who are not eating get extra attention; thus they may also refuse to eat to obtain more interactive time with staff.

Anorexia nervosa can recur in older women who had an episode of this condition as teenagers. Older men and women may develop extremely abnormal attitudes toward eating and an abnormal body image. In some cases, this is related to a desire for immortality and to the belief that calorie restriction or low cholesterol levels will extend life. This disorder has been called anorexia tardive. Recognition of these abnormal attitudes about eating is essential for appropriate management. In addition to depression, other psychiatric disorders may also be related to poor nutritional intake. Late-life paranoia can present with refusal to eat because of the belief that the food is poisoned. Mania can result in weight loss due to increased energy utilization.

In some NH residents, failure to eat is related to a perception of life as an overwhelming burden and as such represents a form of passive suicide. In these residents, treatable depression must be excluded. At present, there is no single clear ethical principle that determines whether a NH resident who can make decisions for herself or himself should be allowed to starve to death. In the case of the severely demented individual, a written advance directive authorizing withholding or withdrawal of feeding appears legally necessary. Passive suicide should be distinguished from the normal failure to eat that is often noted in the last few weeks of life in very old individuals. Ethical issues surrounding artificial feeding and hydration are discussed further in Chapter 27.

Several medical disorders and medications can contribute to weight loss (**Table 13-3**). Among the medical causes of weight loss, apathetic hyperthyroidism should not be missed. Among NH residents with severe weight loss in whom hypertension is difficult to control, the presence of pheochromocytoma should be considered. Malnutrition occurs in 25 percent of residents on digoxin, and anorexia improves when this drug is discontinued. High doses of psychotropics often result in malnutrition. On the other hand, withdrawal of psychotropic medications from residents who need them can result in dramatic weight loss. Sometimes this is the only indication of the need to restart psychotropic therapy. Severe wasting may occur when residents are treated with fluoxetine for depression. Early satiation may represent a presentation of nitrioxide (NO) deficiency. NO is the neurotransmitter responsible for dilation of the fundus of the stomach in response to eating a meal. This condition may respond to nitroglycerine being swallowed instead of placed under the tongue. Gallstones are another cause of early satiation. Cholecystectomy can result in dramatic weight gain in residents with weight loss and gallstones. Residents with chronic obstructive pulmonary disease often become dyspneic when eating. These residents should have several (at least six) small meals a day.

Difficulties with swallowing are a major problem in NH residents. Besides leading to aspiration pneumonia, swallowing disorders can also result in a conditioned aversion to feeding. The single most important management strategy for dysphagic individuals is an upright posture, allowing maximum use of gravity. Feeding in a nondistracting environment is another important feature of the management of swallowing disorders such as dysphagia. Other techniques for feeding residents with dysphagia are outlined in **Table 13-6**. All dysphagic NH residents should have a modified barium swallow and evaluation by a speech therapist. Some success has been obtained with giving liquid supplements in place of water at the time of medication passes to help with the swallowing of drugs.

Management

Tables 13-6 and **13-7** outline the resident assessment protocol (RAPs) for nutritional status and feeding tube status. The management of protein–energy malnutrition involves the early and aggressive use of supplements. Caloric supplements for weight loss should be given between meals, at least 1½ hours before the next meal. Liquid supplements are preferred as they empty from the stomach much more quickly than solids. Before the institution of tube feeding, documentation that both hand feedings and swallowing therapy have been

Table 13-6 Summary of resident assessment protocol (RAP) for nutritional status

Trigger	Guidelines	Care plan
The following suggest malnutrition: • Weight loss (57. in 1 month, 107. in 6 months)[a] • Complains about taste of food[b] • Leaves 25 percent or more of food uneaten at most meals[c] • Parenteral/IV feeding[d] • Mechanically altered diet • Syringe feeding • Therapeutic diet[e] • Pressure ulcer	**Factors impeding ability to consume food:** • Reduced ability to self-feed • Ostomy losses • Chewing problems • Possible medical causes	**Enhance oral intake:** • Review food preferences • Assistance in feeding • Adaptive utensils • Modify nutrient consistency • Optimize dining atmosphere • Fortify diet • Add caloric supplements • Make sure food intake is adequate • Stop therapeutic diets
	Problems related to nutritional status problems: • Mental problems –fear food is poisoned –dementia –anxiety –depression • Behavior problems –pacing –wandering –throwing food –slowness in self-feeding –withdrawal from activities • Inability to communicate • Functional problems • Loss of upper extremity or amputation	**Tube Feeding:** • Initiate tube feeding when oral intake insufficient to meet needs *or* • Document resident/family referral of tube feeding
		Nutrition counseling: • Provide appropriate education for resident, family and health care team members

[a]Weights are often wrong. Weights that differ from previous month should be rechecked.

[b]Consider zinc deficiency or drug nutrient interaction.

[c]Food left on plate is consistently underestimated. This parameter will miss many residents with anorexia.

[d]Peripheral parenteral nutrition can be used to maintain nutritional status during acute illnesses, where slowed gastrointestinal transit may decrease ability to tube feed.

[e]There is little indication for therapeutic diets in nursing homes and these should be avoided whenever possible.

Table 13-7 Summary of the resident assessment protocol (RAP) for feeding tube status

Trigger	Guidelines	Care plan
Consider efficacy and need for feeding tube if a feeding tube is present	**Factor that may impede removal of tube:** • Coma • Failure to eat and resists assistance in eating • Stroke • Gastric bleeding or ulcers • Chewing or swallowing problems • Mouth pain • Length of time feeding tube has been in use	**Prevent misplaced tubes:** • Used weighted tube • Utilize radiological confirmation of placement • Check PM • Auscultate over stomach when all is injected • Assess for signs of respiratory difficulty • Use ostomy tube whenever possible
	Potential complications of tube feeding: • Recurrent lung aspiration/ infections • Self-extubation and/or physical restraints to prevent self-extubation • Side effects of enteral products: diarrhea, constipation, fecal impaction, abdominal distension pain, dehydration • Respiratory problems • Cardiac distress • Abnormal laboratory values • Negative values nitrogen balance	**Prevent aspiration pneumonia:** • Elevate head of bed to 45° • Check gastric residual prior to feeding (> 100 ml needs evaluation) • Monitor for signs of respiratory distress • Avoid too rapid rates of infusion
		Assess lab values: • BUN and creatinine ratio for dehydration • Hyponatremia • Hemoglobin for GI bleeding • Liver functions

attempted must appear in the resident's record. A number of drugs have been utilized to enhance appetite, although in general the results have been somewhat disappointing. Most studies suggest that enteral feedings usually produce only weight maintenance, not weight gain. These data suggest the need for early introduction of enteral feeding to prevent malnutrition. Alternatively, the calories

Table 13-8 Key aspects of the resident assessment protocol for dental care

Factors	Problems to be considered
Cognitive	• Does resident need reminders to clean teeth/dentures? • Does resident remember the steps necessary to complete oral hygiene? • Can resident follow verbal directions or demonstrations of mouth care?
Vision	• Is resident's vision adequate for performing mouth care?
ADL Function	• Has resident been assessed to see if he/she could perform dental care independently?
Motivation/ knowledge	• Is resident brushing adequately? • Has resident been instructed to brush near the gumline? • Does resident resist mouth care? • Does resident require reinforcement for maintaining good hygiene?
Equipment	• Would resident benefit from using a built-up, long-handled, or electric toothbrush, or suction brush for cleaning teeth?
Diagnosis/ conditions medication	• Is resident taking any medications that can cause dry mouth (e.g., decongestants, antihistamines, diuretics, antihypertensives, antidepressants, antipsychotics, antineoplastics)?
Pain and conditions	• Does resident have mouth pain or sensitivity? • Does resident have candidiasis (white areas that appear to be able to be removed) in mouth or on tongue? • Are teeth in good repair? • Does resident use his/her dentures (or partial plate)? • Are dentures comfortable to wear when eating or drinking? • Does resident like the way he/she looks when wearing dentures? • Is there a need for dental hygienist to assess resident regarding oral hygiene care? • Has dental examination been performed by a dentist? • Is resident on coumadin or heparin which would put resident at risk for bleeding if dental work is necessary? • Does resident have valvular heart disease or prosthesis (e.g., heart valve, pacemaker) which might indicate need for antimicrobial prophylaxis? • Does resident have presence of lesions, ulcers, inflammation, bleeding, swelling or rashes?

administered need to be increased to more than 2000 per day until weight gain occurs. For reimbursement, this requires documentation that lower levels of calories failed to produce weight gain. Attention to dental status and its impacts on the resident's ability to take in adequate calories is critical. **Table 13-8** outlines key aspects of the dental care RAP.

The indications for tube feeding are outlined in **Table 13-9**, and the major complications of enteral feeding are outlined in **Table 13-10**. Before switching from elemental to blenderized formulas, the presence of diarrhea should be documented. **Table 13-11** lists other potential approaches to diarrhea associated with tube feeding. **Table 13-12** gives the composition of some of the commonly

Table 13-9 Indications for enteral nutrition in long-term care setting

Protein–energy malnutrition with inadequate oral intake for 5 days
Less than 50% of required nutrient intake for 7 to 10 days
Severe dysphagia
Radiation or chemotherapy with anorexia
Organ failure with anorexia

Table 13-10 Potential complications of enteral feeding

Problems with tube placement
Intolerance of tube
Aspiration
Gastric erosions
Diarrhea
Selenium deficiency
Fluid intolerance
Hypotension (with bolus feeding)
Glucose intolerance
Electrolyte imbalance (low blood levels of potassium, phosphorus, calcium, sodium, magnesium)

Table 13-11 Management of diarrhea among tube-fed residents

Rule out treatable causes of diarrhea
Medication side effects
Antibiotic-associated enterocolitis
Fecal impaction
Other
Dilution of formula may work, but results in decreased intake of calories
Switch to a lactose-free feeding
Switch to blenderized formula
Give banana chips orally
Try a high-fiber diet among those who take food orally

used enteral products. The feeding tube may be placed through the nose or through the skin, or it can be implanted surgically. It appears that overall there is little difference in complications regardless of the method of placement. Thus the choice should be dictated by resident and/or staff preference. There is no clear advantage to percutaneous gastrostomy tube placement over jejunostomy tube placement. Tubes placed in the stomach pose a greater risk of aspiration than tubes placed in the small intestine. They have the advantage, however, of allowing bolus feedings. Aspiration from endogenous secretions continues to occur after tube placement, no matter what type of tube is placed. Placing a soft small-bore tube in ice before insertion may facilitate placement by the nasogastric route. Alternatively, a small-bore tube may be attached to a larger

Table 13-12 Composition of some commonly used enteral feeding products

	Calories (per ml)	Protein (g/liter)	Sodium (meq/liter)
Ensure (Ross)	1.1	37	37
Isocal (Mead-Johnson)	1.1	34	23
Osmolite (Ross)	1.1	37	28
Replete (Clinitec-Nutrition)	1.0	62	22
Sustacal (Mead-Johnson)	1.5	49	36
Resource (Sandoz)	1.1	37	37
Jevity (Ross)[a]	1.1	45	40
Sustacal with fiber[a] (Mead-Johnson)	1.1	46	31
Compleat (Sandoz)[b]	1.1	43	57
Mentene Liquid (Sandoz)[b]	1.0	69	48
Ensure Plus (Ross)	1.5	55	50
Isocal MN (Mead-Johnson)	2.0	75	35
Nutren 2.0 (Clinitec Nutrition)	2.0	80	43
Two Cal MN (Ross)	2.0	84	46
Sustagen (Mead-Johnson)[b]	1.7	112	55

[a]Contains fiber.
[b]Contains lactose.

nasogastric tube, either by holding the two together with a gelatin capsule or placing the small-bore tube inside the larger tube after it has been split open lengthwise. Both these techniques are associated with a greater rate of mechanical complication during insertion.

Among the methods of tube feeding, bolus feedings are the most poorly tolerated, are most likely to result in missed feedings, and involve the most staff time. Cyclical feeding at night frees the resident from being attached to a pump during the day and allows him or her optimal opportunity to eat. Cyclical feeding is often better tolerated psychologically as well. Continuous feedings have better gastrointestinal tolerance and more easily achieve adequate calorie delivery than do cyclical feedings. They also smooth metabolic control. Their major disadvantage is that the resident is "tube tied" throughout the day and night.

Elemental formulas containing 1.0 to 1.5 calories/ml should be sufficient for most NH residents (see **Table 13-12**). Residents who develop infections should be switched to high-protein formulas. Low-protein formulas are used for residents with renal failure. High-fat formulas can be used for residents with chronic obstructive pulmonary disease, because they decrease the amount of oxygen needed for the metabolism of the food and may smooth the control of patients with diabetes mellitus. High-fiber formulas should be given only to residents who are ambulatory, because they can produce constipation in immobile residents. All residents receiving tube feeding should be supplemented with 100 ;gmg of sodium selenite daily unless the formula contains selenium.

VITAMIN DEFICIENCY

Vitamin deficiency is not rare in the NH population. The presence of vitamin deficiency closely parallels that of protein–energy malnutrition. Individuals with cheilosis, angular stomatitis, and a magenta tongue have vitamin B_{12} (riboflavin) deficiency. Pyridoxine (B_{16}) deficiency may present similarly but without the magenta tongue. Individuals with vitamin $B_{11,12}$ (cobalamin) deficiency often have a beefy red, large tongue. Dermatological findings suggestive of these vitamin deficiencies that can be seen in NH residents include cheilosis and dermatoses. It therefore appears prudent to give a B-complex vitamin to any NH resident with a low caloric (less than 1200 calories per day) intake.

Pernicious anemia occurs in 1 percent to 2.5 percent of persons over 60 years of age. Vitamin B_{12} deficiency is classically associated with megaloblastic anemia, subacute combined degeneration of the spinal cord, and/or dementia. It is now recognized that in individuals with both iron and vitamin $B_{11,12}$ deficiencies, the anemia may be either normo- or microcytic. Dementia can occur in the face of vitamin B_{12} deficiency without the development of anemia. In residents who have borderline normal levels of vitamin B_{12}, it may be useful to obtain a serum methylmalonic acid level, which if elevated makes the diagnosis of vitamin B_{12} deficiency. However, this is an expensive test and its use may not be cost-effective. NH residents with dementia may also develop a secondary vitamin B_{12} deficiency associated with malnutrition. In these cases, some cognitive improvement may be obtained by treatment with vitamin B_{12}. If this approach is taken, a vitamin B_{12} level below the normal range should be documented. The resident's cognitive status should also be documented, and this should be repeated every 3 months, using a standard scale to measure improvement.

Vitamin C (500 mg per day) may be useful for NH residents with pressure sores or other poorly healing skin lesions. Higher doses of vitamin C appear to offer no benefit. Vitamin C must be withdrawn at least 72 h before testing for blood in the stool, as it can cause false-negative occult blood tests. **Table 13-13** summarizes the controlled trials of vitamin deficiency treatment in older persons. Vitamin D deficiency is discussed in Chapter 18.

Table 13-13 Vitamins in nursing homes: interventional studies

Study	Outcome
Multivitamin	• Fewer skin hemorrhages and capillary fragility • No change in tongue or in capillary fragility • Decrease in excitement
Vitamin B_6	• Improved clock drawing in deficient subjects
Vitamin C	• Weight gain and improved nurse assessment • Weight gain, improved albumin levels, and decrease in purpura • No decrease in purpura or hemorrhage

Table 13-14 Putative effects of zinc deficiency

Anorexia
Hypogeusia
Poor wound healing
Immune dysfunction
Age-related macular degeneration

MINERAL DEFICIENCY

NH residents often have a borderline zinc status. This is especially true among those receiving thiazide diuretics and those with diabetes mellitus or liver disease. The putative effects of zinc deficiency are outlined in **Table 13-14**. The major indications for zinc supplementation in a NH resident are poorly healing skin ulcers and anorexia without an obvious cause. Age-related macular degeneration may also be slowed by administration of zinc. The preferred dosage is zinc sulfate 220 mg three times a day with meals. The sulfate may cause gastrointestinal distress. Breaking the zinc capsule and mixing the contents with water may alleviate the gastrointestinal distress.

Selenium deficiency may occur in tube-fed NH residents and can be associated with muscle weakness and/or pain and nail changes (i.e., thickened and fragile, with rough, ridged surfaces). Residents with selenium deficiency can also have humoral and cellular immune dysfunction and may have a greater propensity to develop candidiasis. Treatment consists of supplementation with 100 μg of sodium selenite daily.

WATER

Water is the single most abundant part of the body's composition yet it is most likely to be forgotten. Screening for dehydration can be carried out by identifying all residents with a blood urea nitrogen to creatinine ratio of greater than 20:1. Further diagnosis then depends on demonstrating a postural blood pressure drop or an increasing pulse rate in response to standing for 2 minutes. Several factors make NH residents susceptible to dehydration. Older individuals do not recognize thirst as readily as younger ones do. In addition, older individuals may have impaired access to fluids because of physical restraints or because of inherent impaired mobility. Incontinent residents sometimes self-limit fluid intake in an attempt to decrease urinary frequency. Increased fluid loss occurs with fever; special attention must be paid to the fluid needs of such residents. For these reasons, it is essential that NH residents be offered fluids at regular intervals. Key elements of the resident assessment protocol (RAP) for dehydration is given in **Table 13-15**.

Table 13-15 Summary of the resident assessment protocol (RAP) for dehydration/fluid maintenance

Trigger	Guidelines	Care plan
Dehydrated insufficient fluid/ did not consume all liquids provided Urinary tract infection Weight fluctuation of greater than 3 lbs Fever Internal bleeding Parenteral/IV Feeding tube Taking diuretic	**Factors impeding ability to maintain fluid balance:** • Delirium • Impaired decision making capacity • Comprehension/ communication problem • Body control problems • Hand dexterity problem • Constipation • Fecal impaction • Swallowing problem • Recent deterioration in ADLs	• Provide and encourage intake of appropriate amount of fluids • Replace GI losses and those due to excessive sweating • Consider dehydration with weight loss • Check for orthostasis • Add adequate free water when resident is tube fed • Record fluid intake in at risk residents • Provide extra fluid in hot weather • Consider short term IV fluids when resident has fever • Educate resident, family, caregivers, about importance of fluid
	Resident dehydration risk factors: • Purposeful restriction of fluids • Diarrhea, presence of infection • Fever, vomiting, nausea • Excessive sweating • Frequent laxative/enema/ diuretic use • Excessive urine output • Dry oral mucus membranes • [Diabetes mellitus][a] • [Hypercalcemia][a]	

[a]Not included in MDS 2.0.

SUGGESTED READINGS

Abbasi AA, Rudman D: Undernutrition in the nursing home: Prevalence, consequences, causes and prevention. *Nutrition Rev* 52:113–122, 1994.

Abbasi AA, Rudman D: Observations on the prevalence of protein-calorie undernutrition in VA nursing homes. *J Am Geriatr Soc* 41:117–121, 1993.

Blaum CS, Fries BE, Fiatarone MA: Factors associated with low body mass index and weight loss in nursing home residents. *J Gerontol* 50:M162–168, 1995.

Katz IR, Beaston-Wimmer P, Parmelee P, Friedman E, Lawton MP: Failure to thrive in the elderly: Exploration of the concept and delineation of psychiatric components. *J Geriatr Psy & Neurol* 6:161–169, 1993.

Lindenbaum J, Healton EB, Savage DG, Brust JCM, et al: Neuropsychiatric disorders caused by cobalamin deficiency in the absence of anemia or macrocytosis. *N Engl J Med* 318:1720–1728, 1988.

Martin DC, Francis J, Protetch J, Huff FJ: The dependency of cognitive recovery with cobalamin replacement: Report of a pilot study. *J Am Geriatr Soc* 40:168–172, 1992.

Miller M, Morley JE, Rubenstein LZ: Hyponatremia in a nursing home population. *J Am Geriatr Soc* 43:1410–1413, 1995.

Morley JE, Silver AJ: Nutritional issues in nursing home care. *Ann Intern Med* 123:850–859, 1995.

Morley JE, Kraenzle D: Causes of weight loss in a community nursing home (see comments). Comment in: *J Am Geriatr Soc* 43:82–83, 1995. *J Am Geriatr Soc* 42:583–585, 1994.

Morley JE: Nutritional status of the elderly. *Am J Med* 81:679–695, 1986.

Morley JE, Glick Z, Rubenstein LZ: *Geriatric Nutrition: A Comprehensive Review.* New York, Raven Press, 1990.

Morley JE, Mooradian AD, Silver AJ, et al: Nutrition in the elderly. *Ann Intern Med* 109:890–904, 1988.

Rabeneck L, Wray NP, Petersen NJ: Long-term outcomes of patients receiving percutaneous endoscopic gastrostomy tubes. *J Gen Intern Med* 11:287–293, 1996.

Ship JA, Duffy V, Jones JA, Langmore S: Geriatric oral health and its impact on eating. *J Am Geriatr Soc* 44:456–464, 1996.

Stabler SP: Screening the older population for cobalamin (Vitamin B_{12}) deficiency. *J Am Geriatr Soc* 43:1290–1297, 1995.

Yao Y, Yao S-L, Yao S-S, Yao G, et al: Prevalence of Vitamin B_{12} deficiency among geriatric outpatients. *J Fam Pract* 35:524–528, 1992.

CHAPTER

FOURTEEN

PRESSURE SORES AND OTHER SKIN DISORDERS

PRESSURE SORES

Pressure sores and other skin disorders are prevalent among nursing home (NH) residents and present a challenge for both prevention and management. Pressure sores are commonly used as indicators of poor quality of care. Most studies have been conducted among older hospitalized patients in acute care hospitals and report prevalence rates of between 20 and 30 percent. The true incidence of pressure sores in NHs is not known. One prospective study found a 25 percent incidence of pressure sores in two Veterans Administration NHs over 1–4 weeks; another found an incidence of close to 25 percent for nonblanchable erythema (Stage 1 pressure sore) over a 60-day period of time. It is estimated that 60,000 people die per year from complications of pressure sores. In addition to the human toll, the financial aspects are significant. Nursing time per NH resident doubles for the resident with a pressure sore. Cost estimates to heal each pressure sore range from \$5000 to \$40,000. The annual national cost of care for pressure sores is estimated at \$3.5 to \$7 billion. In addition, medical outcomes associated with pressure sores can be devastating. For example, a fourfold risk of death has been reported for institutionalized patients who develop pressure sores.

Etiology and Pathogenesis

Table 14-1 describes primary and secondary factors associated with the development and healing of pressure sores. As their name implies, pressure is the causative factor leading to these lesions. Normal capillary pressure in humans is

Table 14-1 Factors associated with the development of pressure sores

Primary factors	Secondary factors
Pressure over bony prominences	Malnutrition
Shearing forces	Immobility
Tissue tolerances	Moisture
	Friction
	Anemia
	Vascular insufficiency
	Diabetes mellitus
	Sensory impairments

about 35 mmHg. Pressure between a bony prominence and a hard resting surface can exceed 300 mmHg. The concentration of pressure over a limited area reduces capillary blood flow to near zero at the point of pressure. High pressure can be tolerated, but only if it is relieved intermittently. Mobile people with intact sensation can sense the ischemia as discomfort and shift their position periodically. Thus, NH residents with impaired mobility are at increased risk for developing pressures that produce pressure sores. Pressure as low as 70 mmHg can produce irreversible tissue damage if it is applied for more than 2 h. Microscopic examination of damaged tissue shows characteristic ischemic changes of cellular infiltration, extravasation, and hyaline degeneration. A cone-shaped area of ischemia develops from the point of pressure to a wider area in the deeper tissues. The skin itself may be the last tissue layer to demonstrate ischemic changes. Ischemia and subsequent inflammatory changes therefore show a predilection for sites overlying bony prominences, particularly below the belt line. Most pressure sores develop on the sacrum, ischial tuberosities, greater trochanters, heels, and lateral malleoli (**Fig. 14-1**).

Another primary factor implicated in the development of pressure sores is the shearing forces caused by sliding adjacent surfaces. These forces are encountered clinically when the head of a bed is raised, causing the patient's torso to slide down while the sacral skin remains fixed. This can cause stretching and agitation of small blood vessels, with subsequent thrombosis. Friction also contributes to the development of pressure sores by removing the skin's outer protective layer. Moisture, regardless of the source, also promotes maceration and skin breakdown.

With continued pressure on skin that has become ischemic, a dermatitis-like picture develops. Edema and softening of the skin allow further damage due to friction. Bacterial invasion of damaged tissue can take place when the epithelium is disrupted. Infection can cause major delay in healing because of tissue damage and bacterial competition for oxygen.

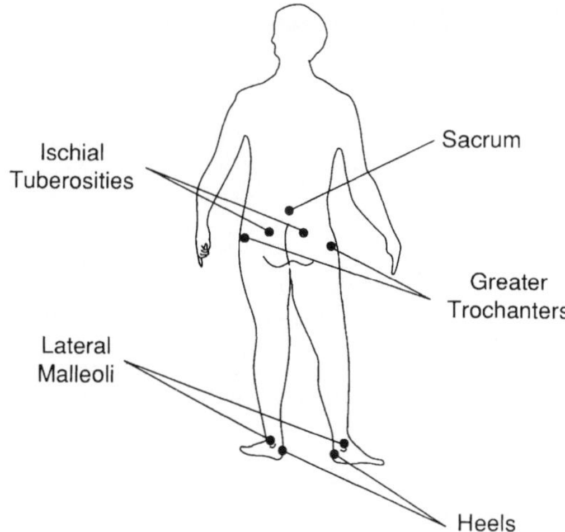

Figure 14-1 Most common sites of development of pressure sores in NH residents.

There remains some disagreement regarding risk factors and their role in the development of pressure sores. One study identified hypoalbuminemia, fecal incontinence, and hip fracture as independent risk factors for developing pressure sores. Other reported risk factors include immobility, weight loss, and hypotension. All these factors are common among NH residents, making them especially vulnerable to pressure sores.

Assessment

Proper assessment of pressure sores requires careful examination of the sore. Most sores cannot be accurately assessed until all eschar and purulent material has been removed. Several descriptive assessment tools can be found in the literature. All use depth of the lesion as a grading criterion. The classification of Shea, which describes four stages, is used most often and helped form the basis of the National Pressure Ulcer Advisory Panel's Consensus Conference Statement in 1989 (**Table 14-2**). Current recommendations discourage "reverse staging" of healing ulcers. This is because the Shea stage measures extent of initial tissue injury, but as full thickness wounds heal they fill in with different tissue types than were originally present, so a tool used to measure extent of injury in normal tissues cannot be used to assess this. Currently the Minimum Data Set (MDS) supports reverse staging but the Health Care Financing Administration (HCFA) plans to revise this in the future. The Sessing Scale has been shown to reliably describe pressure ulcer healing (**Table 14-3**).

Determining the stage of the pressure sore is only one aspect of assessment. The wound should also be assessed for location, size (length and width in centimeters), depth, undermining or tunneling, exudate (type, amount), odor,

Table 14-2 The staging of pressure sores

Stage I	Nonblanchable erytheme on intact skin; the heralding lesions of skin ulceration
Stage II	Partial-thickness skin loss involving epidermis and/or dermis. The ulcer is superficial and present clinically as an abrasion, blister, or shallow crater
Stage III	Full-thickness skin loss involving damage or necrosis of subcutaneous tissue; this may extend down to but not through underlying fascia. The ulcer presents clinically as a deep crater with or without undermining of adjacent tissue
Stage IV	Full-thickness skin loss with extensive destruction, tissue necrosis, or damage to muscle, bone, or supporting structures (e.g., tendon, joint capsule, etc.)

Source: National Pressure Sore Advisory Panel Consensus Conference Statement (1989).

Table 14-3 The Sessing Scale used to assess pressure sore healing[a]

Stage	Description
0	Normal skin, but at risk
1	Skin completely closed May lack pigmentation or may be reddened
2	Wound edges and center are filled in Surrounding tissues are intact and not reddened
3	Wound bed filling with pink granulating tissue Slough present Free of necrotic tissue Minimum drainage and color
4	Moderate to minimal granulating tissue Slough and minimal necrotic tissue Moderate drainage and odor
5	Presence of heavy drainage and odor, eschar, and slough Surrounding skin reddened or discolored
6	Breaks in skin around primary ulcer Purulent drainage, foul odor, necrotic tissue and/or eschar May have septic symptoms

[a]The scale is cored by calculating the change in numerical values over successive wound assessments over time. Positive scores indicate ulcer improvement and negative scores indicate worsening ulcers.

color of wound bed, surrounding tissue status, necrotic tissue (type, color, and amount), and granulation tissue. It is important to review previous treatment strategies and to identify contributing factors that may also affect the progress of healing.

Closed pressure sores, usually covered by eschar, may involve large areas of destruction under the skin, with only a small area of overlying skin appearing to be involved. These sores can be deceptive and may require debridement or

SECTION M. SKIN CONDITION

1.	**ULCERS** (Due to any cause)	*(Record the number of ulcers at each ulcer stage—regardless of cause. If none present at a stage, record "0" (zero). Code all that apply during* ***last 7 days****. Code 9 = 9 or more.)* ***[Requires full body exam.]***	Number at Stage
		a. Stage 1. A persistent area of skin redness (without a break in the skin) that does not disappear when pressure is relieved.	
		b. Stage 2. A partial thickness loss of skin layers that presents clinically as an abrasion, blister, or shallow crater.	
		c. Stage 3. A full thickness of skin is lost, exposing the subcutaneous tissues - presents as a deep crater with or without undermining adjacent tissue.	
		d. Stage 4. A full thickness of skin and subcutaneous tissue is lost, exposing muscle or bone.	
2.	**TYPE OF ULCER**	*(For each type of ulcer,* ***code for the highest stage in the last 7 days*** *using scale in item M1—i.e., 0=none; stages 1, 2, 3, 4)*	
		a. Pressure ulcer—any lesion caused by pressure resulting in damage of underlying tissue	
		b. Stasis ulcer—open lesion caused by poor circulation in the lower extremities	
3.	**HISTORY OF RESOLVED ULCERS**	Resident had an ulcer that was resolved or cured **in LAST 90 DAYS** 0. No 1. Yes	
4.	**OTHER SKIN PROBLEMS OR LESIONS PRESENT**	***(Check all that apply*** *during* ***last 7 days****)*	
		Abrasions, bruises	a.
		Burns (second or third degree)	b.
		Open lesions other than ulcers, rashes, cuts (e.g., cancer lesions)	c.
		Rashes—e.g., intertrigo, eczema, drug rash, heat rash, herpes zoster	d.
		Skin desensitized to pain or pressure	e.
		Skin tears or cuts (other than surgery)	f.
		Surgical wounds	g.
		NONE OF ABOVE	h.
5.	**SKIN TREAT-MENTS**	***(Check all that apply*** *during* ***last 7 days)***	
		Pressure relieving device(s) for chair	a.
		Pressure relieving device(s) for bed	b.
		Turning/repositioning program	c.
		Nutrition or hydration intervention to manage skin problems	d.
		Ulcer care	e.
		Surgical wound care	f.
		Application of dressings (with or without topical medications) other than to feet	g.
		Application of ointments/medications (other than to feet)	h.
		Other preventative or protective skin care (other than to feet)	i.
		NONE OF ABOVE	j.
6.	**FOOT PROBLEMS AND CARE**	***(Check all that apply*** *during* ***last 7 days)***	
		Resident has one or more foot problems—e.g., corns, callouses, bunions, hammer toes, overlapping toes, pain, structural problems	a.
		Infection of the foot—e.g., cellulitis, purulent drainage	b.
		Open lesions on the foot	c.
		Nails/calluses trimmed during **last 90 days**	d.
		Received preventative or protective foot care (e.g., used special shoes, inserts, pads, toe separators)	e.
		Application of dressings (with or without topical medications)	f.
		NONE OF ABOVE	g.

Figure 14-2 Skin assessment contained in the Minimum Data Set (MDS).

Table 14-4 Key aspects of the pressure sore resident assessment protocol (RAP)

Factors	Problems to be considered
Diagnosis	• Does the resident have a pressure ulcer? • Is the resident exhibiting conditions that would place him/her at higher risk of developing pressure ulcers or complicate treatment (e.g. peripheral vascular disease, diabetes mellitus, dementia)?
Medications	• Is resident taking medication, antidepressants, antianxiety/ hypnotics, or antipsychotics?
ADL Function	• Does resident have impaired ability to reposition self at regular intervals? • Is resident confined to bed or chair? • Does resident have poor skin integrity? • Is resident's skin desensitized? • Does resident have urinary or bowel incontinence? • Are restraints being used? • Does resident have a history of pressure sores?
Nutrition	• Has resident had a significant weight loss?

radiological evaluation (computed tomography (CT), magnetic resonance imaging (MRI), or sinography) for accurate assessment.

Figure 14-2 illustrates the skin assessment section of the MDS. The pressure ulcer resident assessment protocol (RAP), outlined in **Table 14-4**, provides a road map for further assessment of NH residents admitted with selected risk factors for pressure sores. Systematic monitoring of protocol implementation and outcomes, such as the number of new pressure ulcers, should be part of regular quality improvement activities. Any negative trends, such as an increase in number of pressure ulcers or failure to heal, should be examined case by case.

Management of Pressure Sores

The best strategy for preventing the development of pressure sores is to avoid immobility and pressure. High-quality nursing care is critical. A reliable risk-assessment or screening tool to identify high-risk NH residents has yet to be perfected. The Agency for Health Care Policy and Research (AHCPR) guidelines for pressure in adults prediction and prevention (1992) recommends that all bed-bound or chair-bound patients be assessed utilizing one of two risk assessment scales for conducting this systematic assessment: the Norton Scale or the Braden Scale for predicting pressure ulcer risk. Both scales are sensitive, but have limited predictive validity. Utilizing them in conjunction with other risk factors such as diastolic blood pressure, body temperature, immobility,

Table 14-5 Guidelines for the prevention of pressure sores

A. Reduce and/or relieve pressure

Rationale: In providing effective pressure relief, both pressure and time must be considered.

1. Pressure relieving devices

   Rationale: Capillary closing pressure is 25 to 32 mmHg. *Pressure relieving* devices are those which *consistently* reduce pressure below this level and can be used to prevent pressure breakdown.

   Candidates

   Residents who cannot tolerate turning

   Residents who have skin breakdown or who are at risk for skin breakdown involving multiple surfaces.

   Examples

   Low airloss bed therapy.

   Air fluidized bed therapy.

2. Pressure reducing devices

   Rationale: Pressure reducing devices lower pressure, as compared to standard hospital mattresses or chair surfaces. They *do not* reduce pressure below capillary closing levels on a constant basis and must be used in conjunction with a turning or position change schedule.

   Candidates

   Residents who *can* be turned.

   Residents with skin breakdown or at risk for skin breakdown involving only one surface.

   Examples

   Dynamic—pressure reducing devices, which *move* (e.g., alternating air mattress), reduce pressure locally.

   Static—pressure reducing devices, which are stationary (such as foam mattresses, gel cushions, water beds, and air mattresses), also reduce pressure locally.

3. Establish schedule for major position changes and weight shifts. Generally turning every 2 h is sufficient, but some individuals may require more frequent turning.

B. Reduce and/or relieve shearing

Rational: Shearing is caused when tissue layers slide against each other and results in angulation or disruption of blood vessels, usually at the fascial level.

1. When not contraindicated, keep head of bed at or below 30° angle and flat.
2. If not contraindicated, use knee gatch when head of bed is elevated.
3. Use padded foot board.

C. Reduce and/or relieve friction

Rationale: Friction—caused when the skin rubs against another surface—can cause superficial skin damage.

1. Use assistive devices and/or techniques—such as turning sheets, trapeze bar, lifts, transfer boards—to facilitate movement.
2. Use powder or cornstarch on surfaces contacting skin to reduce surface friction and absorb moisture.

D. Reduce excessive moisture

Rationale: Excessive moisture and/or contact with urine or stool causes maceration and/or chemical erosion of the skin.

1. Institute measures to contain fecal and/or urinary incontinence and to protect the skin.

E. Evaluate nutritional and hydration status

Rationale: Tissue hydration and positive nitrogen balance are critical elements in wound healing.

1. Consult dietician and provide nutrition and hydration support as required.

fecal incontinence, and dietary intake improves the ability to predict pressure ulcer formation. Familiarity with the known risk factors (**Table 14-1**) leads to the development of a preventive strategy, such as the one described in **Table 14-5.** The development of specific protocols for the prevention and treatment of pressure sores can be useful to nursing staff in order to standardize their approach to the problem. **Figure 14-3** displays the AHCPR pressure ulcer prediction and a prevention algorithm.

Staff education and appropriate nursing management techniques are especially important to assure compliance and accountability for proper body positioning and the prevention of immobility (i.e., walking the resident, changing positions), which are critical elements in the prevention of pressure sores. **Figure 14-4** illustrates various body positions relative to pressure sore development. Implementation of management strategies should integrate skin prevention with other core protocols (i.e., urinary incontinence, mobility to increase efficiency and increase staff compliance. More specific administrative and management considerations regarding quality assurance are described in Chapter 8.

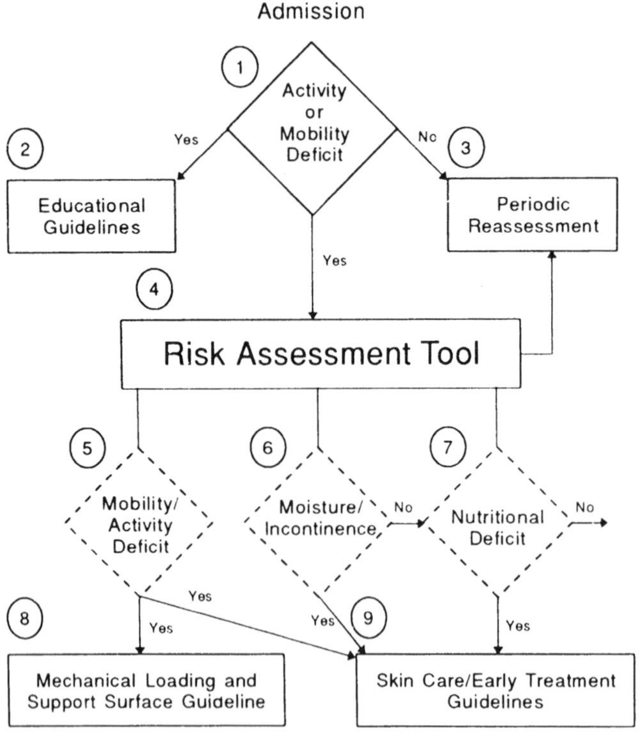

Figure 14-3 Pressure ulcer prediction and prevention algorithm from the Agency for Health Care Policy and Research (AHCPR) clinical practice guidelines.

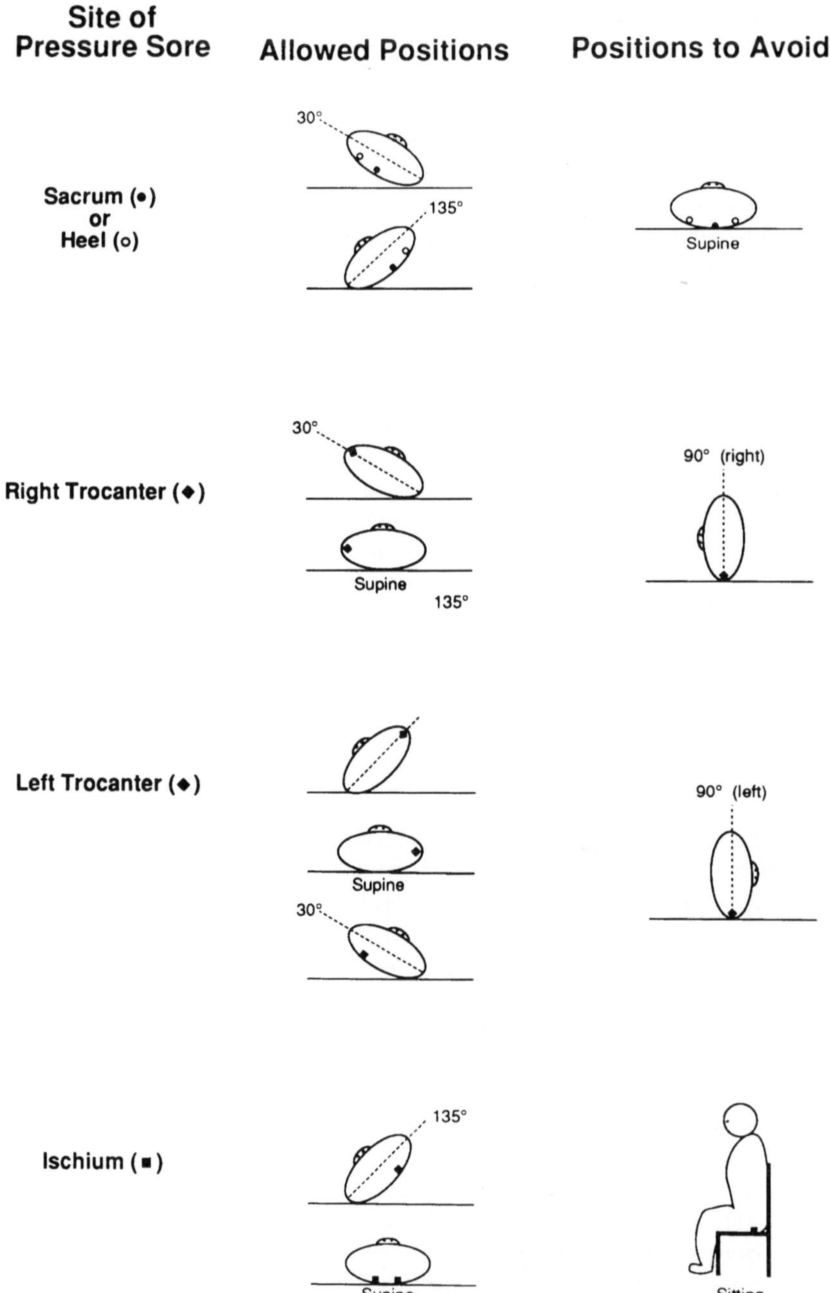

Figure 14-4 Body position and the prevention of pressure sores. Modified from Sieler WO, Stahelin HS: *Geriatrics* 40(7):53–60, 1985.

Primary physicians should work with nursing staff to carefully and systematically observe NH residents at high risk for pressure sores and to identify and treat early sores before they become deeper. The use of enterostomal therapy (ET) nurses, who have special education in pressure sore management, or other nurse consultants in NHs can enhance pressure sore care and staff education. The management of medical conditions that place residents at high risk for pressure sores should be optimized (e.g., malnutrition, anemia, vascular disease, diabetes). It is important to note that many pressure sores develop during an acute hospital stay; it is the NH staff that then has to deal with them. It has unfortunately been the practice of long-term care regulatory agencies to penalize NHs for the presence or aggravation of pressure sores. Effective prevention and management of pressure sores must therefore involve a cooperative effort between acute hospital and NH staffs. Regulatory agencies should focus on assisting such cooperative efforts rather than trying to find someone to blame for the development of individual pressure sores. Relief of pressure should be viewed as a preventive strategy for high risk NH residents, and is further discussed later in this chapter. Pressure sores differ little from other skin wounds, and general principles of wound care are applicable to their management. Although not specifically discussed in this chapter, the general principles of managing lower extremity venous and arterial ulcers are similar to those of managing pressure sores. General medical care should focus on nutritional repletion to reverse protein catabolism and promote wound healing. **Table 14-6** reviews the functions of nutritional elements in wound healing. (For more detailed information on wound healing, see "Suggested Readings.") Correction of anemia, control of underlying medical conditions such as diabetes, and improvement in oxygenation and tissue perfusion may also enhance wound healing.

The objectives of managing pressure sores include the relief of pressure, prevention of further tissue damage, wound debridement and the elimination of local infection, and the promotion of a healing environment. In severe cases, excision and closure of defects may be necessary. Some 70 to 90 percent of pressure sores are superficial (stage II or less) and may be managed with conservative therapy.

Relief of pressure can be accomplished in a variety of ways, including frequent turning in order to prevent prolonged exposure to one area (see **Fig. 14-1**) and the use of local padding or pressure-reducing beds. It is important to note that use of local skin padding such as "donuts" should be avoided because of their propensity to impede circulation, and worsen the already present ischemia. Heel protectors are useful in preventing friction and shearing, but they require monitoring to ensure that they do not cause undue pressure. Several types of pressure-reducing support surfaces are available. Foam mattresses are probably the least expensive and most convenient. Their advantages are offset by the fact that they offer the least pressure reduction and are generally considered devices that serve only to enhance comfort if the foam-rubber projections are less than 4 in. high (including bases and peaks). Water beds provide modest pressure

Table 14-6 Function of various nutritional elements in wound healing

Element	Function	Effect of deficiency
Protein	Cell proliferation, collagen metabolism	Delayed healing
Carbohydrate	Energy source	Altered leukocyte function
Fats	Membrane function	Not known
Vitamin C	Enzyme cofactor in collagen metabolism	Rickets, altered collagen formation, delayed healing
Vitamin A	Antagonizing effect of steroids	Not well known
Thiamine	Energy metabolism	Decreased cell proliferation and collagen metabolism
Vitamin E	Membrane stabilization	None known
Vitamin K	Coagulation cofactor	Excessive bleeding, hematoma, wound disruption
Water and salts (sodium, potassium, chlorine)	Membrane function, hydration	Volume depletion, decreased tissue profusion
Phosphorus	ATP metabolism	Altered cell replication and protein metabolism
Calcium, magnesium, manganese	Enzyme cofactors in collagen metabolism	Altered collagen formation, delayed healing
Zinc	RNA metabolism	Altered cell replication, delayed healing
Iron, copper	Enzyme cofactors in collagen metabolism	Delayed healing, anemia

reduction, but their inflation pressure is critical. Over- or underinflation results in less than optimal pressure reduction. The materials used for these mattresses is usually plastic or rubber, and moisture may become a problem. Air mattresses provide better pressure reduction, and aerated models also help to decrease moisture. Air fluidized and low airloss beds provide a levitation medium (air or fiberglass spheres). These units provide adequate pressure dispersion, pressure relief, and labor conservation (requiring less turning and changes of linen). They provide a dry environment, decreasing the effect of perspiration and incontinence, and a freely movable surface that may decrease the forces of friction and shear. Reports suggest these beds—as opposed to foam mattresses—may have a significant positive effect on large pressure sores during the first week of wound care. The average NH cannot afford the cost of these beds unless supplemental coverage by insurance is available. Until recently, because air fluidized/low-air-loss beds are costly, their use was considered only for residents with large stage III and stage IV wounds for whom positioning was difficult. However, one study showed that treatment of pressure ulcers utilizing low-air-loss beds is even more effective for the population with mild stage II or early stage III ulcers with better healing characteristics. Another study analyzed the cost-effectiveness of pressure ulcer prevention and treatment. Outcomes were measured as patient days of ulcer-free life. It demonstrated that the cost of prevention (utilizing regular care) as $1.36 per ulcer-free day and $26 for treatment utilizing low-air-loss beds. With proper staff and physician documentation, the NH can fill out a treatment authorization request and be reimbursed for the use of the bed by some Medicaid programs. Medicare Part A recognizes the selective need for this modality and frequently authorizes its use, reimbursing the cost through the NH's cost reporting mechanism.

Table 14-7 provides examples of protocols for the management of various types of pressure sores. Many NH nurses have their own favorite protocols. Many of these protocols do work, but none has been adequately tested in randomized controlled trials. The effective management of stage I and stage II pressure sores involves pressure relief, the optimization of nutrition, treatment of underlying medical conditions, and excellent local care. Superficial cultures have no role in the management of stage I and stage II sores and should not be ordered routinely (see Chapter 19). Debridement must be added to management protocols for stage III and stage IV sores, for which removal of necrotic tissue is essential. Debridement is done mechanically or enzymatically. Mechanical debridement may include surgical (sharp debridement), physical means such as use of a whirlpool, or by using saline wet or dry dressings. The latter are painful, require considerable nursing time, and may remove new granulating tissue. Sharp debridement is generally preferred for deeper necrotic wounds as long as there is an adequate arterial circulation. If whirlpool is used in persons with significant arterial vascular disease, it is important to keep the water temperature tepid and not warm. Alternatively, one may use "slow" chemical debridement using proteolytic enzymes to help liquify the necrotic tissue. Collagenase is capable of digesting undenatured collagen, which is found in most eschar. Semiocclusive dressings (e.g., hydrocolloid) may be applied after a wound is cleaned and debrided. This provides an environment conducive to healing. Topical antibiotics or oxidizing agents offer no advantage and may actually retard healing by being toxic to new cells or by encouraging the growth of resistant bacteria. The reduction of moisture and fecal contamination is also essential. Absorptive pads are preferable to indwelling catheters to manage incontinence because of the risk of sepsis, although the temporary use of an indwelling catheter may be necessary to help heal some pressure sores. Adequate staffing and intensive nursing care are necessary to provide the frequent cleaning that may be required for incontinent residents with pressure sores.

Control of infection is achieved mostly by debridement and removal of necrotic material. Use of systemic antibiotics should be limited to lesions

Table 14-7 Examples of protocols for the management of various stages of pressure sores[a]

A. Pressure sore classification: stage I, epidermis intact

1. Wound cleansing
   a. No special cleansing necessary
2. Topical treatment: goal—protect and maintain intact epidermis
   a. Transparent semipermeable membrane
      Rationale: Protects intact epidermis yet allows visualization of area.
      Procedure: Apply to clean, dry skin. Change every 7 days in p.m.
   b. Skin barrier film
      Rationale: Protects intact epidermis yet allows visualization of area.
      Procedure: Available as wipes or spray. Apply to clean, dry area once a day.

B. Pressure sore classification: stage II, partial-thickness wounds and/or stage III, shallow, full-thickness wounds with little exudate

1. Wound cleansing
   a. Normal saline
      Rationale: Normal saline is physiologic and has no deleterious effects on the wound-healing process. Wound cleansing promotes removal of wound debris and bacteria from wound surface.
2. Topical treatment: goal—keep wound surface clean, moist, and free of secondary infection.
   a. Transparent semipermeable membrane
      Rationale: Provides a moist wound-healing environment by trapping wound exudate under dressing; allows visualization of wound.
      Procedure: Apply to clean wound with at least 2 cm of dressing extending beyond wound. Dressing should be changed every 7 days and/or whenever wound fluid leaks from underneath dressing.
   b. Hydrocolloid dressing
      Rationale: Provides a moist wound-healing environment by trapping wound exudate under dressing. Many encourage angiogenesis as most are occlusive dressings.
      Procedure: Apply to clean wound with at least 2 cm of dressing extending beyond wound. Dressing should be changed every 7 days and/or whenever wound fluid leaks from underneath dressing. If more frequent dressing changes are needed, use smaller dressing with less extending around wound.
   c. Gel dressing
      Rationale: Provides a moist wound-healing environment. May absorb some wound exudate. Used with other dressings (transparent semipermeable membrane, hydrocolloid, or gauze).
      Procedure: Apply gel to clean wound and cover with secondary dressing of choice (transparent semipermeable membrane, hydrocolloid, gauze). Change according to secondary dressing used (usually every 3 to 4 days). If gauze is used, change every day or every other day.
   d. Calcium alginate dressing
      Rationale: Provides a moist wound-healing environment. Absorbs wound exudate.
      Procedure: Apply enough to cover wound bed on clean wound. If wound is fairly dry, moisten dressing with small amount of normal saline. After application, cover with gauze dressing and change when drainage strikes through cover dressing, generally every 3 to 5 days. Alternatively, cover with transparent semipermeable membrane and change every 7 days and/or when there is leakage of exudate from underneath dressing.

Table 14-7 (*Continued*)

e. Moist gauze dressing

Rationale: If applied correctly, will provide a moist wound-healing environment. Absorbs small amount of wound exudate.

Procedure: Use gauze instead of cover sponges. Moisten gauze with normal saline, fluff, and apply to clean wound. Cover with dry cover sponge. Change every 4 h. Gauze should not be allowed to dry out, as this will retard wound healing.

f. Lubricating spray

Rationale: Provides a moist wound healing environment.

Procedure: Spray in clean wound bed and cover with gauze dressing. Change dressing every day to every shift, depending on amount of wound exudate.

C. Pressure sore classification: stage III and/or stage IV; full thickness wounds, deep craters, or wounds with excessive or pooled exudate

1. Culture and sensitivity, after cleansing of the wound base, in the following circumstances: symptoms or signs of clinical infection (e.g., cellulitis) bone/joint involvement; sepsis when doing the etiology is unknown

Rationale: *All* dermal wounds are contaminated; culture is indicated *only* for evidence of clinical infection or potential for osteomyelitis. Surface swab cultures are of *no* value; culture should be taken from deep necrotic tissue or bone.

2. Wound cleansing

Rationale: Thorough cleansing at each dressing promotes removal of wound debris and bacteria from wound surface. Many commonly used solutions have deleterious effects on the wound healing process and should be used with caution if used at all. For example:

Povidone-iodine—inhibits and/or destroys macrophages and fibroblasts

Hydrogen peroxide—provides mechanical cleansing through effervescence but also destroys fibroblasts even when diluted

Dakin's solution (*potassium hypochlorite*)—controls odor, is effective for staphylococcal and streptococcal infections, helps liquify necrotic tissue, but also destroys fibroblasts.

Acetic acid—appropriate for *psuedomonas* infections, but also destroys fibroblasts even when diluted.

a. Normal saline

Rationale: Normal saline is physiologic and has no deleterious effects on the wound healing process. It is appropriate for all wounds.

Procedure: May be used for irrigation or for less aggressive cleansing.

3. Topical treatments: Goal—keep wound surface clean, moist, and free of secondary infection; pack wound to obliterate dead space without damaging tissue.

a. Absorption dressing—copolymer starches and dextranomers

Rationale: Absorption dressings absorb excess exudate, obliterate dead space, and provide a moist wound-healing environment.

Procedure: Mix or prepare dressing according to manufacturer's guidelines and apply to clean wound bed, taking care to pack dead space. Cover with gauze dressing and change once a day or more frequently depending on wound exudate.

Table 14-7 (*Continued*)

b. Absorption dressing—calcium alginates

Rationale: Absorbs excess exudate, obliterates dead space, and provides a moist wound-healing environment.

Procedure: Gently pack dead space and apply to clean wound bed. Cover with gauze dressing and change when drainage strikes through dressing. (In heavily exudating wounds, this may be once or twice a day; less frequently for wounds with less exudate.)

c. Absorption dressing—moist gauze

Rationale: Absorbs excess exudate, obliterates dead space, and provides a moist wound-healing environment.

Procedure: Use gauze instead of cover sponges. When packing wounds with large amounts of dead space, it is best to use rolled gauze for easy removal. Moisten gauze with desired solution; normal saline is appropriate for all wounds (see notes on wound cleansing solutions and C2, above.) Gently pack dead space and fluff to apply to clean wound bed.

D. Pressure sore classification: stage III and/or stage IV, with necrotic tissue present

1. Topical treatments: Goal—debridement of necrotic tissue

Rationale: Necrotic tissue is an impediment to wound healing and must be removed

a. Conservative instrumental debridement

Rationale: Conservative debridement can be used in conjunction with other topical therapy to enhance the process without the risks involved in surgical debridement.

Procedure: May be done by enterostomal therapy (ET) nurses and/or other nurse specialists depending on state nurse practice acts and education. Removal of tissue is done by scalpel or sharp scissors and is limited to clearly identified necrotic tissue.

b. Enzymatic debriding ointments

Rationale: Enzymatic agents chemically break down necrotic tissue; effectiveness is dependent on appropriate use.

Procedure: Many wound cleaning solutions interfere with the action of enzymatic debriding ointments; if used, they must be thoroughly rinsed from wound bed with normal saline. Apply ointment to necrotic tissue only and cover with gauze dressing. Some ointments work better with a moist gauze dressing. Most should be changed every 8 h (check manufacturer's guidelines for duration of action). If the necrotic tissue is hard or eschar is present, scoring or cross-hatching of the hard eschar may be required prior to use of enzymatic ointment.

c. Physiologic debridement using transparent semipermeable membrane dressings

Rationale: Transparent semipermeable membrane dressing enhance leukocyte migration and resultant autolysis of necrotic tissue.

Procedure: Especially effective on hard eschar necrotic tissue. Apply to clean wound with at least 2 cm of dressing extending beyond wound. Change every 7 days or whenever wound fluid leaks from underneath dressing.

d. Mechanical debridement using wet-to-dry dressings and/or water propulsion therapy

Rationale: Wet-to-dry dressings are a nonselective debriding approach; granulation tissue may be removed in addition to necrotic tissue. Water propulsion provides mechanical removal of *loose* necrotic tissue.

Table 14-7 (*Continued*)

Procedure:	Moisten gauze (not cover sponges), fluff; apply to wound bed and cover with cover sponge: allow gauze to dry prior to next dressing change (usually 4 h) and pull dry gauze out of wound bed. Gauze should not be moistened to ease removal, as this contradicts the purpose of the dressing. This debridement method can be painful, and pain medication may be needed prior to dressing changes. Water propulsion can be performed by needle and syringe, Water Pik, or whirlpool therapy. Water propulsion will remove only necrotic tissue that is already loose.

e. Once debridement of necrotic tissue is accomplished, topical treatments include those identified in C, above.

[a]All protocols should be accompanied by prevention strategies (see Table 14-3) and optimization of nutrition and management of other medical conditions.

Source: International Association for Enterostomal Therapy: *Standards of Care Dermal Wounds: Pressure Sores*. Irvine, California, 1987.

complicated by cellulitis, osteomyelitis, bacteremia, or sepsis. The management of infected pressure sores is discussed in detail in Chapter 19.

A number of studies have demonstrated a marked improvement in pressure ulcers healing with pulsed low-intensity direct current (300 to 600 μA). Alterations in calcium homeostasis enhance fibroblast and keratinocyte growth. Pressure sores heal twice as fast when electrical current is used for stage 2 and 3 pressure ulcers.

Recently topically applied recombinant basic fibroblast growth factor (BFGF) has been used to treat pressure ulcers. BFGF increases fibroblasts and capillaries in the wound. A double-blind placebo controlled trial has found that BFGF has a greater ability to produce wound closure and decrease pressure ulcer volume.

OTHER SKIN DISORDERS

Dry Skin (Xerosis)

Dry skin is one of the most common dermatologic problems affecting the elderly. It usually occurs on exposed surfaces, including the hands, feet, and face. The sides of the torso are also frequently involved. The clinical signs of xerosis include scaling, flaking, cracks, and fissures. Symptomatically, xerosis manifests itself by pruritus, which may be intense and can cause excoriations complicated by superinfection. Since many other skin disorders (e.g., contact dermatitis, seborrheic dermatitis, allergic reactions, psoriasis) as well as some medical conditions (e.g., renal failure, cholestasis) can cause pruritus, a careful assessment should be done before pruritus is ascribed simply to dry skin.

Table 14-8 Strategies to prevent dry skin and pruritus

1. Encourage adequate fluid intake.
2. Use tepid baths and bath oils to preserve skin moisture.
3. Apply moisturizing creams or lotions after baths and two to three times per day.
4. Use soft, absorbent clothing.
5. Prescribe topical steroid creams sparingly to avoid skin atrophy.
6. Whenever possible, avoid antihistamines unless severe pruritus is causing excoriations or disrupting sleep.

Prevention of xerosis is largely dependent upon retarding the loss of moisture from the surface of the stratum corneum. **Table 14-8** lists some general guidelines for the prevention of dry skin. Many NH residents develop dry skin in winter because indoor heated air is very low in humidity, and forced-air heating systems keep air currents moving past exposed skin. Use of a humidifier to maintain adequate humidity (i.e., above 40 percent) may be important in preventing xerosis, pruritus, and other complications. Sebum from sebaceous glands helps preserve epithelial hydration. When combined with sweat, sebum forms an emulsion that coats the skin, forming a barrier against transdermal water loss. Commercial moisturizing creams, lotions, and oils act by producing an occlusive or semiocclusive film that coats the surface and helps the sebaceous glands to reduce evaporation. These products also lubricate the skin, making rough, dry, scaly skin smoother and less irritated. Any treatment for dry skin should be supplemented by an effort to replace the moisture lost through perspiration and evaporation. Nursing home residents should be encouraged to drink several glasses of water per day. This will help to prevent not only dry skin but also dehydration and its complications.

Dermatitis and Eczema

The terms dermatitis and eczema are often used interchangeably or in combination. Both imply superficial inflammation of the skin due to irritant exposure, allergic sensitization, and/or other factors that contribute to skin irritation. Pruritus can result in erythema and edema of the skin, which may progress to vesicle formation, oozing, crusting, and scaling. **Table 14-9** describes several types of dermatitis that are seen in the NH population. Many NH residents develop a dermatitis of unknown etiology. Treatment consists of avoiding the excessive use of products that might irritate the skin, such as drying soaps and detergents. Clothing made of nonirritant materials such as cotton should be worn next to the skin. Emollients should be used liberally, especially after bathing. Corticosteroid creams or ointments should be applied two to three times daily to affected areas. Once symptoms are alleviated, use of the topical corticosteroid can be reduced and often discontinued in favor of emollients alone. Antihistamines may be necessary to reduce severe pruritus and help the resident

Table 14-9 Types of dermatitis seen in the nursing home population

Condition	Description/characteristics	Management
Idiopathic eczema of the hand	Persistent erythema and scaling of the palms or lateral digits without an obvious precipitating cause.	Emollients, topical steroids; overnight occlusion to intensify steroid absorption.
Contact dermatitis	Skin inflammation caused by contact with irritant or allergic substance.	Avoid contact with irritant such as soaps, detergents, solvents. Acute eczema with blister formation should be referred to a dermatologists.
Stasis dermatitis	Inflammation occurring as a result of venous hypertension in the lower leg.	Well fitting support stockings to control edema; keep limb elevated as much as possible.
Drug-caused eruptions	Eruption of the skin that occurs after administration of a drug. Starts 1 to 10 days after the resident first takes the drug and may last for 14 days after it is discontinued.	Drug should be removed; symptomatic treatment of lesions; severe reactions may require the use of systemic corticosteroids.
Toxic epidermal necrolysis	Severe eruption that begins with general malaise, skin tenderness, and erytheme; rapidly progresses to blistering.	Remove drug (NSAID, sulfa, penicillin); systemic steroids; diphenylhydantoin; severe reactions may require care in a burn unit.
Psoriasis	Well-defined erythematous plaques covered with a silver scale. Affects especially knees, elbows, scalp, and buttocks.	Coal tar or cream or paste (0.1% to 0.4%); topical corticosteroids; phototherapy; methotrexate.
Seborrheic dermatitis	Scaly erythematous eruption affecting face, eyebrows, eyelids, scalp, nasolabial folds, and body flexures. May cause blepharitis and conjunctivitis.	Topical hydrocortisone creams or ointments; tar-containing shampoos for scalp involvement.

sleep. However, these agents must be used with caution in elderly NH residents, since they have anticholinergic effects and may produce urinary retention, paradoxical agitation, and other side effects.

Herpes Zoster ("Shingles")

Herpes zoster is a cutaneous eruption caused by the reactivation of a varicella zoster viral infection. The lesions begin as pustules and then rupture, with resultant crusting in a unilateral dermatomal distribution. Occasionally secondary bacterial infection becomes a serious problem. After 2 to 4 weeks, the skin lesions resolve, sometimes leaving some scarring. Pain in the dermatome may precede the onset of the lesions and persist for weeks or months after the skin lesions heal (postherpetic neuralgia). The management of herpes zoster is discussed in Chapter 19.

Scabies

Scabies is an eruption caused by the mite *Sarcoptes scabiei.* The female mite burrows into the skin and deposits eggs, which hatch into larvae in a few days. Scabies is transmitted by skin-to-skin contact and can rapidly spread throughout a NH. Scabies may present less typically and may mimic eczema or exfoliative dermatitis, with thick crusted lesions. Erythroderma and generalized lymphadenopathy may be present. The mite must be excavated with a needle or a scalpel blade in order to make the diagnosis. In long-standing cases with widespread excoriation, a mite may be impossible to find. In these cases, treatment based on a presumptive diagnosis may be the best option in order to prevent an outbreak. The management of scabies is discussed in Chapter 19.

Pediculosis (Lice)

Lice may infest the head (pediculosis capitis) and/or the body (pediculosis corporis). NH residents are at risk for head and body lice. Pediculosis capitis is transmitted through personal contact or through hairbrushes and head wear. Infected individuals develop severe itching of the scalp, often with secondary eczematous changes and impetiginization. Cervical lymphadenopathy may also be present. On examination, small gray or white mites (ova) are seen on the hair shafts. Unlike scales, they cannot easily be removed. Pediculosis corporis produces intense generalized itching that, in turn, can lead to the development of eczematous changes, excoriations, and secondary bacterial infections. Lice or mites may be found in the seams of clothing.

For head lice, shampoo containing 1 percent lindane is applied to the scalp and left in place for 4 to 6 min. After rinsing, the hair should be combed with a fine tooth comb. The procedure should be repeated in 10 days to destroy any remaining mites. Combs and brushes should be soaked in the shampoo for 1 hour. For body lice, the resident's clothing should be dry-cleaned or washed in a machine (hot cycle). The seams of the clothing should be pressed with a hot iron. Alternatively, the clothing can be disinfected with an insecticidal powder such as DDT 10 percent or malathion 1 percent. Eczema and/or infection that develops as a result of the infestation should be treated appropriately.

Bullous Pemphigoid

Bullous pemphigoid is an autoimmune disorder of the skin that occurs most commonly in the elderly. Pathologically, immunoglobulin (IgG) is deposited

Table 14-10 Examples of malignant skin tumors seen in the geriatric nursing home population

	Description	Treatment
Basal cell carcinoma	Lesion on sun-exposed areas of fair-skinned individuals. Slow-growing, superficial, reddened or pearly with irregular border. Metastases are rare.	Superficial lesions: topical 5-fluorousracil. Small tumors: curettage and cauterization cryotherapy. Larger tumors: excision with closure or split-thickness skin graft; radiotherapy.
Squamous cell carcinoma	A rise in sun-damaged skin in fair-skinned people. Commonly a shallow ulcer surrounded by a wide, elevated, indurated border. Ulcer may be covered by crust, which conceals the red base. May present as a persistent nonhealing ulcer. Lesions on lips or genitals are likely to metastasize.	Well differentiated: surgical treatment. Poorly differentiated: radiotherapy. Cryotherapy used for multiple lesions.
Malignant melanoma	Pigmented macular lesion with irregular border on sun-exposed areas.	Wide local excision. Close follow-up for irregular pigmentation, nodularity, or bleeding.
Superficial spreading melanoma	Accounts for about 60% of all melanomas. Can occur on any part of the body. Irregular border with pigmentation.	Wide local excision. Close follow-up for irregular pigmentation, nodularity, or bleeding.
Kaposi's sarcoma	An indolent tumor in elderly men of central European origin. One or more purple or dark blue macules on legs; these slowly enlarge to nodules and ulcers.	Simple excision or radiotherapy.

along the basement membrane of the skin. Sometimes the mucosa is also involved. Clinically, bullous pemphigoid presents as intact tense blisters that occur on normal or erythematous skin. Crusting occurs after the bullae rupture. This disorder is usually well controlled by systemic corticosteroid therapy. Other immunosuppressive drugs such as azathioprine and methotrexate are also used in some cases. Some reports have linked bullous pemphigoid with malignant neoplasms, but there is no evidence that individuals with bullous pemphigoid have a higher rate of cancer than the general elderly population. Other bullous diseases may present similarly. Skin biopsies with immunoflurescent studies are usually diagnostic—when they are not, serum antibody tests to pemphigoid/pemphigus are often helpful, although only certain laboratories perform them.

Skin Tumors

Skin malignancies are strongly related to aging and are therefore common in the NH population. Virtually all skin cancers can be recognized early. Most can be cured with appropriate medical or surgical therapy. **Table 14-10** describes several malignant skin tumors. It is important for primary care physicians to recognize these lesions and refer residents for dermatologic evaluation when a malignant lesion is suspected. In addition to malignant skin tumors, benign and premalignant lesions are also commonly seen in the geriatric population. The most common benign lesions are seborrheic keratoses. These are brown, sharply demarcated, slightly raised lesions that are found in areas where sebaceous glands are plentiful, such as the trunk, face, and extremities. They do not need treatment unless they become irritated and are bothersome. The rapid appearance or increase in size of seborrheic keratoses in a previously blemish-free area (sign of Leser-Trelat) is associated with internal malignancy. Actinic keratoses are well demarcated, scaly, rough papules on sun exposed areas. These are premalignant lesions and can be managed by a number of different techniques e.g., cryotherapy, curettage, topical 5-fluorouracil (5FU), or excisional surgery. Bowen's disease is a form of squamous cell carcinoma in situ. Lesions are often multiple and appear as slowly enlarging erythematous patches with sharp but irregular borders and crusting. These lesions are treated in a manner similar to squamous cell carcinoma (see Table 14-10).

SUGGESTED READINGS

Allman, RM, Goode, PS, Patrick MM, et al. Pressure ulcer risk factors among hospitalized patients with activity limitation. *JAMA* 273:865–870, 1995.

Allman RM: Pressure ulcers among the elderly. *N Engl J Med* 320:850, 1989.

Allman RM, Laparda CA, Noel LB, et al: Pressure sores among the elderly. *Ann Intern Med* 105:377, 1986.

Balin AK: Aging of the human skin, in Hazzard WR, Andres R, Bierman EL, Blass JP (eds): *Principles of Geriatric Medicine and Gerontology.* New York, McGraw-Hill, 1990, pp 383–412.

Bergstrom, N, Braden, B: A prospective study of pressure sore risk among institutionalized elderly. *J Am Geriatr Soc* 40:747–758, 1992.

Bergstrom N, Braden B, Kemp M, Champagne M, Ruby E: Multi-site study of incidence of pressure ulcers and the relationship between risk level, demographic characteristics, diagnoses, and prescription to preventive interventions. *J Am Geriatr Soc* 44:22–30, 1996.

Brandeis, GH, Ooi, WL, Hossain, M, et al. A longitudinal study of risk factors associated with the formation of pressure ulcers in nursing homes. *J Am Geriatr Soc* 42:388–393, 1994.

Ferrell BA, Osterweil D: Pressure sores and nutrition, in Morley J, Glick Z, Rubenstein LZ (eds): *Geriatric Nutrition.* New York, Raven Press, 1990, pp 363–379.

Ferrell, BA, Keeler, E., Siu, AL, et al. Cost-effectiveness of low-air-loss beds for treatment of pressure ulcers. *J Gerontol* 50A:M141–M146, 1995.

Ferrell, BA, Artinian, BM, Sessing, D. The Sessing Scale for assessment of pressure ulcer healing. *J Am Geriatr Soc* 43:37–40, 1995.

Phillips TJ, Gilchrest BA: Skin changes and disorders, in Abrams WB, Berkow R (eds): *The Merck Manual of Geriatrics*. Rahway, New Jersey, Merck Sharp & Dohme Research Laboratories, 1990, pp 1025–1053.

Reuler JB, Cooney TG: The pressure sore: Pathophysiology and principles of management. *Ann Intern Med* 94:661, 1981.

Robson MC, Phillips LG, Lawrence WT, et al: The saftey and effect of topically applied recombinant basic fibroblast growth factor on the healing of chronic pressure sores. *Ann Surg* 216:401–406, 1992.

Stefanowska A, Vodovenek L, Benko M, Tark R: Treatment of chronic wounds by means of electric and electromagnetic field. *Medical & Prological Engineering & Computing* 31:213–220, 1993.

U.S. Dept. of Health & Human Services, PHS, AHCPR. *Pressure ulcers in adults: prediction and prevention*. Clinical Practice Guideline, No. 3, May, 1992.

Wood JM, Evans PE, III, Schallreutes KA, Jacobson WE, et al: A multicenter study on the use of pulsed low-intensity direct current for healing chronic stage II and stage III decubitus ulcers. *Arch Dermatol* 129:999–1009, 1992.

Xakellis, GC, Frantz, RA, Arteaga, M, et al. A comparison of patient risk for pressure ulcer development with nursing use of preventive interventions. *J Am Geriatr Soc* 40:1250–1254, 1992.

Xakellis, GC, Frantz, RA. The cost-effectiveness of interventions for preventing pressure ulcers. *J Am Board Fam Pract* 9:79–86, 1996.

CHAPTER
FIFTEEN

INCONTINENCE

PREVALENCE AND MORBIDITY

Urinary incontinence (UI) affects approximately half of nursing home (NH) residents. The prevalence varies among individual facilities depending upon case mix; rates may be as low as 40 percent to as high as 70 percent, or even higher in facilities with a very functionally impaired resident population. In contrast to UI among ambulatory community-dwelling geriatric patients, UI among NH residents is more severe and more commonly associated with stool incontinence. Incontinent NH residents generally have multiple episodes of UI throughout the day and night, and approximately half also have stool incontinence more than once per week.

UI in the NH is associated with substantial morbidity and cost. Although data demonstrating a cause-and-effect relationship are lacking, UI has been shown to be associated with several physical conditions including skin irritations, urinary tract infections (UTI), and falls. For those afflicted, UI is uncomfortable; it can lead to skin irritation and make pressure ulcers difficult to heal, it can result in UTI when urinary retention with overflow UI remains undiagnosed or when UI is inappropriately managed by a chronic indwelling catheter, and it may lead to falls among residents with urge UI and impaired balance or gait. The adverse psychological effects of UI have been difficult to document systematically, but incontinent residents who are not severely demented are often embarrassed and frustrated by their condition. The NH staff generally consider UI to be one of the most onerous and difficult conditions for which they care and perceive that they spend a disproportionate amount of time on incontinent residents.

The economic costs of UI in the NH are less difficult to document. Conservative estimates of the costs of managing UI are approximately $3 billion annually, including staff time, laundry, and supplies.

Although it is unrealistic to expect to cure UI or dramatically reduce the costs of its management in the NH, it is realistic and, in fact, appropriate to attempt to diagnose and treat potentially reversible factors which may cause or contribute to UI, to identify selected residents who may benefit from specific therapeutic approaches, to implement reasonable policies and procedures for bladder and bowel management programs and catheter care, and to utilize containment devices such as padding and incontinence undergarments in a cost-effective manner.

BASIC PRINCIPLES OF MANAGING INCONTINENCE IN THE NURSING HOME

As is emphasized throughout this text, NH residents are heterogeneous. A realistic and appropriate goal for one type of resident may be totally unrealistic and inappropriate for another. The approach to UI brings this concept into sharp focus. A resident undergoing active rehabilitation after a hip fracture or a stroke may, after a thorough incontinence assessment, benefit from a specific bladder retraining protocol and/or pharmacologic therapy for detrusor hyperactivity. Incontinence undergarments and indwelling catheters are unlikely to be appropriate for this type of resident. On the other hand, a resident with end-stage dementia and severe agitation may be most appropriately managed by a containment device.

Thus, an extremely important aspect of incontinence care is to determine if a particular resident has the potential to respond to specific interventions for UI. Because even severely impaired residents may respond very well to a prompted voiding program (see the discussion under "Assessment" and "Behavioral Interventions," below), a bias in favor of assessment and a therapeutic trial is appropriate.

Several other basic principles of incontinence management for the NH are outlined in **Table 15-1**. Each of these principles will be discussed in more detail in subsequent sections of this chapter. First, however, a brief review of the basic types and causes of UI will be presented in order to put the specific recommendations into context.

BASIC TYPES AND CAUSES OF URINARY INCONTINENCE

The pathogenesis of UI among NH residents is often multifactorial, involving urological/gynecological conditions, neurological disorders, behavioral and environmental factors, and functional impairments. Thus, the approach to

Table 15-1 Basic principles of managing incontinence in the nursing home

1. Identify a physician and nurse who will oversee an incontinence management program.
2. Develop written policies and procedures where applicable.
3. Provide in-service education on incontinence to medical and nursing staffs.
4. Assess the continence status of all new residents at admission and at least quarterly thereafter as required in the Minimum Data Set (**Fig. 15-1**).
   (a) A legible bladder record should be used (**Fig. 15-2**).
5. Make an interdisciplinary decision about the resident's potential.
   (a) Do not automatically attribute incontinence to functional disability and manage palliatively.
   (b) Develop realistic goals: eg. reduction of frequency of UI (vs cure); elimination of daytime UI with palliative management at night.
6. Perform a basic diagnostic evaluation focusing on the identification of reversible factors (**Table 15-2**).
7. Use specific criteria to refer selected residents for further evaluation (**Table 15-6**).
8. Develop standardized bladder retraining and prompted voiding protocols (**Tables 15-8, 15-9**).
9. Systematically monitor the response to specific therapeutic interventions using a bladder record (**Fig. 15-2**) and modify the approach if necessary.
10. Do not overuse padding, undergarments and indwelling catheters.
    (a) Specific indications for indwelling catheters should be documented (**Table 15-10**).
    (b) Implement a catheter care protocol for residents who are managed by chronic indwelling catheterization (**Table 15-11**).

assessment and treatment must be comprehensive and should include all of these potential factors.

The most important factors to consider are those that are potentially reversible. While identification and management of these reversible factors may not cure the UI, it may reduce its frequency and make the UI more manageable by other interventions (e.g., prompted voiding). Reversible factors are more commonly found among residents with recent-onset incontinence, which may be the situation for many newly admitted NH residents. It is essential to recognize, however, that reversible factors may also be contributing to persistent forms of UI that have been present for months or even years. As outlined in **Table 15-2**, reversible factors can be remembered by using the acronym "DRIP".

Table 15-3 illustrates a basic classification of the types of persistent UI. Three important features of this classification should be noted. First, from a neurourological perspective, this classification is greatly simplified and does not include all the pathophysiological types of UI. Nonetheless, it is helpful in attempting to develop a basic approach to the assessment and treatment of UI in the geriatric population. Second, many incontinent NH residents have mixtures of these types of UI. The predominant abnormality of lower urinary tract functioning found among NH residents is detrusor hyperactivity (involuntary bladder contractions found on cystometry; also termed detrusor instability,

Table 15-2 Reversible factors that may contribute to urinary incontinence "DRIP"

D	Delirium	New onset UI may be associated with delirium due to acute underlying conditions requiring diagnosis and treatment
R	Restricted Mobility	Acute conditions causing immobility may precipitate UI; environmental manipulation and scheduled toileting are appropriate while rehabilitative efforts are undertaken
	Retention	Urinary retention may be precipitated by many drugs (see below), may occur acutely due to anatomic obstruction; immobility and large fecal impactions may also contribute
I	Infection	Acute cystitis may precipitate urge UI Asymptomatic bacteriuria, with or without pyuria, should not be treated in the absence of symptoms of acute urinary tract infection
	Inflammation	Atrophic vaginitis and urethritis can cause irritative voiding symptoms including UI
	Impaction	Fecal impaction may be associated with UI (as well as fecal incontinence)
P	Polyuria	Poorly controlled diabetes with glucosuria can contribute to urinary frequency and UI Excess intake of caffeinated beverages may exacerbate symptoms Edema due to congestive heart failure and/or venous insufficiency can cause nocturia and exacerbate nocturnal UI
	Pharmaceuticals	Rapid acting diuretics (urge UI) Psychotropics (sedation, immobility) Anticholinergics, alpha agonists, calcium channel blockers, narcotics (urinary retention) Alpha antagonists (stress UI) Alcohol (sedation, immobility, polyuria)

unstable bladder, and detrusor hyperreflexia—the latter in the presence of a neurological disorder). Although most often associated with urge-type UI, detrusor hyperactivity is commonly seen in conjunction with sphincter weakness and stress UI among women, obstruction in men with benign or malignant prostatic enlargement, and with impaired bladder contractility resulting in incomplete bladder emptying (termed detrusor hyperactivity with impaired contractility, or DHIC). Thus, depending on the type of therapeutic approach being considered, it may be important to identify these mixed types of UI (see "Assessment," below). Third, and most important, functional-type UI should be a diagnosis of exclusion, because most NH residents have impairments of cognitive and/or physical functioning that may interfere with toileting skills. These residents may also have other potentially treatable conditions contributing to their UI. Thus, a search for reversible factors and other types of UI should be completed before labeling a NH resident's UI as functional.

Table 15-3 Basic types and causes of urinary incontinence

Type	Symptoms	Common causes
Stress	Involuntary loss of urine (usually small amounts) with increases in intra-abdominal pressure (e.g., cough, laugh, or exercise)	Weakness and laxity of pelvic floor musculature Bladder outlet or urethral sphincter weakness
Urge	Leakage of urine (usually larger volumes) because of inability to delay voiding after sensation of bladder fullness is perceived	Detrusor hyperactivity isolated or associated with one or more of the following: Local genitourinary condition such as cystitis, urethritis, tumors, stones, outflow obstruction, impaired bladder contractility Central nervous system disorders such as stroke, dementia, parkinsonism, spinal cord injury or disease
Overflow	Leakage of urine (usually small amounts) resulting from mechanical forces on an over-distended bladder or from other effects of urinary retention on bladder and sphincter function	Anatomic obstruction by prostate, prolapsed cystocele Acontractile bladder associated with diabetes mellitus or spinal cord injury Neurogenic (detrusor–sphincter dyssynergy) associated with multiple sclerosis and other suprasacral spinal cord lesions
Functional[a]	Urinary leakage associated with inability to toilet because of impairment of cognitive and/or physical functioning, psychological unwillingness, or environmental barriers	Severe dementia Immobility Physical restraints Inaccessible toilets Unavailability of regular toileting assistance Depression

[a]Functional incontinence should be a diagnosis of exclusion. Potentially reversible factors should be identified and managed, and appropriate residents should undergo further assessment (see text).

ASSESSMENT

An assessment of bladder and bowel function is a requirement for all newly admitted NH residents, and this assessment must be updated quarterly using the Minimum Data Set (**Fig. 15-1**). A bladder and bowel record such as the one depicted in **Fig. 15-2** is helpful in documenting the continence status of new residents and can also be used as a component of periodic reassessments. A

SECTION H. CONTINENCE IN LAST 14 DAYS

1.	CONTINENCE SELF-CONTROL CATEGORIES (***Code for resident's PERFORMANCE OVER ALL SHIFTS***) 0. *CONTINENT*—Complete control *[includes use of indwelling urinary catheter or ostomy device that does not leak urine or stool]* 1. *USUALLY CONTINENT*—BLADDER, incontinent episodes once a week or less; BOWEL, less than weekly 2. *OCCASIONALLY INCONTINENT*—BLADDER, 2 or more times a week but not daily; BOWEL, once a week 3. *FREQUENTLY INCONTINENT*—BLADDER, tended to be incontinent daily, but some control present (e.g., on day shift); BOWEL, 2-3 times a week 4. *INCONTINENT*—Had inadequate control BLADDER, multiple daily episodes; BOWEL, all (or almost all) of the time				
a.	**BOWEL CONTI-NENCE**	Control of bowel movement, with appliance or bowel continence programs, if employed			
b.	**BLADDER CONTI-NENCE**	Control of urinary bladder function (if dribbles, volume insufficient to soak through underpants), with appliances (e.g., foley) or continence programs, if employed			
2.	**BOWEL ELIMINATION PATTERN**	Bowel elimination pattern regular—at least one movement every three days	a.	Diarrhea	c.
				Fecal impaction	d.
		Constipation	b.	*NONE OF ABOVE*	e.
3.	**APPLIANCES AND PROGRAMS**	Any scheduled toileting plan	a.	Did not use toilet room/ commode/urinal	f.
		Bladder retraining program	b.	Pads/briefs used	g.
		External (condom) catheter	c.	Enemas/irrigation	h.
		Indwelling catheter	d.	Ostomy present	i.
		Intermittent catheter	e.	*NONE OF ABOVE*	j.
4.	**CHANGE IN URINARY CONTI-NENCE**	Resident's urinary continence has changed as compared to status of **90 days ago** (or since last assessment if less than 90 days) 0. No change 1. Improved 2. Deteriorated			

Figure 15-1 Minimum Data Set (MDS) assessment of continence status.

3- to 5-day monitoring period is enough to document the timing, amount, and situations associated with any incontinence. The specific symbols used are not important, but there should be a simple way of documenting wetness, dryness, appropriate toileting, bowel status, and comments. Records such as the one shown in **Fig. 15-2** can be reduced photographically so that several records can fit on one page. This type of record is also helpful in monitoring responses to therapeutic interventions.

Because many newly admitted residents come from acute-care hospitals, they frequently arrive at the NH with an indwelling bladder catheter. In this situation it is essential to determine why the catheter was placed (i.e., to monitor urinary output versus urinary retention versus management of UI) and to consider the resident for a bladder retraining program, as described under "Behavioral Interventions," below. The catheter should be removed unless there is an appropriate indication for keeping it in place (see "Catheters and Catheter Care," below).

After this initial assessment and documentation, an interdisciplinary decision should be made about whether the resident should undergo further assessment or

INCONTINENCE MONITORING RECORD

INSTRUCTIONS: EACH TIME THE PATIENT IS CHECKED:
1) Mark *one* of the circles in the BLADDER section at the hour closest to the time the patient is checked.
2) Make an X in the BOWEL section if the patient has had an incontinent or normal bowel movement.

● = Incontinent, small amount | Ø = Dry | X = Incontinent BOWEL
● = Incontinent, large amount | △ = Voided correctly | X = Normal BOWEL

PATIENT NAME ______________ ROOM # ________ DATE ________

	BLADDER			BOWEL			
	INCONTINENT OF URINE	DRY	VOIDED CORRECTLY	INCONTINENT X	NORMAL X	INITIALS	COMMENTS
12 am	● ●	○	△ cc ___				
1	● ●	○	△ cc ___				
2	● ●	○	△ cc ___				
3	● ●	○	△ cc ___				
4	● ●	○	△ cc ___				
5	● ●	○	△ cc ___				
6	● ●	○	△ cc ___				
7	● ●	○	△ cc ___				
8	● ●	○	△ cc ___				
9	● ●	○	△ cc ___				
10	● ●	○	△ cc ___				
11	● ●	○	△ cc ___				
12 pm	● ●	○	△ cc ___				
1	● ●	○	△ cc ___				
2	● ●	○	△ cc ___				
3	● ●	○	△ cc ___				
4	● ●	○	△ cc ___				
5	● ●	○	△ cc ___				
6	● ●	○	△ cc ___				
7	● ●	○	△ cc ___				
8	● ●	○	△ cc ___				
9	● ●	○	△ cc ___				
10	● ●	○	△ cc ___				
11	● ●	○	△ cc ___				
TOTALS:							

Figure 15-2 Example of a NH bladder and bowel record for assessing and following response to therapy. (Copyright, Regents of University of California, 1984; reprinted with permission.)

be managed palliatively with containment devices. Even if the decision is made to manage the UI palliatively, an assessment for the potentially reversible factors listed in **Table 15-2** should be undertaken, because identification and management of these conditions may have quality of life benefits beyond those related specifically to UI. It is also important to reemphasize in this regard that UI should not automatically be attributed to functional disability for at least two reasons: (1) although functional disability may be contributing to the UI, specifically treatable conditions can also be detected; and (2) many very functionally impaired NH residents respond well to a simple prompted voiding program. Specific predictors of responsiveness to prompted voiding are outlined later in this chapter.

Table 15-4 presents the basic approach to urinary incontinence and indwelling catheters recommended in the resident assessment protocol (RAP). While the approach we recommend is consistent with the RAP, we do not agree

Table 15-4 Basic approach to urinary incontinence and indwelling catheters recommended in the the resident assessment protocol (RAP)[a]

1. Identify reversible problems
   (a) Many potentially reversible causes and contributing factors can be identified by the MDS, e.g.:
   Symptomatic UTI, fecal impaction, delirium, lack of toilet access, immobility, depression, congestive heart failure, edema, recent stroke, diabetes, medications
2. Search for other potential causes or contributing factors
   (a) If the resident has no memory recall, requires extensive assistance in self-transfer and is free of pain, identifying these factors may not be beneficial
   (b) Factors include:
      (1) Pain
      (2) Excessive or inadequate urine output
      (3) Atrophic vaginitis
      (4) Abnormal lab values (blood calcium, glucose, urea nitrogen, creatinine, vitamin B_{12})
   (c) Serious conditions that cause or accompany incontinence, e.g.:
   Bladder cancer or stones, prostate cancer, spinal cord or brain lesions, poor bladder compliance, and tabes dorsales
3. Final evaluation if incontinence persists
   (a) If a resident has no memory recall, is extensively dependent in self-transfer, and the facility's ability to toilet the resident on a regular schedule is limited, then the resident may not benefit from this part of the evaluation
   (b) Recommended procedures
      (1) Post-void residual determination (PVR)
      (2) Kidney ultrasound for men with PVR >100 ml
      (3) Bladder stress tests for women
4. Final evaluation for residents with indwelling catheters
   (a) Unless the resident meets exclusionary criteria, a voiding trial can be attempted (see **Tables 15-8 and 15-10**)

[a]The authors do not agree with all of the specific recommendations in the RAPs (see text).

Identified As Incontinent on MDS Assessment

BASIC ASSESSMENT

History
Medical record review
Physical exam

Potentially reversible conditions identified? **(Table 15 -2)**

Yes → Manage → Still incontinent? → Yes

No ↓

Unable to state or recognize name; irreversible immobility requiring 2-person transfer; or severe pain with repeated transfer

Yes → Manage supportively with check and change program

No ↓

3-DAY TRIAL OF PROMPTED VOIDING

- mobility and behavioral assessments
- monitor wet and toileting rates
- bladder stress tests
- urine specimen collection
- post-void residual determination

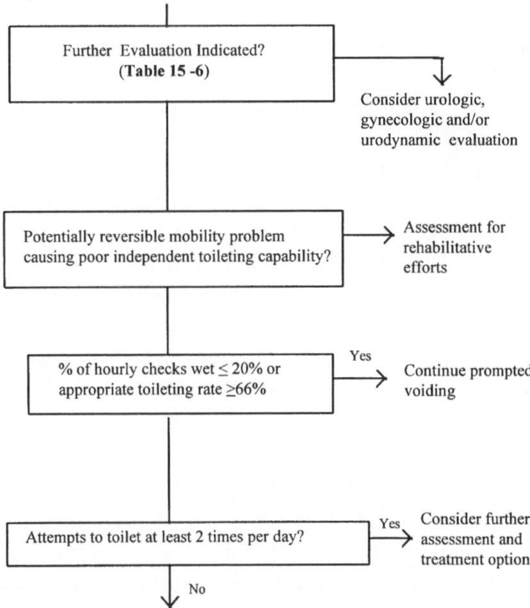
Further Evaluation Indicated?
(Table 15 -6)
Consider urologic, gynecologic and/or urodynamic evaluation
Potentially reversible mobility problem causing poor independent toileting capability?
Assessment for rehabilitative efforts
% of hourly checks wet ≤ 20% or appropriate toileting rate ≥66%
Yes
Continue prompted voiding
Attempts to toilet at least 2 times per day?
Yes
Consider further assessment and treatment options
No
Check and change program

Figure 15-3 General strategy for diagnostic assessment and management of incontinence among NH residents.

with some of the specific recommendations. For example, we believe that some of the laboratory tests recommended in the RAP (blood calcium, urea nitrogen, creatinine, and vitamin B_{12}) should only be done in carefully selected residents in the evaluation of incontinence, and that a kidney ultrasound is not necessary in all men with a post-void residual greater than 100 ml. In addition we believe that a bladder stress test is technically difficult to perform in many residents, and that the results are not helpful in identifying those who respond well to prompted voiding—which we believe should be the initial therapeutic approach for the vast majority of residents.

Figure 15-3 illustrates our recommended approach to assessment and management. **Table 15-5** outlines key aspects of the clinical assessment. The objectives of this assessment include the following:

1. Identification of potentially reversible factors (**Table 15-2**).
2. Identification of conditions that may require further urological, gynecological, and/or urodynamic evaluation (see below and **Table 15-6**).
3. Identification of residents who may benefit from rehabilitative efforts targeted at enhancing independence in toileting skills.
4. Determining responsiveness to prompted voiding and whether the resident should be:
   (a) Continued on a prompted voiding program
   (b) Further assessed for other treatments such as drug or surgical therapy
   (c) Managed supportively with a check and change program.

The history, medical record review and physical examination can identify most of the potentially reversible causes and contributing factors (**Table 15-2**). We recommend that all residents undergo a 3-day trial of prompted voiding unless they are so severely demented that they cannot state or respond to their name, have irreversible immobility which requires a two-person transfer onto a commode, or have a terminal illness or end-stage musculoskeletal disease which makes regular toileting painful.

A 3-day prompted voiding trial facilitates the performance of the bladder stress tests and post-void residual determination (PVR), as well as the collection of a urine specimen. These procedures can be time consuming and the repeated opportunities to toilet during the prompted voiding trial provide an efficient opportunity to accomplish them. We recommend that the PVR be done by portable ultrasound if one is available in the NH. We also recommend that the resident not be catheterized to collect a clean urine specimens unless catheterization is necessary for the PVR. The techniques outlined in **Table 15-5** will yield accurate urine specimens if performed properly.

If the resident meets any of the criteria outlined in **Table 15-6**, then consideration should be given to further evaluation. In addition, if during the prompted voiding trial the resident is noted to have mobility impairment due to deconditioning or a gait/balance disorder, consideration should be given to

Table 15-5 Key aspects of the clinical assessment of incontinence in the nursing home

History

1. Often difficult to obtain from the resident
2. Important symptoms
   - (a) Irritative (suggestive of urge UI and detrusor hyperactivity): frequency, urgency, nocturia, bed-wetting, leakage without warning
   - (b) Voiding difficulty (suggestive of obstruction and/or bladder contractility problem): hesitancy, poor or intermittent stream, straining to finish voiding.
   - (c) Stress incontinence: leaks with straining, coughing, changing position, or leaks continuously
3. Nursing observations can be helpful in detecting signs of urgency, stress incontinence, or voiding difficulty

Physical examination

1. Functional status (can be assessed during trial of prompted voiding—see **Table 15-9**)
   - (a) Ability to locate toilet and initiate voiding appropriately
   - (b) Ability to respond appropriately to a prompt to void
   - (c) Ability to use a toilet or toilet substitute, manage cleaning and clothing
2. Lumbosacral innervation
   - (a) Detection of focal finding or neuropathy
3. Abdominal
   - (a) Suprapubic palpation after voiding (may not be sensitive in detecting significant urinary retention)
4. Rectal for fecal impaction and prostate exam
5. Pelvic
   - (a) Significant prolapse (see **Fig. 15-4**)
   - (b) Atrophic vaginitis (patchy erythema, telangiectasias, friability, bleeding)

Urinalysis and urine culture

1. Urinalysis can detect glucosuria and sterile hematuria
2. Urine culture should only be done if resident has symptoms of UTI *other than* stable incontinence
3. May be difficult to obtain a clean specimen
   - (a) Urine can be collected during prompted voiding assessment (**see Table 15-9**)
   - (b) For women, clean urethra and perineal area with antiseptic and have them void into a disinfected bed pan to avoid catheterizing
   - (c) For men, clean penis with antiseptic, apply a clean condom catheter, and collect specimen from first void
   - (d) If catheterization is necessary to collect clean urine it should be done in conjunction with post-void residual determination

Post-void residual determination

1. Can be measured during prompted voiding assessment (**Table 15-9**)
2. Can be done by portable ultrasound device if available

Bladder stress test (women)

1. Not helpful in identifying responders to prompted voiding, but important if further treatment is considered
2. May be difficult to perform due to inability of resident to stand and cough forcefully, and difficulty in timing the test when resident has adequate bladder volume
   - (a) Performing this test during the trial of prompted voiding (**Table 15-9**) can facilitate repeated tests before voiding

Table 15-6 Criteria for referral of incontinent nursing home residents for further urological, gynecological, and/or urodynamic evaluation

Criteria	Definition	Rationale
History		
Recent history of lower urinary tract or pelvic surgery or irradiation	Surgery or irradiation involving the pelvic area or lower urinary tract within the past 6 to 12 months	A structural abnormality relating to the recent procedure should be sought
Relapse or rapid recurrence of a symptomatic urinary tract infection	Onset of dysuria, new or worsened irritative voiding symptoms, fever, suprapubic or flank pain associated with significant growth of a urinary pathogen; symptoms and bacteriuria return within 4 weeks of treatment	A structural abnormality or pathologic condition in the urinary tract predisposing to infection should be excluded
Physical examination		
Marked pelvic prolapse in a woman who would consider a pessary or surgery (see **Fig. 15-4**)	Pronounced uterine descensus to or through the introitus or a prominent cystocele that descends the entire height of the vaginal vault with coughing during speculum examination	Anatomic abnormality may underlie the pathophysiology of the incontinence and may require surgical repair
Marked prostatic enlargement and/or suspicion of cancer in a man who is candidate	Gross enlargement of the prostate on digital exam; prominent induration or asymmetry of the lobes	An evaluation to exclude prostate cancer that requires curative or palliative therapy should be undertaken
Post void residual		
Post void residual volume >200 ml	Volume of urine remaining in the bladder within 5 to 10 minutes after the patient voids spontaneously in as normal a fashion as possible	Anatomic or neurogenic obstruction or poor bladder contractility may be present and resident may be at risk for complications
Urinalysis		
Hematuria (sterile) in a resident who is a candidate for evaluation and treatment	Greater than five red blood cells per high power field on repeated microscopic exams in the absence of infection	A pathologic condition in the urinary tract should be excluded
Uncertain diagnosis	After the assessment and prompted voiding trial, the resident remains frequently wet despite attempting to toilet at least twice per day, and the type of incontinence is uncertain based on symptoms, stress tests and PVR determination	A urodynamic evaluation may help better define and reproduce the symptoms associated with the incontinence and target specific treatment approaches

referring then for a physical therapy evaluation. Our experience in over 25 NHs suggests that 25–40 percent of residents respond well to daytime prompted voiding and reduce their wetness frequency to once per day or less. If the resident repeatedly attempts to toilet but remains wet, they should be considered for further evaluation and other treatments. On the other hand, if they attempt to toilet infrequently, then additional treatment is probably not warranted and the most appropriate management is a regular checking and changing program.

APPROACHES TO THERAPY

Reversible Factors

The first step in treating incontinence is to manage the potentially reversible causes and contributing factors (**Table 15-2**). While an acute urinary tract infection may precipitate or exacerbate UI, several studies suggest that treating asymptomatic bacteriuria (with or without pyuria) in NH residents has no effect on morbidity, mortality or the severity of the UI. Thus, a urine culture should only be ordered if the resident has symptoms of a urinary tract infection other than chronic stable UI (e.g., new onset or recent worsening of UI, dysuria, unexplained fever, or recent unexplained change in mental or functional status).

Atrophic vaginitis should be treated by either vaginal estrogen cream (1–2 g to be applied 3 to 5 nights per week) or oral conjugated estrogen at a dose of 0.3–0.625 mg/day. There is no standard treatment protocol, but we recommend a 1- to 2-month trial. The goal is not necessarily to cure the UI but to reduce its frequency and possibly make the resident more responsive to other forms of treatment. If there is a clear response, estrogen therapy can either be continued or alternatively withdrawn and reinstituted if symptoms and signs recur. Estrogen is contraindicated in women with a history of breast cancer, and women given estrogen for long periods of time should have mammography if they have not already had routine mammography in the past year.

Fecal impaction is a common and often a recurrent problem which can cause or contribute to both UI and fecal incontinence. The management of constipation is discussed in Chapter 22.

Factors contributing to polyuria and/or nocturia should be addressed. Although it may be difficult to control diabetes tightly in some NH residents (see Chapter 18), the osmotic diuresis induced by glucosuria can certainly exacerbate UI and an attempt should be made at achieving better glucose control. Edema due to congestive heart failure and/or venous insufficiency may be mobilized in the evening and night hours and cause bothersome nocturia. This may even be hazardous in some residents who are prone to falls. It is therefore reasonable, in some situations, to initially manage the UI by adding (or increasing the dose of) a rapid-acting diuretic in the morning to reduce the edema and to make the resident urinate more often when there is better access to a commode.

Mobility impairment is common among incontinent NH residents. The potential reversibility of some of these impairments can be assessed during the 3–day trial of prompted voiding. If, for example, the resident is noted to be weak or deconditioned, or to have a new or worsening gait or balance disorder, consideration should be given to a physical therapy assessment.

Drugs which may be contributing to the UI should be removed whenever possible, especially if urinary retention is present. If it is not possible to discontinue them, reducing the dose may help manage the UI. The latter is most relevant to furosemide and other rapid acting diuretics.

Behavioral Interventions

Most NHs have “bladder training” protocols which consist of simple scheduled toileting on an every-2-hour basis. While this is practical for staff and may help some residents, it is probably not the most efficient procedure and should be combined with other techniques whenever feasible.

Behavioral interventions can be divided into two basic types, “patient-dependent” and “caregiver-dependent” (**Table 15-7**). Patient-dependent procedures such as bladder retraining require highly functional and motivated individuals and are most relevant for residents with recent-onset UI, especially those who are admitted to the NH with an indwelling catheter. An example of a bladder retraining protocol is depicted in **Table 15-8**. The precise protocol will depend on the resident’s bladder function. If the catheter was placed to measure urine output or to manage UI during a hospitalization, the bladder is likely to be irritable and of small capacity; in this instance an attempt can be made to progressively increase the intervoiding interval. In highly functional residents, pelvic muscle exercises and other behavioral techniques may be helpful during this period of bladder retraining. If the catheter was placed for urinary retention, the bladder muscle may be decompensated; in this situation regular attempts to void should be combined with routine post-void or intermittent catheterizations. It may take weeks for the bladder to begin refunctioning. If post-void residuals remain elevated and the resident remains incontinent, a urological and urodynamic evaluation should be considered. Note that in either situation clamping the catheter before removal is not necessary; it has never been shown to be beneficial and may be harmful to residents who already have a decompensated bladder after urinary retention. Other patient-dependent procedures, such as pelvic muscle exercises and biofeedback for stress incontinence, are relevant only to a small number of NH residents. Electrical stimulation, which can be used as an adjunct to these techniques, appears promising, but it has not been adequately tested in the NH population.

Although all the caregiver-dependent techniques have been shown to be effective, we recommend prompted voiding because it is the most practical, efficient, and well-studied technique. An example of a prompted voiding protocol is depicted in **Table 15-9**. As opposed to bladder retraining (**Table 15-8**), the goal

Table 15-7 Examples of behavioral interventions for urinary incontinence

Procedure	Definition	Types of Incontinence	Comments
Patient-dependent			
Pelvic muscle (Kegel) exercises	Repetitive contraction of pelvic muscles	Stress and urge	Requires adequate functioning and motivation Biofeedback may be useful in teaching the exercises
Biofeedback	Use of bladder, rectal, or vaginal pressure recordings to train resident to contract pelvic floor muscles and relax bladder	Stress and urge	Requires equipment and trained personnel Relatively invasive Requires adequate cognitive and physical function and motivation
Bladder training	Use of pelvic muscle exercises with or without biofeedback and other strategies to manage urgency	Urge	Requires trained therapist, adequate cognitive and physical functioning, and motivation
Bladder retraining (**See Table 15-8**)	Progressive lengthening or shortening of intervoiding interval, with adjunctive techniques[a] such as intermittent catheterization used in residents recovering from bladder overdistension with persistent retention	Acute (e.g., postcatheterization with urge or overflow, poststroke)	Goal is to restore normal pattern of voiding and continence Requires adequate cognitive and physical function and motivation
Caregiver-dependent			
Prompted voiding (**See Table 15-9**)	Regular (every 2 h during the day 7 a.m.–7 p.m.) prompts to void with positive reinforcement	Urge, stress and functional	Goal is to prevent wetting episodes Can be used in residents with impaired cognitive or physical functioning Requires staff/caregiver availability and motivation
Habit training	Variable toileting schedule based on pattern with of voiding with positive reinforcement	As above	As above
Scheduling toileting	Fixed toileting schedule	As above	As above

[a]Techniques to trigger voiding (running water, stroking thigh, suprapubic tapping), empty bladder completely (bending forward, suprapubic pressure), and alteration of fluid or diuretic intake patterns.

Table 15-8 Bladder retraining protocol for use after the removal of on indwelling catheter[a]

Goal: To restore a normal pattern of voiding and continence after the removal of an indwelling catheter

1. Monitor the resident's urine output every 8 hours for 1 or 2 days
2. Remove the indwelling catheter (clamping the catheter before removal is not necessary)[a,b]
3. Initiate a toileting schedule
   (a) Begin by taking the resident to the toileting:
      (1) Every 2 hours during the day and evening
      (2) Before getting into bed
      (3) Every 4 hours at night
   (b) Instruct the resident on techniques to trigger voiding (e.g., running water, stroking inner thigh, suprapubic tapping) and to help completely empty bladder (e.g., bending forward, suprapubic pressure, double voiding)
4. If the resident is unable to void by the time the expected bladder volume is 800 ml (on the basis of monitoring in Step (1), or if the post-void residual is >400 ml, reinsert the catheter and consider a urodynamic evaluation or the use of a permanent catheter
5. If the post-void residuals are 100–400 ml, continue to monitor until they are consistently less than 200 ml[c]
6. Monitor the resident's voiding and continence pattern with a systemic record (see **Fig. 15-2**) that allows the recording of:
   (a) Frequency, timing, and amount of incontinence episodes
   (b) Fluid intake pattern
   (c) Post-void or intermittent catheter volume
7. If the resident is voiding frequently (that is, more often than every 2 hours), encourage the resident to delay voiding as long as possible and instruct him/her (if possible) to use pelvic muscle exercises and techniques to help empty bladder completely, and consider the use of biofeedback if available
8. If the resident continues to have incontinence:
   (a) Rule out reversible causes (**Table 15-2**)
   (b) Consider urodynamic evaluation to determine cause and appropriate treatment

[a] Indwelling catheters should be removed from all residents who do not have an indication for their short- or long-term use. For those who have had significant retention (>400 ml), the catheter should be kept in for several days to decompress the bladder.

[b] Clamping routines have never been shown to be helpful and are not appropriate for residents who have had overdistended bladders.

[c] A precise value cannot be recommended on the basis of available data. Residual volumes <200 ml generally do not cause upper urinary tract complications.

is not necessarily to restore a normal pattern of voiding and continence; it is, rather, to prevent wetness. When motivated staff implement it properly, prompted voiding has been shown to be highly effective in reducing incontinence frequency during the day and evening hours. Because it appears to be effective in NH residents with different types of lower urinary tract dysfunction and is virtually free of side effects, it is a reasonable initial approach to managing most incontinent NH residents (**Fig. 15-3**). Note that the best results from prompted

Table 15-9 Prompted voiding protocol

Goal: To reduce the frequency of wetness in selected residents from 7 a.m.–7 p.m.

Assessment period (3 days)

1. Contact the resident every 2 hours from 7 a.m. to 7 p.m.
2. Focus their attention on voiding by asking them whether they are wet or dry.
3. Check them for wetness, record on bladder record, and give feedback on whether they are correct or incorrect.
4. Whether wet or dry, ask the resident if they would like to use the toilet, bedpan, or urinal.
   (a) If they say yes:
      (1) Assist them
      (2) Record the results on the bladder record
      (3) Give them positive reinforcement by spending on extra minute or two talking with them
   (b) If they say no, prompt and encourage them to toilet 2 more times
   (c) If they continue to say no, inform them that you will be back in an hour and request they try to delay voiding until then
5. Offer the resident a drink of fluid before leaving.
6. Every other hour check the resident for wetness (without prompting them) and record results on a bladder record.
   (a) If the resident spontaneously requests toileting assistance, provide it and record the results on the bladder record.
   (b) Offer the resident a drink of fluid before leaving.
7. During the 3-day assessment period:
   (a) Collect a clean urine specimen for urinalysis and culture (if indicated).
   (b) Perform a post-void residual (PVR) determination.
   (c) Perform bladder stress tests in women until either the test is positive, or the test is negative and the resident's total bladder volume (voided volume plus PVR) exceeds 150–200mL.

Targeting

1. Prompted voiding is more effective in some residents then others. Between 25% and 40% of residents respond well.
2. The best candidates for a long-term prompted voiding program are residents who show the following characteristics during the assessment period:
   (a) Have an average of one or less episode of UI per day
   (b) Have an hourly wet check % of ≤20%
   (c) Have an appropriate toileting rate of >66% (calculated by no. of voids into toilet divided by total no. of voids)
3. Residents who do not meet these criteria but who attempt to toilet at least twice per day should be considered for further evaluation and other more specific treatments.
4. Residents who fail to respond and attempt to toilet infrequently should be considered for a supportive check and change program.

Prompted voiding (ongoing protocol)

1. Contact the resident every 2 hours from 7 a.m. to 7 p.m.
2. Use same procedures as for the assessment period (See 1–4 above).
3. For nighttime management, use either a modified prompted voiding schedule or a containment device.
4. A quality assurance nurse should perform random wet checks to ensure that responsive residents are maintaining expected levels of dryness.
5. If a resident who has been responding well has an increase in incontinence frequency despite adequate staff implementation of the protocol, they should be evaluated for reversible factors (**Table 15-2**).

voiding have been documented when the protocol is implemented from 7 a.m. to 7 p.m. It is not clear whether the potential benefits of regular toileting throughout the nighttime hours are outweighed by disruption of the resident's sleep. In addition, staffing patterns at night may preclude an effective prompted voiding program, even in targeted residents. Thus, until further data are available, NHs should modify the protocol for nighttime hours and/or use incontinence undergarments.

Responders to prompted voiding can easily be identified by a 3-day trial of the intervention. Residents who achieve either a 20 percent or lower wet rate (based on hourly checks) or an appropriate toileting rate of at least 66 percent (number of times resident voided into a toilet divided by total number of voids) are the best candidates for long term prompted voiding. Our experience suggests that 25–40 percent of residents respond well. Targeting the prompted voiding to the responders makes the intervention more efficient and cost-effective, and also provides an expected level of dryness which can be used as an outcome measure in a quality assurance program based on principles of continuous quality improvement.

Drug Therapy

Because of the close association between functional disability and UI among NH residents, drug therapy for UI is generally an adjunct to some form of toileting program such as prompted voiding. Unless the resident demonstrates some willingness to attempt to toilet during a prompted voiding trial, we would not recommend a trial of drug therapy.

Drug therapy for UI in the NH is directed at one of two abnormalities of lower urinary tract functioning or a combination of both. Detrusor hyperactivity (involuntary bladder contractions on urodynamic testing) is the most common urodynamic abnormality found in incontinent NH residents and is generally associated with urge-type UI. Drug treatment for detrusor hyperactivity involves an anticholinergic agent. Although several are available, none have been adequately studied in the NH setting. New types of drugs and long-acting preparations (e.g., slow-release capsules, skin patches) are under investigation but are not currently available. Until better data are available, we recommend that detrusor hyperactivity in NH residents with urge-type UI be treated with oxybutynin. The starting dose should be 2.5 mg two or three times per day (and/or at bedtime for nocturnal UI); this can be increased to 5 mg three to four times per day. Two to four weeks is an adequate therapeutic trial. Careful observation for anticholinergic side effects (dry mouth, constipation or fecal impaction, blurry vision, worsening cognitive function, urinary retention) should be undertaken. Men with irritative voiding symptoms including urgency and urge incontinence may benefit from a careful trial of an alpha antagonist such as prazosin, terazosin or doxazosin.

For sphincter weakness with stress-type UI in women, drug treatment involves a combination of estrogen and an alpha agonist. Estrogen can be given in the form of vaginal cream (1–2 g at bedtime) or as an oral tablet (0.3–0.625 mg conjugated estrogen daily). Either pseudoephedrine (30 to 60 mg three times per day) or phenylpropanolamine (75 mg twice daily) can be used as the alpha agonist. Drug treatment for stress UI should be combined with a toileting program (to keep the bladder volume as low as possible) and pelvic muscle exercises (for residents who can cooperate). Women who have prominent pelvic prolapse or who fail a 3– to 6–month trial of drug and/or behavioral therapy should be considered for surgical intervention (see **Table 15-5** and under "Surgery," below).

For women with mixed urge and stress UI, a combination of the above approaches can be used. Imipramine (10–25 mg three times per day) may be used as a combination anticholinergic-alpha agonist. This drug is, however, contraindicated in the presence of cardiac conduction abnormalities and can, in addition to its anticholinergic side effects, cause significant postural hypotension.

Drug treatment for overflow UI is usually not effective on a chronic basis. Cholinergic agonists (e.g., bethanechol) have been used in patients with poor bladder contractility, and alpha antagonists have been used for increased sphincter tone. Neither of these pharmacologic approaches is, however, generally recommended for the chronic therapy of overflow UI in the NH setting.

Surgery

Surgical intervention for UI is a consideration for a small but important subgroup of incontinent NH residents. Since UI is not a life-threatening problem, it must be bothersome enough to the resident to justify the pursuit of elective surgical treatment.

Surgery for UI is basically of two types. Women with stress UI associated with significant pelvic prolapse (**Fig. 15-4**) may benefit from bladder neck suspension and repair of the pelvic prolapse if indicated. In properly selected cases, the short-term (1 to 5 years) success of this type of surgery by an experienced surgeon is high (probably in the range of 75 percent for significant reduction or elimination of wetness). Women with stress incontinence associated with intrinsic urethral sphincter weakness (diagnosed urodynamically) may benefit from periurethral injections of collagen. Thus, NH residents who have bothersome stress UI and who fail to respond adequately to nonsurgical approaches might be referred for further evaluation if an experienced surgeon is available.

The other type of surgical intervention for UI is the removal of anatomic obstruction, most commonly an enlarged prostate in males or a urethral stricture or bladder neck contracture. Incontinent male NH residents who are suspected of having significant obstruction should be referred for a urologic and urodynamic evaluation, because obstruction may be difficult to diagnose in this population.

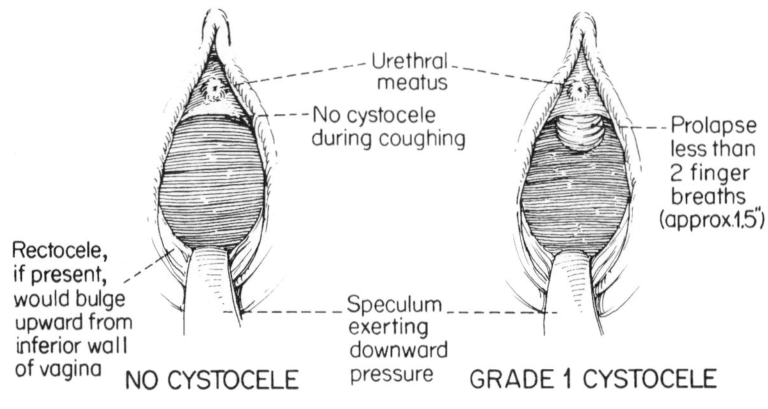

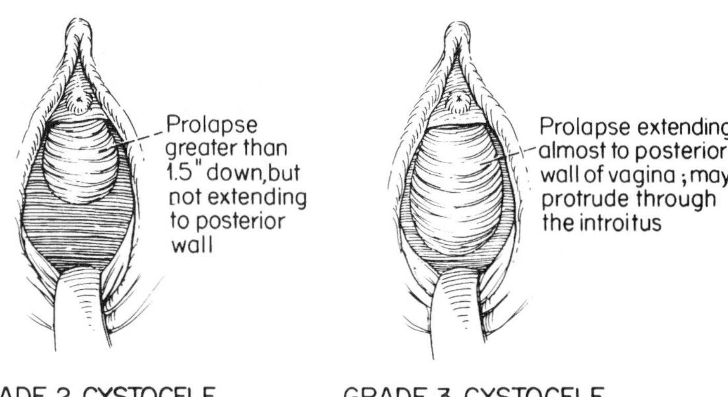

Figure 15-4 Example of a grading system for cystoceles. A grade 3 cystocele would be a criterion for further evaluation. See **Table 15-5**. (Reprinted with permission, *J Am Geriatr Soc* 37:715–724, 1989.)

Pads and Undergarments

Highly absorbent launderable or disposable pads and incontinence undergarments are the most common method of managing UI in the NH. This method of management is certainly appropriate for the subgroup of incontinent NH residents who are identified for supportive incontinence care. Pads and garments may also be very helpful at night for residents who are managed by prompted voiding and/or other interventions during the day and evening. These containment devices should not, however, be used as the sole solution to UI in the NH or in a manner that fosters further dependency. When pads or garments are used, residents should still be regularly checked, toileted, and/or changed if necessary in order to avoid skin irritation and breakdown.

Catheters and Catheter Care

Three basic types of catheters and catheterization procedures are used for the management of urinary incontinence in NHs: external catheters, intermittent straight catheterization, and chronic indwelling catheterization. External catheters consist of some type of condom connected to a drainage system. Improvements in design and observance of proper procedure and skin care when applying the catheter will decrease the risk of skin irritation as well as the frequency with which the catheter falls off. Studies of complications associated with the use of these devices have been limited, but existing data suggest that male NH residents with external catheters are at increased risk of developing symptomatic UTIs. External catheters should therefore be used only to manage intractable incontinence in male residents who do not have urinary retention and who are extremely physically dependent. As with incontinence undergarments and padding, these devices should not be used as a matter of convenience, since they may foster dependency.

Intermittent catheterization is used in the management of urinary retention and overflow incontinence. The procedure involves straight catheterization two to four times daily, depending on residual urine volumes. Studies conducted largely among younger paraplegics have shown that this technique is practical and, as compared with chronic catheterization, reduces the risk of symptomatic infection. Intermittent self-catheterization has also been shown to be feasible for elderly female outpatients who are functional and both willing and able to catheterize themselves. However, studies carried out in young paraplegics and elderly female outpatients cannot automatically be extrapolated to the NH population. The technique may be useful for certain NH residents, such as women who have undergone bladder neck suspension or following removal of an indwelling catheter in a bladder retraining protocol (**Table 15-8**). However, the practicality and safety of this procedure in the NH setting have not been well documented. Elderly NH residents, especially men, may be difficult to catheterize, and the anatomic abnormalities commonly found in the lower urinary tract of NH residents may increase the risk of infection due to repeated straight catheterizations. In addition, using this technique in an institutional setting (which may have an abundance of organisms relatively resistant to many commonly used antimicrobial agents) may pose an unacceptable risk of nosocomial infections. Using sterile catheter trays for these procedures would be very expensive. Thus, it may be extremely difficult to implement such a program in a typical NH setting.

Chronic indwelling catheterization is probably overused in the NH and has been shown to increase the incidence of a number of complications, including chronic bacteriuria, symptomatic UTI, bladder stones, periurethral abscesses, and even bladder cancer. Elderly NH residents, especially men, managed by this technique are at relatively high risk of developing symptomatic UTI. Given these risks, it seems appropriate to recommend that the use of chronic indwelling catheters be limited to specific situations (**Table 15-10**). When indwelling catheterization is used, sound principles of catheter care should be observed in order to minimize complications (**Table 15-11**).

Table 15-10 Indications for a chronic indwelling bladder catheter

1. Urinary retention characterized by the following:
   (a) Causes persistent overflow incontinence, symptomatic infections, or renal dysfunction.
   (b) Cannot be corrected surgically or medically.
   (c) Cannot be managed practically with intermittent catheterization.
2. Skin wounds, pressure sores, or irritations that are being contaminated by incontinent urine.
3. Care of terminally ill or severely impaired persons for whom bed and clothing changes are uncomfortable or disruptive.
4. Preference of patient or caregiver when patient has not responded to more specific treatments.

Table 15-11 Key principles of managing chronic indwelling bladder catheters

1. Maintain sterile, closed, gravity drainage system and avoid breaking the closed system
2. Use clean techniques in emptying and changing the drainage system; wash hands between patients in institutional settings
3. Secure the catheter to the upper thigh or lower abdomen to avoid perineal contamination and urethral irritation due to movement of the catheter
4. Avoid frequent and vigorous cleaning of the catheter entry site; washing with soapy water once per day is sufficient
5. Do not routinely irrigate unless repeated obstructions occur.
6. If bypassing occurs in the absence of obstruction, consider the possibility of a bladder spasm, which can be treated with a bladder relaxant
7. Change the catheter every 4 to 8 weeks to avoid the build-up of encrustations.
8. If catheter obstruction occurs frequently, increase the patient's fluid intake and acidify the urine if possible (dilute acetic acid irrigations may be helpful)
9. Do not routinely use prophylactic or suppressive urinary antiseptics or antimicrobials
10. Do not do routine surveillance cultures to guide management of individual patients because all chronically catheterized patients have bacteriuria (which is often polymicrobial) and the organisms change frequently
11. Do not treat infection unless symptoms develop; symptoms may be nonspecific, and other possible sources of infection should be carefully excluded before symptoms are attributed to the urinary tract
12. If a symptomatic infection occurs, the catheter should be changed before a specimen is collected for culture (specimens obtained from the old catheter may be misleading because of colonization of the catheter lumen)
13. If a symptomatic urinary tract infections frequently develop, a genitourinary evaluation should be considered to rule out pathology conditions such as stones, periurethral or prostatic abscesses, and chronic pyelonephritis

FECAL INCONTINENCE

Fecal incontinence is less common than urinary incontinence, but a large proportion (about 50 percent) of residents with frequent urinary incontinence also have episodes of fecal incontinence. Defecation, like urination, is a physiological process that involves smooth and striated muscles, central and peripheral innervation, coordination of reflex responses, mental awareness, and physical ability to get to a toilet. Disruption of any of these factors can lead to fecal incontinence.

The major causes of fecal incontinence include constipation, excessive laxative use, hyperosmotic enteral feedings, neurological disorders, and colorectal disorders (**Table 15-12**). Constipation is extremely common in the elderly

Table 15-12 Causes of fecal incontinence

Fecal impaction	Colorectal disorders
Laxative overuse/abuse	Diarrheal illnesses (see Chapter 19)
Hyperosmotic enteral feedings	Diabetic autonomic neuropathy
Neurological disorders	Rectal sphincter damage
Dementia	
Stroke	
Spinal cord disease	

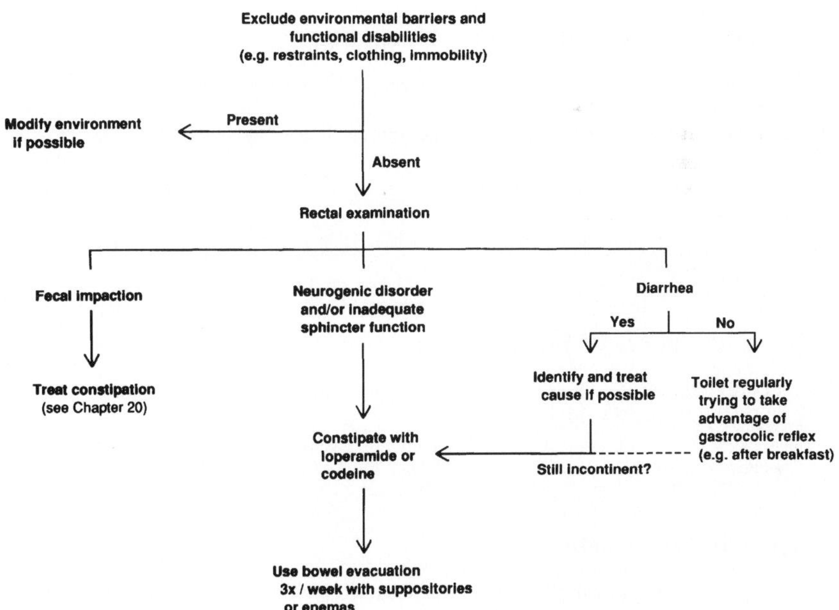

Figure 15-5 Strategy for managing fecal incontinence in the nursing home.

and when chronic can lead to fecal impaction and incontinence. The hard stool (or scybalum) of fecal impaction irritates the rectum and results in the production of mucus and fluid. This fluid leaks around the mass of impacted stool and precipitates incontinence. Appropriate management of constipation will prevent fecal impaction and resultant fecal incontinence. The management of constipation is discussed in Chapter 22.

Fecal incontinence due to neurological disorders is sometimes amenable to biofeedback therapy, although most elderly residents with dementia are unable to cooperate. For those residents with severe dementia, a program of alternating constipating agents (if necessary) and laxatives on a routine schedule (such as giving laxatives and enemas three times a week) is effective in controlling defecation and preventing fecal incontinence. **Fig. 15-5** depicts an approach to managing fecal incontinence in the NH setting.

SUGGESTED READINGS

General

Resnick NM, Ouslander JG (eds): NIH Conference on Urinary Incontinence. *J Am Geriatr Soc* 38:263–386, 1990.

Skelly J: Urinary incontinence associated with dementia. *J Am Geriatr Soc* 43:286–294, 1995.

McCormick K, Scheve A, Leahy E: Nursing management of urinary incontinence in geriatric inpatients. *Nurs Clin North Am* 23:231–264, 1988.

Prevalence, Associated Factors, Morbidity

Ouslander JG, Fowler E: Incontinence in VA nursing home care units. *J Am Geriatr Soc* 33:33–40, 1985.

Ouslander JG, Kane RL: The costs of urinary incontinence in nursing homes. *Med Care* 22:69–79, 1984.

Ouslander JG, Kane RL, Abrass IB: Urinary incontinence in elderly nursing home patients. *JAMA* 248:1194–1198, 1982.

Starer P, Libow LS: Obscuring urinary incontinence: Diapering the elderly. *J Am Geriatr Soc* 12:842–846, 1985.

Types and Causes of Incontinence

Pannill FC III, Williams TF, Davis R: Evaluation and treatment of urinary incontinence in long term care. *J Am Geriatr Soc* 36:902–910, 1988.

Resnick NM, Yalla SV, Laurino E: The pathophysiology of urinary incontinence among institutionalized elderly persons. *N Engl J Med* 320:1–7, 1989.

Diagnostic Assessment

Ouslander JG, Simmons S, Tuico E, et al: Use of a portable ultrasound device to measure post-void residual volume among incontinent nursing home residents. *J Am Geriatr Soc* 42:1189–1192, 1994.

Treatment

Hu T-W, Igou JF, Kaltreider DL, et al: A clinical trial of a behavioral therapy to reduce urinary incontinence in nursing homes. *JAMA* 261:2656–2662, 1989.

Ouslander JG, Greengold BA, Chen S: Complications of chronic indwelling urinary catheters among male nursing home patients: A prospective study. *J Urol* 138:1191–1195, 1987.

Schnelle JF, Sowell VA, Hu T-W, Traughber B: Reduction of urinary incontinence in nursing homes: Does it reduce or increase costs? *J Am Geriatr Soc* 36:34–39, 1988.

Ouslander JG, Schnelle JF, Uman G, Fingold S: Predictors of Successful Prompted Voiding Among Incontinent Nursing Home Residents. *JAMA* 273:1366–1370; 1995.

Ouslander JG, Schnelle JF, Uman G, et al: Does oxybutynin add to the effectiveness of prompted voiding for urinary incontinence among nursing home residents? A placebo-controlled trial. *J Am Geriatr Soc* 43:610–617, 1995.

Ouslander JG, Simmons S, Schnelle JF, Uman G: Effects of prompted voiding on fecal incontinence among nursing home residents. *J Am Geriatr Soc* 44:424–428, 1996.

Schnelle JF, McNees P, Crooks V, Ouslander JG: The use of a computer-based model to implement an incontinence management program. *Gerontologist* 35:656–665, 1995.

CHAPTER

SIXTEEN

GAIT DISORDERS AND FALLS

Falls among nursing home (NH) residents are a monumental problem, accounting for substantial morbidity, mortality, and cost. Falls, which inhibit residents' courage and threaten their independence, are one of the primary justifications for the widespread use of restraints. Falls may also be a marker for preexisting morbidity that requires assessment and management. In this chapter we review the epidemiology of gait instability and falls in the NH, their causes, and approaches to their evaluation and prevention.

PREVALENCE, INCIDENCE, AND MORBIDITY

Forty to 50 percent of residents in NHs have difficulty with walking. Falls are common, even among nonambulatory residents. The estimated annual incidence ranges from 0.6 to 3.6 falls per NH resident or 1600 falls per 1000 beds per year. Four percent of falls (range 1–10) result in fractures; 12 percent (range 1–36) result in serious injury other than fractures such as hematomas, lacerations, and dislocations which require medical care or result in restricted activity for more than a few days. Subdural hematomas or cervical fractures, the most devastating injuries, are rare. A recent study reported differences in the circumstances of injurious falls in nonambulatory and ambulatory residents. Falls in non-ambulatory residents are more likely to involve equipment (wheelchair, bed), and occur when they are seated or during transfer. The incidence of injurious falls in nonambulatory residents is less than half that in ambulatory residents, and those at highest risk are nonambulatory but not bed-bound and with the capacity for independent transfer. Ambulatory residents at highest risk tend to be those using psychotropic drugs. The estimated cost for care of injurious falls in the United States may be as high as $500 million per year. The frequency and lasting morbidity of injuries other than hip fractures have not been studied thoroughly enough to provide accurate estimates in the NH population.

There are approximately 200,000 hip fractures annually in the United States, most due to falls by older persons. Although many hip fractures occur among elderly NH residents, most occur in the community-dwelling geriatric population. Many of these fractures require at least a brief stay in a NH for rehabilitation.

Each year about 1800 fatal falls occur in US nursing homes. One-year mortality from hip fractures is estimated to be 25 percent in the United States (12 to 67 percent elsewhere). In some proportion of hip fractures, the victim falls and fractures his or her hip (traumatic fracture), while in others, the order of events is reversed due to osteoporotic bone (pathologic fracture). The relative proportion of these two types of hip fractures is not known. It is noteworthy that osteoporosis, falling, and hip fractures are more common in elderly women and that somewhat more trauma is generally required for a male to fracture his hip. However, mortality after hip fracture is higher at all ages for males than for females.

NORMAL GAIT

Multiple factors interact to produce a fall. Abnormalities of gait and balance are the leading factors, followed closely by environmental factors. It is important to understand some of the basic biomedical and physiological factors relating to normal gait in the aged in order to understand the pathophysiology of falls.

Figure 16-1 illustrates the normal gait cycle. It begins when the right heel strikes the floor, an event that initiates the "stance phase" for the right leg. The "swing phase" begins when the right toe leaves the floor. The stance phase for the legs overlaps, so that 20 to 25 percent of the time both feet are on the ground (double limb support). Flexor muscles are active in the swing phase and extensor muscles during the stance phase. Modern gait laboratories have helped to assess the elements of this gait cycle. The most important elements appear to be gait velocity, gait cadence, and stride length. The coordination of the complex task of ambulation is mediated by the spinal cord and integrated in the brain. Balance is maintained by keeping the center of gravity over the base of support, an area bounded by foot contact. Adjustments of the trunk and leg muscles occur during stance, beginning roughly 100 ms after a shift in the support surface. The automatic responses in maintaining dynamic equilibrium during walking require reliable afferent information from the visual system, the vestibular system, and the proprioceptors in the lower limbs.

Aging has several potential effects on balance and gait. During normal aging, body sway while standing increases, postural support responses are

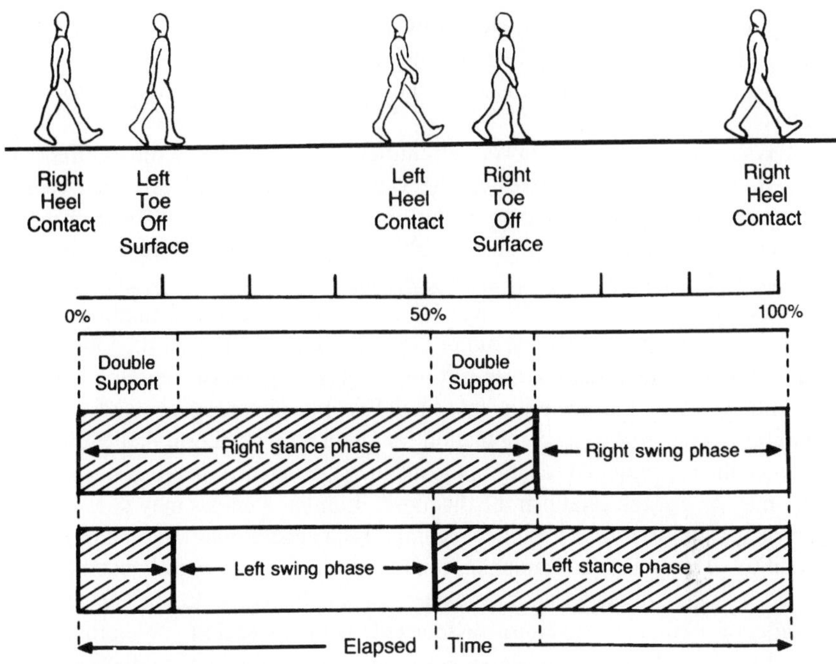

Figure 16-1 The normal gait cycle. (Reprinted from Sudarsky L: Gait disorders in the elderly. *N Engl J Med* 322:1441–1445, 1990.)

slowed, and there is a change in the capacity to integrate sensory information, with greater reliance on proprioception. While the elderly are more dependent on afferent information to maintain balance, these sensory systems are vulnerable to age-related changes and disease. Because so much of the nervous system is called on to support ambulation, changes in gait are often associated with neurological diseases which are common in the elderly. Elderly individuals demonstrate a shorter, broader-based stride, reduced pelvic rotation and joint excursions, and increased reliance on double-limb support. Normal velocity for a fit person at the age of 80 is 1.0 to 1.2 m/s, which represents a 10 to 20 percent decline from the value for younger persons. When the decrease in gait velocity with age is compounded by profound slowness or an abnormal pattern of ambulation, a gait disorder is present.

CAUSES OF INSTABILITY AND FALLING

Intrinsic Factors

Commonly described causes of gait instability and falling are either related to the individual (intrinsic) or are environmental (extrinsic). Instability and falling may result from a single intrinsic or extrinsic cause or, very often among NH residents, from the combined effects of multiple intrinsic and extrinsic factors. **Table 16-1** lists the most common intrinsic risk factors for falling.

Physical changes in the lower extremities and spine have a direct effect on the gait. Osteoarthritic changes in the weight-bearing joints are seen radiographically in 85 percent of the population of age 75 or above. These changes may cause pain, which in turn may result in an antalgic and unsteady gait.

Cervical spondylosis is usually generalized to include any degenerative lesion of the cervical spine. Symptoms include numbness and tingling of the fingers and clumsiness with fine motor tasks such as buttoning shirts. Later there may be mild spastic quadriparesis and impaired perception of vibration because of compression of the posterior columns. The gait abnormalities and postural instability result from a combination of motor dysfunction and impaired proprioception. Computed tomography, magnetic resonance imaging, or myelography may be used to establish the diagnosis. Lumbar stenosis may coexist with cervical spondylosis or occur independently as a cause of gait abnormalities and instability. The most common presenting symptom is pseudoclaudication, defined as pain, numbness, or weakness in the buttocks, thighs, or legs on standing, walking, or exercise associated with extension. Symptoms are generally relieved when the resident is sitting or lying. Physical findings include mild muscle weakness (S1 distribution) and decreased ankle and knee reflexes. Normal-pressure hydrocephalus (NPH) is a syndrome consisting of slowness and paucity of thought and action, unsteadiness of gait, and unwitting incontinence, with hydrocephalus and a cerebrospinal fluid pressure below 180 mmHg. The gait is characterized by reduced cadence ("stuck to the floor") and poor balance; it is similar to the frontal lobe gait. Many elderly persons with gait impairment have enlarged ventricles, so the diagnosis of NPH depends on the demonstration of a dynamic abnormality of cerebrospinal fluid circulation by radioactive scanning techniques. The diagnostic evaluation is aimed at identifying the subgroup of patients with the best chance of responding to a shunt procedure. The clinical response to the removal of 40 to 50 ml of cerebrospinal fluid may be an acceptable screening test among those with a high suspicion for this syndrome.

Some investigators have postulated that specific patterns of central nervous system pathology are associated with gait and balance disorders. Increased ventricular size and white matter loss have been noted with unexplained balance and gait problems. Magnetic resonance imaging has in some cases shown an association between multiple infarcts with gait and balance disorders even among those without a known history of strokes. Gait disorders in hypertensive residents are frequently associated with white matter lesions from small vessel disease (Binswanger's disease). The gait is characterized by hesitation in starting, shuffling, difficulty in picking the feet up off the floor ("magnetic foot response"), difficulty with turns, and poor standing balance. This pattern of

Table 16-1 Intrinsic factors that contribute to falls

Factor	History	Potential etiologies
Sensory		
Vision; near, distant, perception, dark adaptation		Age-related, cataract, glaucoma, macular degeneration
Vestibular	Vertigo; past use of aminoglycosides, furosemide, aspirin; ENT surgery, ear or mastoid infections	Age-related, drugs, tumors, previous surgery, infections, benign positional vertigo
Proprioceptive		
Peripheral nerves, spinal cord	Balance worse in dark, on uneven ground or thick rugs	Age-related, diabetes, vitamin B_{12} deficiency, tabes dorsalis
Cervical	Same as above, worse with head turning, vertigo, history of whiplash injury	Spondylosis, degenerative disease, Paget's disease, rheumatoid arthritis
Central neurological		
Any central nervous system lesion impairing problem solving and judgment	Variable, depends on disease	Variable
Musculoskeletal		
Arthritides, especially of the lower extremities	"Knee gave out," pain, stiffness	Degenerative, inflammatory
Muscle weakness, contractures	Variable	Many
Foot disorders		
Systemic disease		
Postural hypotension	Light-headedness, worse with position change or walking, complaints consistent with predisposing disease (e.g., Parkinson's disease, diabetes)	Age-related, Parkinson's disease, diabetes, autonomic dysfunction, deconditioning, medications
Cardiac, respiratory, metabolic disease	Variable	Any systemic disease
Depression	Vegetative complaints, poor concentration, apathy	Reactive or endofenous
Medications		
All	Confusion, light-headedness, vertigo, fatigue, weakness	Any medication

Source: Tinetti ME: Instability and falling in elderly patients, in Jenkyn L (ed): *Seminars in Neurology.* Volume 9, Number 1, New York, Thieme Medical Publishers, Inc. 1989.

abnormality is also termed frontal gait disorder or gait apraxia. The radiologic abnormality is frequently asymptomatic, and the pathological correlate has not been well characterized. White matter lesions have, however, been associated with recurrent falls in the elderly.

In Parkinson's disease, the gait is characterized by flexed posture, a diminished arm swing, a tendency to festination (starting slowly and gradually becoming more rapid), and difficulty with the initiation of motion and turns. Disturbance of balance occurs later, when postural support responses are compromised. Gait can be improved by drug therapy, but balance is not always restored.

Cerebellar disorders of balance and motor control can present with unsteady gait and a tendency to fall. Gait is characterized by a lateral instability of the trunk, erratic foot placement, and a widened stance. Many balance and gait disorders are related to the afferent systems. Sensory ataxia of tabetic neurosyphilis is a classic but rare example. Neuropathy affecting large-fiber afferents is a "modern" equivalent. The stance in such individuals is destabilized by eye closure (Romberg test). Selective loss of muscle spindle afferents has been proposed as a mechanism for some "senile" gait disorders. Multiple sensory deficits is a syndrome of imbalance resulting from deficits in proprioception, vision, and vestibular sense that impair postural support mechanisms. Age-related changes, such as impaired dark adaptation and lens accommodation, in combination with diseases such as macular degeneration are common and can contribute to the risk of falling. Visual perception (i.e., visual orientation in space) may be more relevant to falling than visual acuity. In view of decreased proprioception and vision, there is a tendency to rely on vestibular senses. Vestibular dysfunction, manifesting as true vertigo or dizziness with specific head movements and worsening instability in the dark, is common among older persons. Hearing and cognitive impairments also tend to increase the number of trips and falls.

The broad category of weakness and gait problems was the most common cause of falls, accounting for one out of four reported cases. Studies have reported 80 percent prevalence of detectable lower extremity weakness in NH residents. Gait and balance disorders, as a group, were found to be a significant risk factor for falls, associated with a three-fold increased risk of falling. A prospective study found three significant and independent risk factors for falls among NH residents: hip weakness, low balance score, and the number of prescription medications taken. Sedating medications, particularly neuroleptic agents and long-acting benzodiazepines, affect postural reflexes and increase the risk of falls. The same applies to vasodilators. Since disorders due to drugs are reversible, their identification should have a high priority. Postural hypotension can be caused by many different drugs and may precipitate falls, but it was not found to independently contribute to the risk of falling in this study. It should be recognized that, even after extensive evaluation, no cause for gait disturbances can be found in 10 to 20 percent of the elderly.

Extrinsic Factors

Accidents, usually implying falls stemming from environmental or extrinsic hazards, constitute a major cause (16–21 percent) of reported falls in the NH. The circumstances of accidents are difficult to verify, and many falls in this category may actually stem from interactions between environmental hazards or hazardous activities and increased individual susceptibility to hazards because of frailty. Environmental or extrinsic causes are implicated in approximately 20 percent of falls in the NH. In a randomized prospective study conducted at the Jewish Homes for the Aging of Greater Los Angeles, most falls occurred in the resident's room. Almost half occurred between the hours of 6 p.m. and 6 a.m., and about 12 percent occurred while the resident was exiting the bed or in the bathroom. **Table 16-2** lists some of the environmental factors that are important in the cause and prevention of falls in the NH. The floor surface is among the environmental hazards most frequently mentioned. Very shiny and smooth floors—as well as a transition from a high-friction surface such as a carpet to a low friction surface such as tile or polished linoleum—may precipitate falls in frail elderly. Spotlights or skylights on these surfaces can cause startle responses and falling in NH residents with Parkinsonism and other gait and balance abnormalities. Lighting plays an important role in providing a safe environment. Very bright and direct sources of light, such as fluorescent bulbs reflected against a highly polished linoleum floor, may be as big a hazard as poorly illuminated areas, since the glare so produced may have a blinding effect on elderly persons with cataracts and poor lens accommodation.

Bedroom falls occur most often at the bedside while the resident is getting in or out of bed. Falls are frequently associated with the use of bed rails. Contrary to common belief and practice, bed rails may increase the seriousness of falls. The same applies to other types of bed or wheelchair restraints. A report describes strangulation resulting in death with the use of "soft restraints." Therefore, bed rails or any other form of physical restraint should not substitute for a more practical and less restrictive approach to safety. Federal regulations (OBRA 1987) require very strict restrictions on the use of restraints. The use of physical restraints in the NH is discussed in more detail in Chapter 12. The features of a safe bedroom include a bed that can be lowered so that its height is approximately 19 in. (62 cm) or less from the top of the mattress to the floor. This will allow for safer transfers. Institutions purchasing beds should seek height-adjustable high-low beds with a frame that is approximately 14 in. (30 cm) in height when the bed is at its lowest position. Other safety features for the bedroom are outlined in **Table 16-2**.

The bathroom is another common site of falls in the NH. Most falls are the result of transferring on or off the toilet, or they occur while the resident is hurrying to urinate or defecate. In addition to appropriate toileting assistance, several environmental designs can improve safety around the bathroom. These include doors that are wide enough to provide entrance for wheelchairs and

Table 16-2 Important environmental safety features in the NH

Interior
Non-slip surfaces
Securely fastened handrails
Sufficient light
Glare-free lights
Low lying objects avoided so as to minimize tripping hazard
Telephone and call-button accessible
Chairs of the proper heights and equipped with armrests to assist in transferring
Time-delayed automatic doors to allow for slow-moving residents
Bathroom
Door wide enough to provide unobstructed entering with or without a device
Skidproof strips or mats in the tub or shower
Toilet and tub/shower grab bars
Elevated toilet seat to assist in transfers
Bedroom
Bedside or night lights for nighttime ambulation
Unobstructed pathway from the bed to the bathroom
Height-adjustable beds to allow safe transfers
Completely recessible bed rails
Sag-resistant mattress edges to provide good sitting support
Closet shelves reachable without standing on tiptoe or chair
Fall-management mobility monitoring devices for bed and wheelchair

walkers, toilet and shower grab bars, appropriate light, and elevated toilet seats which assist with transfers.

An adjunct to bedroom/bathroom/wheelchair safety is an institutional fall management and prevention program involving all levels of staff. Administrative aspects of such programs are discussed at the end of this chapter. Specially designed mobility monitoring devices ("bed alarms") may be a useful addition to fall-prevention programs. **Figure 16-2** illustrates one example of such devices that are designed to alert caregivers when a resident's motion exceeds a predetermined safety zone, indicating that the resident is in danger of falling. The sensor can be used with the nurse-call system or with a separate wireless system, providing local (resident's room) as well as remote (hallway, nurse's station) alarms. One manufacturer provides a sensor that mounts on a wheelchair, which is a common site associated with falls of unattended NH residents. The sensor allows staff to go about their activities while monitoring the resident at risk for falling. Preliminary studies have shown that environmental fall prevention programs geared to residents at risk result in a 25 percent annual decrease in falls. While there are no randomized prospective published studies to document the effectiveness of these approaches, we believe that combining comprehensive fall-management and safety programs with the use of positioning or mobility-monitoring devices is a desirable and promising approach for decreasing falls and injuries in the NH

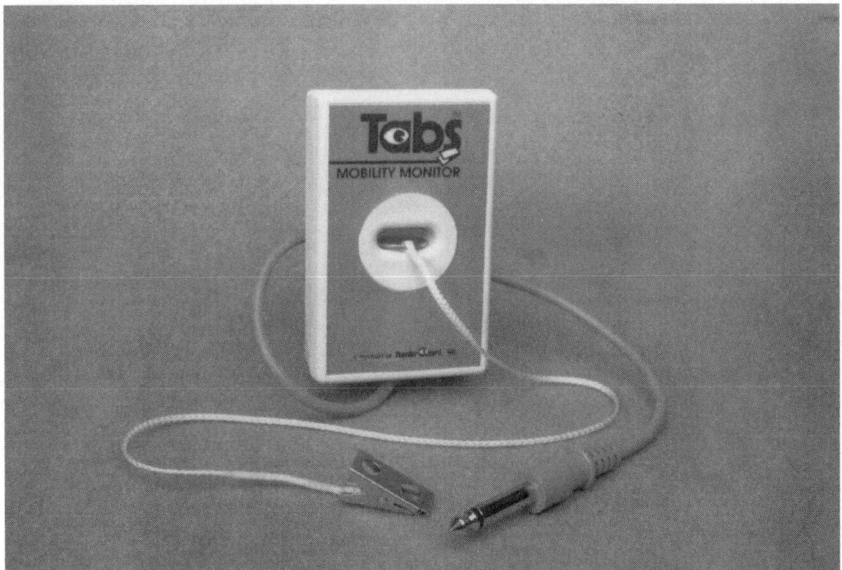

A

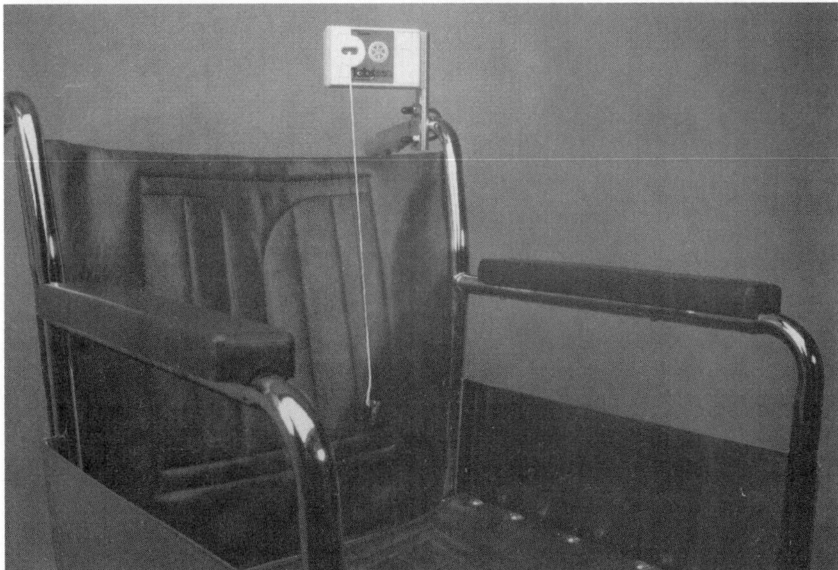

B

Figure 16-2 Examples of sensor devices that detect movement from a bed (A) or a wheelchair (B). These devices can be linked with a call system to alert nursing staff when a high-risk resident is in danger of falling.

Table 16-3 Characteristics of NH residents at high risk for falling

Female	Poor vision (<20/40)
Older than 75	Muscle weakness (hip, ankle dorsiflexors)
Newly admitted	More than four prescription medications
Previous fall within a year	Routine psychotropic drug use
Dementia, moderate and severe	Postural hypotension
Diminished safety awareness	Urinary incontinence
Gait instability, poor balance	Requires assistance with basic ADLs
Multiple physical disabilities	
Inability to carry out more than two basic activities of daily living	

setting. A recent program implementing a restraint-free environment, utilizing such devices as one restraint alternative integrated proactively with a rehabilitation program, showed no increase in injuries, while fall rates kept steady over a 3-year period. Such programs will be most effective if they are targeted to NH residents who are at high risk of falling. **Table 16-3** lists the characteristics of NH residents that are strongly associated with recurrent falls.

ASSESSMENT AND MANAGEMENT

Assessment of Risk

Assessment of mobility and stability is an important aspect of caring for NH residents. A thorough history and gait and balance examination which addresses the ability to transfer safely, and ambulate short distances, as well as safety awareness and potential for injurious falls, is the challenge in evaluating a newly admitted NH resident.

The Minimum Data Set (MDS) includes a section on "Physical Functioning and Structural Problems" **(Fig. 16-3)**, which correlates modestly well with corresponding ADL scales. Responses on this section may trigger the Resident Assessment Protocol (RAP) for falls. (**Table 16-4**) Since sensory impairment may contribute to the fall risk, one may want to consult that appropriate section described in Chapter 17.

Fall prevention and management is discussed later in the chapter. An assessment of safety and mobility utilizing a standardized, validated protocol for safety assessment of frail elderly (SAFE) developed by J. Schnelle and his colleagues. **Table 16-5** describes the key elements of SAFE. (For more details, see the "Suggested Readings.") The test scores help target residents for use of restraints, restraints release and rehabilitative measures. The initial data provide ranges of low injury risk (80–100), moderate risk score (51–79) and high risk score (0–50). Residents at low risk are monitored less frequently (yearly), while those at higher risk are monitored at least monthly. Health outcomes such as

Table 16-4 Key aspects of the fall resident assessment protocol

Factors	Problems to be considered
Multiple falls	• Is there a previous history of falls? • Was the fall an isolated event?
Diagnosis and conditions	• Does resident have a diagnosis, underlying health problem or condition that can cause falls?
Medications	• Is resident receiving psychotropic, cardiovascular or diuretic medication? • Were there any antipsychotics, antianxiety/hypnotics, anti-depressants, cardiovascular medications or diuretics administered prior to fall?
Appliances/devices	• Does the resident experiences problems when using an appliance (i.e. wheelchair, cane, walker)? • Are restraints used? • Were restraints used prior to the fall? • What was resident's mood and behavior prior to fall?
Environmental/ situational hazards and circumstances of recent fall(s)	• Time of day ______________ a.m./p.m. • Time since last meal ______________ • Was resident: a. Doing usual activities? b. Standing still? c. Walking? d. Reaching up? e. Reaching down? f. Reaching out? g. In a crowd of people? h. Responding to bladder/bowel urgency? • Were there changes in resident's environment? • Did this fall follow a similar pattern to resident's previous falls? • Were resident's vital signs taken after fall?

mobility and endurance are also measured when assessing effectiveness of the program. The MDS assessment and RAPs triggers can utilize this approach. The use of SAFE within a total quality management program may assist NH staff to obtain feedback on effectiveness of this process of care. For further discussion on total quality management, see Chapter 8. A fall management and prevention program (integrated with restraint reduction) may use the algorithm adopted from Schnelle et al (**Fig. 16-4**). This approach uses a practical, interdisciplinary strategy for prevention and rehabilitation. Rather than assessing all NH residents who have a known risk factor for injurious falls, a targeted approach to residents at risk is a more effective management technique.

As with any acute or chronic disease, the first steps in caring for fallers involve establishing the cause or causes for falling and setting treatment goals.

SECTION G. PHYSICAL FUNCTIONING AND STRUCTURAL PROBLEMS

1. (A) ADL SELF-PERFORMANCE—(*Code for resident's* ***PERFORMANCE OVER ALL SHIFTS during last 7 days***—*Not including setup*)

0. *INDEPENDENT*—No help or oversight —OR— Help/oversight provided only 1 or 2 times during last 7 days
1. SUPERVISION—Oversight, encouragement or cueing provided 3 or more times during last7 days —OR— Supervision (3 or more times) plus physical assistance provided only 1 or 2 times during last 7 days
2. *LIMITED ASSISTANCE*—Resident highly involved in activity; received physical help in guided maneuvering of limbs or other nonweight bearing assistance 3 or more times —OR—More help provided only 1 or 2 times during last 7 days
3. *EXTENSIVE ASSISTANCE*—While resident performed part of activity, over last 7-day period, help of following type(s) provided 3 or more times:
   — Weight-bearing support
   — Full staff performance during part (but not all) of last 7 days
4. *TOTAL DEPENDENCE*—Full staff performance of activity during entire 7 days
8. *ACTIVITY DID NOT OCCUR* during entire 7 days

(B) ADL SUPPORT PROVIDED—(***Code for MOST SUPPORT PROVIDED OVER ALL SHIFTS during last 7 days; code regardless*** *of resident's self-performance classification*)

0. No setup or physical help from staff
1. Setup help only
2. One person physical assist
3. Two+ persons physical assist
8. ADL activity itself did not occur during entire 7 days

			(A) SELF-PERF	(B) SUPPORT
a.	BED MOBILITY	How resident moves to and from lying position, turns side to side, and positions body while in bed		
b.	TRANSFER	How resident moves between surfaces—to/from: bed, chair, wheelchair, standing position (EXCLUDE to/from bath/toilet)		
c.	WALK IN ROOM	How resident walks between locations in his/her room		
d.	WALK IN CORRIDOR	How resident walks in corridor on unit		
e.	LOCOMOTION ON UNIT	How resident moves between locations in his/her room and adjacent corridor on same floor. If in wheelchair, self-sufficiency once in chair		
f.	LOCOMOTION OFF UNIT	How resident moves to and returns from off unit locations (e.g., areas set aside for dining, activities, or treatments). **If facility has only one floor**, how resident moves to and from distant areas on the floor. If in wheelchair, self-sufficiency once in chair		
g.	DRESSING	How resident puts on, fastens, and takes off all items of **street clothing**, including donning/removing prosthesis		
h.	EATING	How resident eats and drinks (regardless of skill). Includes intake of nourishment by other means (e.g., tube feeding, total parenteral nutrition)		
i.	TOILET USE	How resident uses the toilet room (or commode, bedpan, urinal); transfer on/off toilet, cleanses, changes pad, manages ostomy or catheter, adjusts clothes		
j.	PERSONAL HYGIENE	How resident maintains personal hygiene, including combing hair, brushing teeth, shaving, applying makeup, washing/drying face, hands, and perineum (EXCLUDE baths and showers)		

2. BATHING — How resident takes full-body bath/shower, sponge bath, and transfers in/out of tub/shower (EXCLUDE washing of back and hair.) ***Code for most dependent*** *in self-performance and support.*

(A) BATHING SELF-PERFORMANCE codes appear below — (A) (B)

0. Independent—No help provided
1. Supervision—Oversight help only
2. Physical help limited to transfer only
3. Physical help in part of bathing activity
4. Total dependence
8. Activity itself did not occur during entire 7 days

(*Bathing support codes are as defined in* ***Item 1, code B above***)

Figure 16-3 MDS items on physical functioning and structural problems.

3.	TEST FOR BALANCE (see training manual)	(*Code for ability during test in the* ***last 7 days***) 0. Maintained position as required in test 1. Unsteady, but able to rebalance self without physical support 2. Partial physical support during test; or stands (sits) but does not follow directions for test 3. Not able to attempt test without physical help	
		a. Balance while standing	
		b. Balance while sitting—position, trunk control	
4.	FUNCTIONAL LIMITATION IN RANGE OF MOTION (see training manual)	(*Code for limitations during* ***last 7 days*** *that interfered with daily functions or placed resident at risk of injury*) **(A)** *RANGE OF MOTION*: 0. No limitation; 1. Limitation on one side; 2. Limitation on both sides **(B)** *VOLUNTARY MOVEMENT*: 0. No loss; 1. Partial loss; 2. Full loss	**(A)** **(B)**
		a. Neck	
		b. Arm—Including shoulder or elbow	
		c. Hand—Including wrist or fingers	
		d. Leg—Including hip or knee	
		e. Foot—Including ankle or toes	
		f. Other limitation or loss	
5.	MODES OF LOCOMOTION	(***Check all that apply*** *during* ***last 7 days***) Cane/walker/crutch **a.** Wheeled self **b.** Other person wheeled **c.** Wheelchair primary mode of locomotion **d.** *NONE OF ABOVE* **e.**	
6.	MODES OF TRANSFER	(***Check all that apply*** *during* ***last 7 days***) Bedfast all or most of time **a.** Bed rails used for bed mobility or transfer **b.** Lifted manually **c.** Lifted mechanically **d.** Transfer aid (e.g., slide board, trapeze, cane, walker, brace) **e.** *NONE OF ABOVE* **f.**	
7.	TASK SEGMENTATION	Some or all of ADL activities were broken into subtasks during **last 7 days** so that resident could perform them 0. No 1. Yes	
8.	ADL FUNCTIONAL REHABILITATION POTENTIAL	Resident believes he/she is capable of increased independence in at least some ADLs	**a.**
		Direct care staff believe resident is capable of increased independence in at least some ADLs	**b.**
		Resident able to perform tasks/activity but is very slow	**c.**
		Difference in ADL Self-Performance or ADL Support, comparing mornings to evenings	**d.**
		NONE OF ABOVE	**e.**
9.	CHANGE IN ADL FUNCTION	Resident's ADL self-performance status has changed as compared to status of **90 days ago** (or since last assessment if less than 90 days) 0. No change 1. Improved 2. Deteriorated	

Figure 16-3 (*Continued*)

Ideally, the risk of falling should be minimized without compromising mobility or functional independence. After identifying and treating injuries, a thorough assessment should be undertaken. Recalling that the accumulated effects of multiple diseases and disabilities, as well as the environment, predispose an elderly individual to falling, a fall evaluation should identify all potential contributing factors. Intrinsic risk factors (including sensory impairment, neurological, musculoskeletal, and systemic diseases) should be identified. Specific assessment techniques targeted at these risk factors are outlined in **Table 16-6**. As for almost all geriatric conditions, a review of medications is an important part of the assessment. A wide variety of medications, especially

Table 16-5 Items and scoring ranges from the safety assessment for frail elderly ("SAFE")

	Possible Scoring Range[a]
Transition: Standing up	
1. Does resident lock wheelchair	0–4
2. Does resident move foot pedals	0–4
3. Does resident stand up without use of hands or use device correctly	0–2
4. Can resident stand up	0–3
5. Standing balance	0–3
Walking	
6. Correct use of walking device if applicable	0–2
7. Feet positioning	0–2
8. Body over feet	0–2
9. Walking straight	0–2
10. Hands within correct distance of walking device	0–2
11. Walk at controlled pace	0–2
12. Lift feet off ground	0–2
13. Steps evenly paced	0–2
14. Resident appears stable	0–2
15. Maneuvers around object in path	0–3
16. Picks up object from standing position	0–3
17. Stops steadily	0–2
18. Maintains balance while turning	0–3
Transition: Sitting down	
19. Locks or checks wheelchair for stability	0–4
20. Places hands on chair arms before sitting	0–2
21. Lowers body in controlled manner	0–2
22. Sitting posture	0–2
23. Picks up object (sponge) from floor	0–3
SAFE Percentage Scores[a]	
Transition Factor	0–29
Walk 1 factor (body control)	0–19
Walk 2 factor (use of device/feet)	0–10
Judgement factor	0–25
Total SAFE scores	0–58

Modified with permission from Schnelle et al: Safety assessment for the frail elderly: A comparison of restrained and unrestrained nursing home residents. *J Am Geriatr Soc* 42:586–592, 1995.

[a]Percentage scores calculated by dividing total score achieved by the total score possible on all items applicable to each subject.

cardiovascular and psychotropic agents, can contribute to falls. The environment should be evaluated for potential hazards related to the fall. A careful history should be obtained from the resident (if possible), witnesses, and NH staff. **Table 16-7** outlines the key points of the history. Persons who are chairbound are also at risk for falls. The more functional a chairbound persons is the more likely they

Table 16-6 Assessment and intervention techniques for risk factors for falls among NH residents

Factor	Assessments	Interventions
Vision	Near and distant visual acuity Visual fields Dark adaptation	Appropriate refraction Prescription or adjustment of medications Appropriate lighting
Vestibular	Nystagmus Ear, nose, and throat examination	Avoidance of toxic drugs Surgery if indicated Balance exercises Appropriate lighting
Peripheral nerves and spinal cord	Motor and sensory examination Vitamin B_{12} level if indicated Blood glucose	Treat underlying disease Adequate lighting Appropriate walking aids and footwear
Cervical	Motor and sensory examination for signs of radiculopathy (e.g., clumsiness with fine motor tasks, mild spastic quadriparesis)	Balance exercises Surgery
Central nervous system disorder	Mental status examination to assess judgment (see Chap. 11) Neurological examination to identify focal deficits	Supervised, structured, safe environment
Musculoskeletal		
Arthrides, especially of lower extremities	Joint and periarticular muscle examinations Range of motion	Medical and/or surgical treatment of underlying disease
Muscle weakness, contractures	Strength testing Range of motion	Strengthening exercises; balance and gait training; appropriate adaptive devices
Foot disorders	Podiatric evaluation	Treatment for bunions, calluses, deformities, etc. Appropriate footwear
Systemic diseases		
Postural hypotension	Postural vital signs	Hydration, lowest effective does of necessary medications, reconditioning exercises, stockings (see Chap. 21)
Cardiac, respiratory, metabolic disease	Thorough physical and laboratory evaluation	Optimal medical management
Depression	Psychiatric or psychologic evaluation Depression scale	Nonpharmacologic and pharmacologic treatment (see Chap. 12)
Medications	Medication review Evaluate side effects (e.g., postural hypotension, visual disturbance)	Reduce or eliminate does when possible
Environmental	Environmental assessment	Appropriate modifications where feasible (see Table 16-2)
Safe Score <80	Risk for injurious falls and restraints needed	Walking program Targeted prevention

Table 16-7 Evaluating falls: key points in the history

General medical history focusing on risk factors (see Tables 16-1 and 16-3)

History of previous falls

Medications (especially antihypertensive and psychotropic agents)

Resident's thoughts on the cause of the fall
- Was resident aware of impending fall?
- Was it totally expected?
- Did resident trip or slip?

Circumstances surrounding the fall
- Location and time of day
- Resident's position before the fall (standing, wheelchair, bed)
- Witnesses' accounts
- Relationship to changes in posture, turning of head, cough, urination

Premonitory or associated symptoms
- Light-headedness, dizziness, vertigo
- Palpitations, chest pain, shortness of breath
- Sudden focal neurological symptoms (weakness, sensory disturbance, dysarthria, ataxia, confusion, asphasia)
- Aura
- Incontinence of urine or stool

Loss of consciousness
- What is remembered immediately after the fall?
- Could the resident get up? If so, how long did it take?
- Could loss of consciousness be verified by a witness?

Source: Kane RL, Ouslander JG, Abrass IB: *Essentials of Clinical Geriatrics*, 2d ed. New York, McGraw-Hill, 1989, p 202.

are to fall. A scale for assessing balance in chairbound individuals has been developed and validated (**Table 16-8**).

A very useful technique in the assessment of NH residents who fall is a systematic evaluation of balance and gait. Tinetti has developed an excellent "performance-based" balance and gait evaluation (**Table 16-9**). The overall score on this evaluation is not as important as the identification and description of specific aspects of balance and gait that are abnormal and that might be amenable to rehabilitation or other interventions. We recommend that such a systematic gait evaluation be performed on NH residents who recurrently fall, as well as at the time of admission and at least annually thereafter, so that balance and gait abnormalities can be detected early and intervention implemented.

Based on the results of the assessment, a wide variety of medical, rehabilitative, or environmental interventions might be appropriate (**Table 16-6**). Residents with sensory impairments should be referred for appropriate evaluation and intervention (e.g., refraction, cataract extraction, fitting of hearing aid). Vestibular problems are managed by avoiding ototoxic drugs if possible, providing

Table 16-8 Assessment of balance in chairbound nursing home residents

	Unsteady	Steady
1. Posture: leans to one side	0	1
Leans forward/backward,	0	1
No leaning, upright, steady		
2. Nudge on sternum backward	Eyes opened	Closed
Loses balance	0	0
Moves up to 6 in. forwards with balance maintained	1	1
Maintains balance, solid	2	2
3. Simultaneous nudge forward to posterior aspect of both shoulders	Eyes opened	Closed
Loses balance	0	0
Moves up to 6 in. forwards with balance maintained	1	1
Maintains balance, solid	2	2
4. Nudges in lateral aspect of right shoulder	Eyes opened	Closed
Loses balance	0	0
Moves up to 6 in. to left with balance maintained	1	1
Maintains balance, solid	2	2
5. Nudge to lateral aspect of left shoulder	Eyes opened	Closed
Loses balance	0	0
Moves up to 6 in. to left balanced maintained	1	1
Maintains balance, solid	2	2
6. Reach down with bilateral upper extremities and touch below knee		
Unable = 0		
Holds onto mar with one hand, reaches with other hand = 1		
Both hands down, requires assistance to raise up = 1		
Both hands down, returns to upright unassisted = 2		
7. Raise arms overhead		
Unable = 0		
Raises arms up to shoulder level, maintains balance = 1		
Raises arms beyond shoulder level, maintains balance = 2		
8. Reaching for object at head level, 3 feet from either side		
Loses balance to the left = 0		
Loses balance to the right = 0		
Crosses over midline reaching with opposite arm while supporting with other arm = 1		
Maintains balance both directions while using the arm to other side of the object = 2		
9. Catches thrown ball (approximately 12 in. diameter):		
Unable = 0		
Traps ball against body with one hand while supporting		
10. Throws ball (approximately 12 in. diameter)		
Unable = 0		
Tosses ball underhand or overhand while supporting, with other hand = 1		
Tosses ball underhand or overhand without supporting maintains balance = 2		
11. Don and doff pullover shirt; loses balance while taking off or putting on shirt = 0		
Completes task, but is jerky and slow may need to catch balance = 1		
Completes task, smoothly and efficiently maintains balance = 2		
12. Don and doff shoes and socks:		
Unable = 0		
Loses balance but corrects self, jerky and slow = 1		
Completes task, smoothly and efficiently maintains balance = 2		

After Perry NM, et al: *Nursing Home Medicine* 4:173, 1994.

Table 16-9 Tinetti balance and gait evaluation[a]

Balance

Instructions: The subject begins this assessment seated in a backless (or straight-backed), armless, firm chair. A *walking aid* is defined as a cane or walker. Circle the appropriate score.

1. *Sitting balance*
   Leans or slides down in chair = 0
   Steady, stable, safe = 1

2. *Rising from chair*
   Unable without human assistance = 0
   Able but uses arms (on chair or walking aid) to pull or push up = 1
   Able to rise in a single movement without using arms on chair or walking aid (Note: use of arms on subject's own thighs scores a 2) = 2

3. *Attempts to rise*
   Unable without human assistance = 0
   Able but requires multiple attempts = 1
   Able to rise with one attempt = 2

4. *Immediate standing balance (first 3–5 s)*
   Any sign of *unsteadiness* (defined as grabbing at objects for support, staggering, moving feet, or more than minimal trunk sway) = 0
   Steady but USES WALKING AID or grabs other objects for support = 1
   Steady without holding onto walking aid or other object for support = 2

5. *Standing balance*
   Any sign of unsteadiness regardless of stance, or holds onto object = 0
   Steady but *wide stance* (defined as medial heels more than 4 in. apart) or USES WALKING AID or other support = 1
   Steady with *narrow stance* (defined as medial heels less than 4 in. apart) and without holding onto any object for support = 2

6. *Nudge on sternum* (with subject standing with feet as close together as possible, examiner pushes with light even pressure over sternum three times; reflects ability to withstand displacement)
   Begins to fall or examiner has to help maintain balance = 0
   Needs to move feet but able to maintain balance (e.g., staggers, grabs, but catches self) = 1
   Steady, able to withstand pressure = 2

7. *Balance with eyes closed* (with subject standing with feet as close together as possible with arms at sides, examiner counts out 5 s)
   Any sign of unsteadiness or needs to hold onto an object = 0
   Steady without holding onto any object with feet close together = 0

8. *Turning balance (360°)* (from a standing still position, have the subject turn around in q 360° circle; demonstrate this first and give the subject one chance to practice)
   Steps are *discontinuous* (defined as subject puts one foot completely on the floor before raising the other foot) = 0
   Steps are *continuous* (defined as the turn is a flowing movement = 1
   Any sign of unsteadiness or hold onto an object = 0
   Steady without holding onto any object = 1

Table 16-9 (*Continued*)

9. *Sitting down*	
Unsafe (falls into chair, misjudges distances, lands off-center)	= 0
Needs to use arms to guide self into chair or not a smooth movement	= 1
Able to sit down in one safe, smooth motion	= 2
	Balance Score: /16
Gait	
Instructions: the subject stands with the examiner. They walk down the hallway or across a room (preferably where there are few people or obstacles). The subject should be told to walk at his/her "usual" pace using his/her usual walking aid. Circle the appropriate score.	
10. *Initiation of gait* (subject is asked to begin walking down the hallway immediately after being told to "go")	
Any hesitancy, multiple attempts to start, or initiation of gait not a smooth motion	= 0
Subject begins walking immediately without observable hesitation and initiation of gait is a single, smooth motion	= 1
11. *Step length and height* (Observe distance between toe of stance foot and heel of swing foot, observe from the side, do not judge first few or last few steps, observe one foot at a time)	
Right swing foot does *not* pass left stance foot with each step	= 0
Right swing foot passes left stance foot with each step	= 1
Right swing foot does *not* clear floor completely with each step (may hearing scraping) or is raised markedly high (e.g., due to drop foot)	= 0
Right swing foot completely clears floor but is not markedly high	= 1
Left swing foot does *not* pass right stance foot with each step	= 0
Left swing foot passes right stance foot with each step	= 1
Left swing foot does *not* clear floor completely with each step (may hear scraping) or is raised markedly high (e.g., due to drop foot)	= 0
Left swing foot completely clears floor but is not markedly high	= 1
12. *Stem symmetry* (observe distance between toe of each stance foot and heel of each foot, observe from the side, do not judge first few or last few steps)	
Step length varies between sides or resident advances with same foot with every step	= 0
Step length same or nearly same on both sides for most step cycles	= 1
13. *Step continuity*	
Steps are *discontinuous* (defined as subject places entire foot, heel and toe, on floor before beginning to raise other foot) or subject stops completely between steps	= 0
Steps are *continuous* (defined as subject begins raising heel of one foot as heel of other foot touches the floor) and there are no breaks or stops in subject's stride	= 1
14. *Path deviation* (observe in relation to floor tiles or a line on the floor, observe one foot over several strides—about 10 ft of path length, observe from behind; difficult to assess if subject uses a walking aid)	
Marked deviation of foot from side-to-side or toward one direction	= 0
Mild/moderate deviation, or subject USES A WALKING AID	= 1
Foot follows close to a straight line as subject advances	= 2

Table 16-9 (*Continued*)

15. *Trunk stability* (observe from behind)	
Marked side-to-side trunk sway or subject USES A WALKING AID	= 0
No side-to-side trunk sway, but subject flexes knees or back or subject spreads arms out while walking	= 1
Trunk does not sway, knees and back are not flexed, arms are not abducted in an effort to maintain stability	= 2
16. *Walk stance* (observe from behind)	
Feet apart with stepping	= 0
Feet should almost touch as one foot passes the other	= 1
	Gait score: /12
	Total score: /28

[a]Reprinted with permission from M. Tinetti.

habituation exercises, and identifying and avoiding problem maneuvers. Those with proprioceptive deficits contributing to instability should be evaluated to exclude vitamin B_{12} deficiency and diabetes. Rehabilitative approaches include balance exercises, assistive devices for walking, appropriate footwear (e.g., firm soles provide better proprioceptive input than bare feet or slippers). Any central nervous system process can contribute to instability and falling. A neurologic examination is therefore an important component of the evaluation of instability and falling. The focus should be on mental status, strength, sensation, tone, and coordination. A formal gait and balance assessment can be done utilizing the Tinetti scale mentioned above (**Table 16-9**). The goal of this evaluation is to reproduce the positional changes and gait maneuvers used during the resident's daily activities, especially those that have been associated with falls. The evaluation can be used to determine the rehabilitative and environmental interventions that may improve gait and mobility and decrease the risk of falling.

Rehabilitative recommendations for residents with proximal muscle weakness, commonly associated with arthritis or deconditioning, include strengthening exercises and the use of firm high chairs and a raised toilet seat. For residents with a balance problem, bright lights, night lights, and an appropriate walking aid should be considered. For residents with abnormal gait patterns such as decreased step height or step length, gait training by a physical therapist should be recommended, as well as an environmental assessment to eliminate tripping hazards. Environmental assessment in NHs should be an ongoing process and should be targeted particularly to residents at risk (see **Tables 16-2** and **16-3**). Potential hazards to look for include cords and wires, inadequate lighting, slippery floors, inadequate or missing grab bars, and inaccessible switches and call buttons. Closet shelves and drawers should be designed so that they are reachable without forcing unsteady residents to stand on tiptoe or on chairs to reach them.

Growing evidence in the scientific literature suggests that assessment and multifactorial interventions for fallers and those at risk for falling can reduce the potential to fall and subsequent morbidity. A large cooperative study supported by the National Institute on Aging (Frailty and Injuries: Cooperative Studies of Intervention Techniques; “FICSIT”) has been completed and early data suggest that interventions ranging from Tai Chi to strength training may be of benefit among frail elderly NH residents (see “Suggested Readings”).

ADMINISTRATIVE CONSIDERATIONS

A careful assessment of NH residents with gait instability and falls can reduce morbidity and, in turn, reduce health care costs. Clinicians practicing in NHs, as well as the administrator, should become familiar with the problem, so that strategies can be developed to deal with the prevention of falls and to avoid potential undesired consequences, such as citations by regulatory agencies or legal action by residents and their families.

A fall that results in injury is an incident reportable to the health department. This requires a systematic approach to falls in each institution that will stand the scrutiny of medical standards as well as administrative survey. Most NHs use a generic “incident report form” that provides information on the time, outcome, and corrective action or other interventions (i.e., resident education, medication change, or environmental modification) for falls. An example of the form developed at the Jewish Home for the Aging of Greater Los Angeles for computer data entry and quality assurance is included in the “Appendix”. This form can provide epidemiological data on the frequency, timing, and factors associated with and outcomes of falls in the institution. This information may then be used by administration for quality-assurance and risk-management purposes. For example, comparing trends of falls with staffing ratios or time of day may help pinpoint specific problems that may play a role in causing falls. Since some studies have shown that falls tend to occur in times of peak activity when most staff is on duty, effective utilization of staff at peak periods is essential for resident safety. Information gathered via other established mechanisms, such as drug regimen review, may also provide data pertinent to the risk and prevention of falls. For example, residents on a high number of medications or who frequently use hypnotics or other psychotropics are at high risk. These data may be used to modify clinical practice and potentially prevent falls. Resident case mix may play a role, since falls are more likely in a predominantly ambulatory NH resident population than among those who are predominantly bed-bound.

The administrator should use specific epidemiological and quality-assurance data in decisions related to safety measures. For example, a predominantly ambulatory demented NH population may require more monitoring devices (**Fig. 16-2**) than a physically disabled but cognitively intact population. Similarly, a

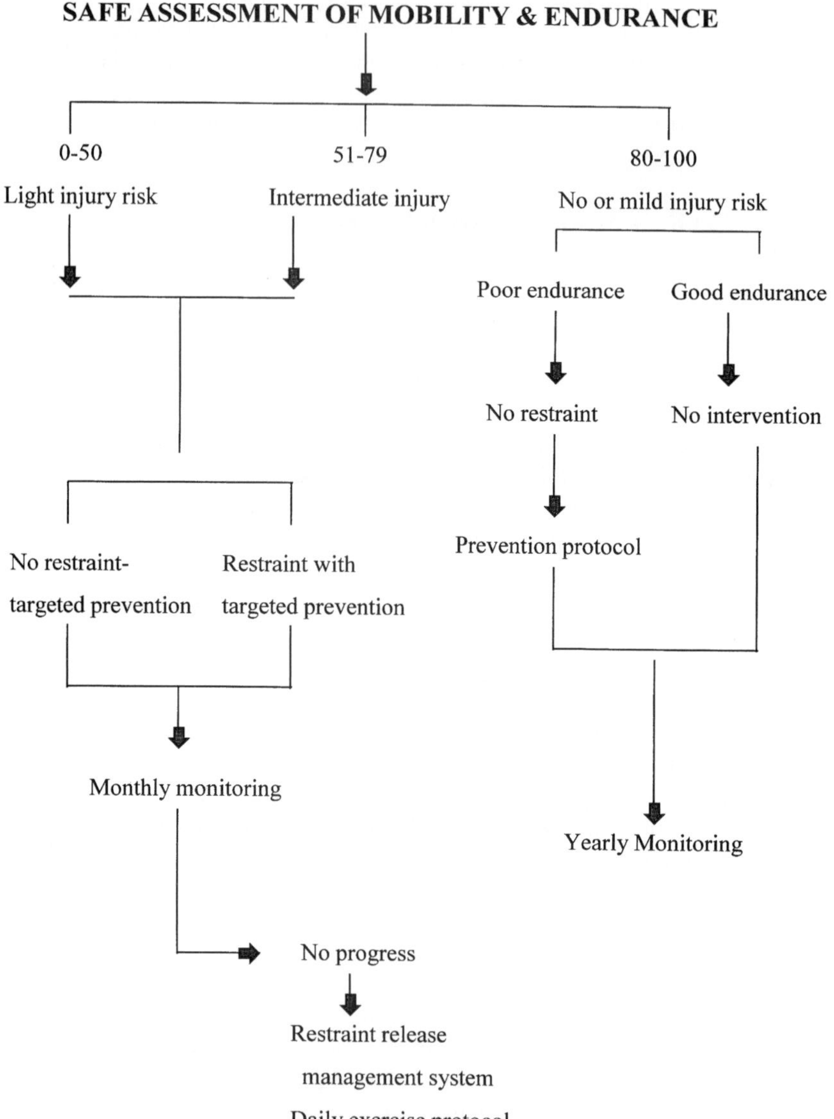

Figure 16-4 Example of an algorithm for a restraint reduction continuous quality improvement system. *Source*: Schnelle JF: Total quality management and the medical director: Medical direction in long term care. *Clin Geriatr Med* 11(3):433–448, 1995.

population with the majority of residents ambulatory and eating in a main dining room requires more staff at meals and thereafter to assist with transfers than does a population of predominantly bed-bound residents.

Policies related to restraints, such as side rails or "postural supports," should be consistent with regulations contained in OBRA (see Chapter 12). Keeping safety at the top of the agenda of staff meetings is also part of an effective fall-management and prevention program. Gathering information on how well the staff is complying with policies and procedures, offering them feedback, and letting them know how their compliance affects outcomes are critical to successful quality-assurance activities related to the prevention of falls and injuries.

In the authors' opinion, principles of total quality management (TQM) seems appropriate to apply in NH fall management and risk reduction programs. The steps in establishing TQM programs include developing an algorithm (process), monitoring compliance with process implementation, describing the nature of the outcomes, and providing feedback to staff. Information on falls can be presented in control charts which provide information on consistency and point out when falls and/or injuries exceed a "warning limit" (see Chapter 8). If that occurs, a further analysis can be conducted to identify how many residents were released from restraints during the past month and what the SAFE scores of these residents were. Such ongoing analysis, triggered by unusual variations in the data, can facilitate the identification of factors that influence injury rates and eventually lead to modification of the algorithm (**Fig. 16-4**) It is critical that NH leadership provide support for this program.

SUGGESTED READINGS

Alexander NB: Gait disorders in older adults. *J Am Geriatr Soc* 44:434–451, 1996.

Fiatarone M, O'Neill E, Ryan ND, et al: Exercise training and nutritional supplementation for physical frailty in very elderly people. *N Engl J Med* 330:1769–1775, 1994.

Kapoor WN: Syncope in older persons. *J Am Geriatr Soc* 42:426–436, 1994.

Levine, JM, Marchello, V, Totolos, E: Progress toward a restraint-free environment in a large academic nursing facility. *J Am Geriatr Soc* 43:914–918, 1995.

Luukinen, H, Koski, K, Honkanen, et al: Incidence of injury-causing falls among older adults by place of residents: A population-based study. *J Am Geriatri Soc* 43:871–876, 1995.

Province MA, Hadley EC, Hornbrook MC, Lipsitz LA, et al: The effects of exercise on falls in elderly patients: A preplanned meta-analysis of the FICSIT trials. *JAMA* 273:1341–1347, 1995.

Rader, J: Guidelines for assessing use of position change alarms. *Nursing Homes*, 42(4), 22–23, 1993.

Robbins A, Rubenstein LZ, Josephson K, Schulman B, Osterweil D: Predictors of falls among elderly people. *Arch Intern Med* 149:1628–1633, 1989.

Rubenstein, LZ, Josephson, KR, Robbins AS: Falls in the nursing home. *Ann Intern Med* 121:442–451, 1994.

Rubenstein LZ, Robbins A, Josephson K, Schulman B, Osterweil D: The value of assessing falls in an elderly population: A randomized clinical trial. *Ann Intern Med* 113:308–316, 1990.

Rubenstein LZ, Robbins AS, Schulman B, et al: Falls and instability in the elderly. *J Am Geriatr Soc* 36:266–278, 1988.

Schmid NA: Reducing patient falls: A research-based comprehensive fall prevention program. *Military Med* 155:202–07, 1990.

Schnelle, JF: Total quality management and the medical director. Medical direction in long term care. *Clin Geriatr Med* 11(3) 433–448, 1995.

Schnelle, JF, Mac Rae, PG, Simmons, SF, et al: Safety assessment for the frail elderly: A comparison of restrained and unrestrained nursing home residents. *J Am Geriatr Soc* 42:586–592, 1994

Schnelle JF, Simmons, SF, Ory MG: Risk factors that predict staff failure to release nursing home residents from restraints. *Gerontologist* 32:767–767, 1992.

Sudarsky L: Gait disorders in the elderly. *N Engl J Med* 322:1441–1445, 1990.

Thapa, PB, Brockman, KG, Gideon, P. et al: Injurious falls in nonambulatory nursing home residents: A comparative study of circumstances, incidence, and risk factors. *J Am Geriatr Soc* 44:273–278, 1996.

Tideiksaar R: Alarm systems, in *Falling in Old Age*. Springer Publishing Co, 1989, pp 175–177.

Tideiksaar R, Osterweil D: Prevention of bed falls: The Sepulveda GRECC method. *Geriatr Med Today* 8:70–78, 1989.

Tinetti ME: A performance-oriented assessment of mobility problems in the elderly. *J Am Geriatr Soc* 34:119–126, 1986.

Tinetti ME, Baker DI, McAvay G, et al: A multifactorial intervention to reduce the risk of falling among elderly people living in the community. *N Engl J Med* 331:821–827, 1994.

Tinetti ME, Williams TF, Mayewsky R: Fall risk index for elderly patients based on number of chronic disabilities. *Am J Med* 80:429–434, 1986.

Wolf SL, Barnhart HX, Kutner NG, McNeely E, Coogler C, Xu T, Atlanta FICSIT Group: Reducing frailty and falls in older persons: An investigation of Tai Chi and computerized balance training. *J Am Geriatr Soc* 44:489–497, 1996.

Wolfson LI, Whipple R, Amerman P, Kleinberg A: Stressing the postural response: A quantitative method for testing balance. *J Am Geriatr Soc* 34:845–850, 1986.

CHAPTER

SEVENTEEN

SENSORY DEPRIVATION

We live in an environment in which our senses are constantly being bombarded by a series of stimuli. Woodburn Heron demonstrated that when college students were placed in an environment devoid of sensory stimuli, their cognitive abilities deteriorated within 24 hours. The students were also more likely to accept the arguments of others. By 48 hours they developed hallucinations and perceptual distortions in this environment. Even the best of long-term care institutions tend to promote states of inactivity that can interact with age-related perceptual changes to result in the development of a sensory deprivation syndrome. **Table 17-1** lists the major features of the sensory deprivation syndrome, which occurs because of lack of stimulation of one or more of the senses: hearing, vision, touch, kinesthesis, smell, and taste. Loss of these senses is often coupled with

Table 17-1 Features of the sensory deprivation syndrome

Decreased quality of life	Inappropriate sexual behavior
Decreased cognition	Withdrawal
Hallucinations	Altered body image
Perceptual distortions	Agitation
Delusions	Incontinence
Emotional lability	Muscle atrophy
Submissiveness	Constipation
Dependent behaviour	Osteopenia
Decreased attention span	Decreased immune system responsiveness
Decreased sociability	Fear of abandonment and death

forced physical inactivity or excessive dependence on others to carry out activities of daily living (ADL).

Little formal information is available on the sensory deprivation syndrome in nursing homes (NHs). Oster developed a program that included brief psychotherapy focused on the prevention of regression and development of increasing independence. The program included reality orientation, enhanced environmental stimuli, ludotherapy (therapy to promote group cohesiveness and interpersonal relations), proprioceptive stimulation, musical therapy for auditory stimulation, bedside visiting, a fiscal responsibility program, intensive concentration on improving activities of daily living, and an active resident council. This comprehensive intervention subjectively improved cognition, memory, attention span, and orientation; it also enhanced interpersonal interactions and increased critical and challenging behaviors by the resident.

In this chapter the major sensory impairments that affect NH residents will be discussed. Taste and its effects on nutritional status are discussed briefly in Chapter 13.

HEARING

Approximately one in four persons over the age of 65 suffers from hearing impairment. Ninety percent of persons over 90 years of age have a hearing deficit. The reported prevalence of hearing impairment in NHs averages 70 percent (range 46 to 100 percent). Hearing impairment has been associated with significant emotional, social, and communication deficits as well as with social isolation. Cognitive impairment may be mistakenly identified when mental status tests are administered verbally to hearing-impaired individuals. Hearing loss can result in irritable or unsociable behavior and apparent inattentiveness. Paranoid ideation has also been associated with hearing loss.

The common causes of hearing loss in older NH residents are listed in **Table 17-2**. There is no change in cerumen production with advancing age. Cerumen impaction occurs in older persons because of a decrease in the cerumen-producing glands, which results in a reduction in moisture in the external auditory canal. In men, large vibrissae (hairs) may also become entangled with the wax. Cerumen impaction can be prevented by regularly placing mineral oil or 6.5 percent carbamide peroxide drops in the ear. This approach is contraindicated when there is a history of tympanic membrane perforation or chronic ear disease.

Middle ear diseases such as otitis media occur no more commonly in older than in younger individuals. Arthritic changes of the ossicular chain are extremely common in persons over age 70 but have not been shown to correlate with conductive hearing loss.

Major causes of inner ear hearing loss in the older population include presbycusis, vascular insufficiency, neoplasms, Meniere's disease, and ototox-

Table 17-2 Causes of hearing loss in the nursing home

Conductive	Sensorineural
External auditory canal	Presbycusis
Cerumen impaction	Vascular insufficiency
Foreign bodies	Meniere's disease
Otitis externa	Acoustic neuroma
Tumors	Hypothyroidism
Middle ear	Collagen-vascular disorders
Otitis media	Ototoxicity
Tympanic membrane perforation	Aminoglycoside antibodies
Otosclerosis	Nonsteroidal anti-inflammatory drugs
Cholesteatoma	Salicylates
	Quinine
	Quinidine
	Furosemide, ethacrynic acid, and bumetanide
	Topical aural antibiotics

icity. Presbycusis is the most common cause of hearing loss with advancing age. It primarily affects high tones and is bilateral. For many NH residents with hearing impairment, consonants with energy in the range 2000–8000 Hz, such as "s," "sh," "v," "t," and "b" are frequently misheard. As a result, residents often conclude that other people are not speaking clearly when, in reality, the problem is faulty consonant perception. Asymmetric sensorineural hearing loss should be evaluated in order to exclude an acoustic neuroma. Sudden sensorineural hearing loss is usually vascular in origin and should be treated as an emergency with a combination of histamine, niacin, propantheline bromide, and prednisone; this regimen may sometimes preserve some hearing. Full evaluation is then carried out after 2 weeks of steroid therapy. This saves an extensive workup in those who have either mild vascular disease or who recover spontaneously. Those who have previously undergone stapes surgery require exploration for a perilymphatic fistula.

Two tools are available for identifying hearing-impaired older persons: the Hearing Handicap Inventory for the Elderly (HHIE) and the Welch–Allyn audioscope. We have adapted the HHIE for use in the NH (**Table 17-3**). A score of 0 to 4 suggests an extremely low likelihood of hearing impairment, while a score above 13 suggests a very high probability of hearing impairment. The hand-held Welch–Allyn audioscope (**Fig. 17-1**) is an excellent instrument with which to screen for hearing impairment. It delivers a 40 dB tone at frequencies of 500, 1000, 2000, and 4000 Hz. Hearing impairment can be defined as a 40 dB loss at the 1000 or 2000 Hz frequency in both ears or a 40 dB loss at the 1000 and 2000 Hz frequencies in one ear. The audioscope has approximately a 94 percent sensitivity and a 72 percent specificity for the detection of hearing loss when it is used in a quiet room.

Table 17-3 Hearing handicap inventory for the elderly (adapted for nursing home residents)

Does a hearing problem cause you to feel embarrassed or upset when you meet new people?
Does a hearing problem cause you to feel frustrated when you are talking?
Do you have difficulty in hearing when someone speaks in a whisper?
Do you feel handicapped by a hearing problem?
Does a hearing problem cause you difficulty when you are talking to friends, family, or staff?
Does a hearing problem cause you to go to religious services less often than you would like?
Does a hearing problem cause you to have arguments?
Does a hearing problem cause you difficulty when you are listening to television or radio?
Do you feel that any difficulty with your hearing limits or hampers your social life with other residents?
Does a hearing problem cause you difficulty when you are in the nursing home dining room?

Note: All responses can be scored "yes" (2 points), "sometimes" (1 point), or "no" (0 points). A score of 13 suggests hearing impairment.

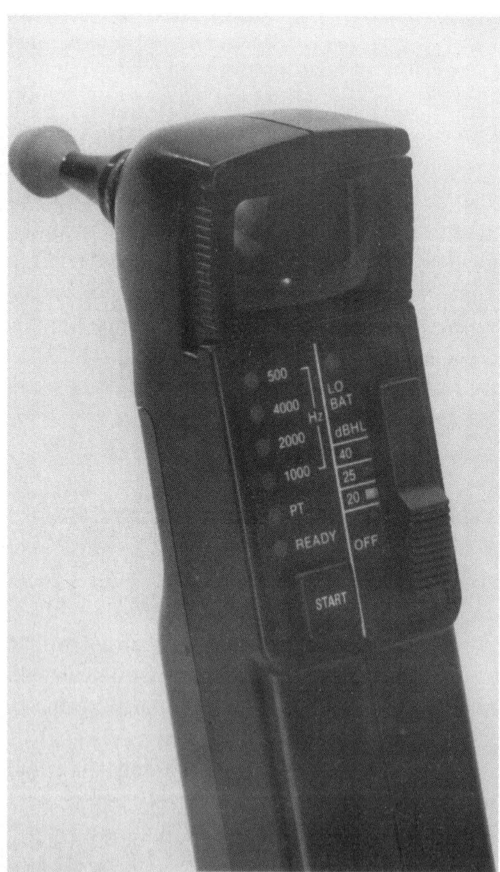

Figure 17-1 The Welch–Allyn audioscope. This device delivers a 400 dB tone at frequencies of 500, 1000, 2000, and 4000 Hz. It is useful in screening for hearing impairment.

A screening program utilizing the Welch–Allyn audioscope in a Veterans Administration (VA) NH yielded the following results: hearing was found to be impaired in 38 percent of the residents screened; of these 25 percent had cerumen impaction. After removal of cerumen, 47 percent had improved hearing. Morale scores were increased in 65 percent of the residents after removal of the cerumen. These data illustrate the importance of regular hearing evaluations and wax removal in the NH setting.

All residents with hearing impairment should be evaluated for the potential to benefit from hearing aids. There are three basic types of hearing aids: canal, in-the-ear, and behind-the-ear. In general, the worse the hearing, the larger the hearing aid needed. Some residents will do very well with a simple amplification device (e.g., a Pocketalker). Those with profound hearing impairment may benefit from cochlear implants.

The Minimum Data Set (MDS) Assessment of Communications and Hearing

Assessment of residents' communication and hearing patterns are done upon admission, with hearing aids where applicable, indicating whether the individual hears adequately, has minimal difficulty when not in a quiet setting, or the speaker has to adjust tonal quality and speak distinctly. Absence of useful hearing indicates the highest impairment. **Fig. 17-2** lists the other elements on the MDS addressing techniques of communication and ability to understand.

Physicians should address their findings along these four levels of impairment so the team can develop an appropriate plan of care including aural rehabilitation when appropriate. Communication difficulty will trigger a resident assessment protocol (**Table 17-4**) that may require a physician evaluation and/or referral to an audiologist and/or speech pathologist. Speech pathologists are excellent resources for evaluation of language disorders (e.g., aphasia) which may lead to practical interventions, such as use of a communication board, and caregiver training and education.

Table 17-5 lists examples of assistive devices that may be useful in the NH. A telephone should be available in the NH with a handset amplifier, and hearing impaired residents should be instructed in its use. Classes in speech-reading may be helpful for some NH residents. **Table 17-6** provides suggestions for improving communication in the hearing-impaired NH resident.

VISION

Changes in vision do not cause as great a decrease in social interaction as do hearing impairments. Nevertheless, vision impairment does increase feelings of vulnerability and social isolation, and interferes with some ADLs in the NH population. Legal blindness is defined as a corrected visual acuity in the better

SECTION C. COMMUNICATION/HEARING PATTERNS

1.	HEARING	*(With hearing appliance, if used)* 0. *HEARS ADEQUATELY*—normal talk, TV, phone 1. *MINIMAL DIFFICULTY* when not in quiet setting 2. *HEARS IN SPECIAL SITUATIONS ONLY*—speaker has to adjust tonal quality and speak distinctly 3. *HIGHLY IMPAIRED*/absence of useful hearing	
2.	COMMUNI-CATION DEVICES/ TECH-NIQUES	***(Check all that apply** during last 7 days)* Hearing aid, present and used Hearing aid, present and not used regularly Other receptive comm. techniques used (e.g., lip reading) *NONE OF ABOVE*	a. b. c. d.
3.	MODES OF EXPRESSION	***(Check all used** by resident to make needs known)* Speech a. — Signs/gestures/sounds d. Writing messages to express or clarify needs b. — Communication board e. American sign language or Braille c. — Other f. *NONE OF ABOVE* g.	
4.	MAKING SELF UNDER-STOOD	*(Expressing information content—however able)* 0. *UNDERSTOOD* 1. *USUALLY UNDERSTOOD*—difficulty finding words or finishing thoughts 2. *SOMETIMES UNDERSTOOD*—ability is limited to making concrete requests 3. *RARELY/NEVER UNDERSTOOD*	
5.	SPEECH CLARITY	*(Code for speech in the **last 7 days**)* 0. *CLEAR SPEECH*—distinct, intelligible words 1. *UNCLEAR SPEECH*—slurred, mumbled words 2. *NO SPEECH*—absence of spoken words	
6.	ABILITY TO UNDER-STAND OTHERS	*(Understanding verbal information content—however able)* 0. *UNDERSTANDS* 1. *USUALLY UNDERSTANDS*—may miss some part/intent of message 2. *SOMETIMES UNDERSTANDS*—responds adequately to simple, direct communication 3. *RARELY/NEVER UNDERSTANDS*	
7.	CHANGE IN COMMUNI-CATION/ HEARING	Resident's ability to express, understand, or hear information has changed as compared to status of **90 days ago** (or since last assessment if less than 90 days) 0. No change 1. Improved 2. Deteriorated	

Figure 17-2 MDS assessment of communication and hearing patterns.

eye of 20/200 or worse or when vision is restricted to 20 diopters in its widest diameter. Three percent of persons over the age of 85 in the United States are blind. In NHs approximately 25 percent of the residents are legally blind.

Presbyopia is the commonest eye complaint of older persons. Presbyopia is the inability to focus clearly at normal reading distances due to thickening of the anteroposterior diameter of the lens. Some persons with presbyopia may be able to read again without bifocals ("second sight"). This is due to the development of myopia, which is often related to the development of cataracts.

Sudden visual loss is an ophthalmic emergency. Individuals with sudden visual loss will have a Marcus–Gunn pupillary response (i.e., illumination of the nonblind eye will result in bilateral pupillary constriction, while illumination of the blind eye immediately thereafter will result in apparent bilateral pupillary dilatation). If this is not present, hysterical blindness is a possibility. The causes of sudden visual loss are listed in **Table 17-7**. Care should be taken not to use

Table 17-4 Key aspects of the communication resident assessment protocol (RAP)

Factors	Problems to be considered
Cognitive	Within last 90 days has there been a decline in: a. Level of consciousness? b. Cognitive skill for daily decision making? c. Short or long term memory? d. Thinking/awareness and/or recall?
ADL function	Within last 90 days has there been a decrease in: a. Self performance? b. Amount of support needed? c. Body control problems? d. ADL potential?
Mood	Within last 90 days has there been an increase in mood problems?
Components of communication	Hearing a. Hears adequately b. Hears with minimal difficulty c. Hears in special situations only d. Has highly impaired hearing Vision a. Has visual limitations b. Has visual appliances Communication devices a. Hearing aid, present and used b. Hearing aid, present and not used c. Reading lips Modes of expression a. Speech b. Writing c. Signs/gestures/sounds d. Communication board Within last 90 days has there been: a. Change in the resident's ability to express, understand or hear information? b. Any discharge or cerumen accumulation?
Chronic conditions	Does resident have a chronic condition that causes a communication deficit?
Transitory conditions	Does resident have an acute or temporary condition that causes a communication deficit (e.g., delirium, depression)?
Medications	Are there medications in use that could cause or complicate communication deficit (e.g., psychotropics)?
Communication	Is resident communicating at level and frequency of ability?
Treatment or evaluation history	Has resident received an evaluation by an audiologist and/or speech/language pathologist? Did evaluation result in a plan of care? Has resident's condition deteriorated since the most recent evaluation?

Table 17-5 Assistive devices for the hearing impaired

Telephone handset amplifiers
Television
- Television caption units
- Infrared sensor with individual volume control (Sennheister, Sound Plus; resident wears headset that picks up sound anywhere in the room; no connection to TV set)
- TV listening loop (allow individual to plug in listening device at different parts of room)
- Direct audio input connection (connected to TV)
- Dynamic pillow speaker

Personal amplification devices
- Electronic stethoscopes
- Pocket talker
- Direct audio input
- Multipurpose communicator (for group meetings)
- Hand-held communicator (allows directional input)

Table 17-6 Improving communication for hearing-impaired nursing home residents

Between resident and caregiver
- Screen all residents for hearing impairment
- Reduce or eliminate background noise. Close doors and turn off TV or running water.
- Face the listener. Keep your face at the level of the listener's eyes. Maintain eye contact.
- Allow adequate light to fall on your face.
- Give the listener a clear view of your face. Keep hands or other objects down. Avoid chewing gum. Beards or mustaches should be well trimmed so as not to interfere with speech reading.
- Use facial expression and gestures to convey meaning.
- Avoid talking while writing or walking around the room.
- Gain the person's attention before beginning to speak.
- Speak in a normal tone of voice or slightly louder.
- Shouting does not help because loss is not simply a reduction in loudness. Making voice slightly deeper sometimes improves hearing.
- Speak clearly, a little more slowly, in short sentences, using simple words.
- Because the person may not admit to a handicap, have the person repeat to be sure the message was understood.
- Be redundant: repeat or rephrase in a different way. Write key words if the person can read.
- If the individual has a hearing aid, learn how to help him or her with it.
- Learn how to use assistive listening devices. Have an amplifier available for important communications.
- Arrange for the individual to have a vision exam.
- Teach lip reading.

In the environment
- Consult with your audiologist for evaluation of background noise in social gathering areas and request ideas on how to reduce or eliminate competing noise.
- Arrange seating in small groups, preferably in circles or at round tables.
- In large meetings, have speakers provide outlines for residents to review.
- Seek help from outside resources such as a local SHHH (Self-Help for Hard-of-Hearing People, Inc.).[a]

[a]These groups encourage identification of persons with hearing losses, provide education, foster public programs, engage hearing-impaired participants in communication, urge participation in daily activities, and help hearing-aid users cope because hearing aids do not do the entire job.

Source: Voeks et al: *J Am Geriatr Soc* 38:141, 1990, with minor modifications.

Table 17-7 Causes of sudden visual loss

Monocular loss
- Painless
  - Subretinal hemorrhage (macular degeneration)
  - Occlusion of central retinal or vein
  - Retinal detachment
  - Ischermic optic neuritis
  - Vitreous hemorrhage (diabetic retinopathy)
- Painful
  - Glaucoma (angle-closure)
  - Temporal arteritis

Binocular loss
- Bilateral occipital lobe infarcts

Table 17-8 Potential causes of common visual complaints in nursing home residents

Blepharoptosis
- Myasthenia gravis
- Horner's syndrome (Pancoast tumor or tuberculosis)
- Hyperhtyroidism
- Normal aging

Periocular pain
- Sinusitis
- Herpes zoster
- Tic douloreux
- Migraine
- Intracranial aneurysm

Painful red eye
- Angle-closure glaucoma
- Bacterial corneal ulcers
- Herpes simplex (may not be painful)

Painless red eye
- Viral conjunctivitis
- Chamydial conjunctivitis
- Bacterial conjunctivitis
- Allergy
- Subconjunctival hemorrhage

Diplopia
- III, IV, VI cranial nerve palsies
- Cataracts (monocular diplopia)
- Vertebrobasilar artery insufficiency
- Myasthenia gravis
- Eaton-Lambert syndrome

Flashing lights/floaters
- Vitreous detachment
- Retinal tear

Visual hallucinations
- Brain tumor
- Cortical ischemia
- Sensory deprivation
- Schizophrenia

Purulent discharge
- Bacterial conjunctivitis

topical steroids in patients with red eyes. Examples of other common visual complaints of NH residents and their causes are listed in **Table 17-8.**

The major causes of gradual visual loss in older people are cataracts, glaucoma, macular degeneration, and diabetic retinopathy. Individuals with cataracts complain of generalized blurred vision; those with glaucoma have blurred peripheral vision; and those with macular degeneration have blurred central vision.

The diagnosis of glaucoma is made by the combination of an increased intraocular pressure (greater than 23 mmHg), an increase in the optic cup-to-disk ratio, and the presence of visual field defects. All NH residents should have their intraocular pressure measured on a yearly basis with a Schiotz indentation tonometer after the eye has been anesthetized with a local anesthetic. The vast majority of individuals with glaucoma have the open-angle version, which is best treated with a combination of eye drops (e.g., timolol, which decreases aqueous humor formation, and/or pilocarpine, a miotic which decreases resistance to the outflow of aqueous humor). Systemic medications that include carbonic anhydrase inhibitors are also sometimes used. It should be remembered that instillation of eye drops into the conjunctival sac is the equivalent of an intravenous infusion of the drug and can result in systemic side effects such as bradycardia. Paresthesias, anorexia, confusion, depression, and drowsiness can all be side effects of carbonic anhydrase inhibitors.

Age-related macular degeneration is diagnosed by the presence of macular degeneration and multiple pale-yellow spots (drusen). Residents with macular degeneration should be referred to an ophthalmologist, as some may benefit from laser photocoagulation. Although there is some controversy, it appears that the rate of deterioration of macular degeneration may be slowed by the administration of zinc sulfate 220 mg three times per day.

Visuospatial abnormalities and the inability to distinguish moving objects clearly have been identified in patients with Alzheimer's disease. These deficits can result in startle reactions. Following stroke, the presence of homonymous hemianopia may be associated with hemineglect. Hemineglect may result in behaviors such as failing to shave one side of the face. Hemineglect may also lead to falls due to ignoring objects in the way of the neglected side. NH residents with hemineglect require intensive stimulation, frequent reminders, and occupational therapy to help restore care for the neglected side.

Age-related changes in the lens (yellowing and opacity) and diabetes mellitus may result in problems with color vision. This can cause residents to dress in poorly coordinated clothes. Changes in color vision with age can also interfere with the ability of NH residents to follow simple color codes. Cataracts can result in severe glare in bright light, which may further impair color vision.

A number of strategies that may help to compensate for visual problems among NH residents are outlined in **Table 17-9. Table 17-10** lists some of the adaptive devices that may be useful to the visually impaired.

Minimum Data Set (MDS) Assessment of Vision Patterns

This assessment is conducted in the best conditions with residents' corrective lenses and adequate light. It uses newspaper print in lieu of formal vision charts, and indicates four degrees of visual functioning/impairment (**Fig. 17-3**). Preliminary studies show poor correlation between MDS vision assessment and

Table 17-9 Adaptive strategies to compensate for visual problems in the nursing home

Object placement

Avoid a cluttered environment.
Keep furniture in same placement. If changes are made, inform residents.
Place food and utensils in the same place on the tray every day.
Keep clothes and objects in the resident's room in the same place.

Lighting

Make sure light is consistent throughout the building and evenly distributed throughout each room.
Use increased bulb wattage.
Have dimmer switches in rooms for residents with cataracts.
Use window blinds to control light.
Have night lights available.
Use fluorescent or brightly colored tape around electrical outlets, light switches, and doorknobs.
Use cups and glasses with contrasting rims.

Color

Light objects should be placed on dark surfaces, and vice versa.
Contrasting color coding may be useful (use distinctly different colors).

Other

Offer residents repeated and unhurried orientation to surroundings.
Identify yourself when you are approaching the resident.

Source: Adapted from Hooyman NR, Lustbader W: *Taking Care of Your Aging Family Members*. New York, The Free Press, 1986.

Table 17.10 Adaptive devices available for residents with visual impairments

- Magnifying glasses
- Large-print books and newspapers
- Magnifying television screen systems
- Talking books[a]
- Computer-operated voice synthesizers that read from books
- Audiotape cassettes for correspondence
- Radio stations with special programming for the visually impaired
- Large-print telephone directories
- Self-threading needles
- Adaptive clothing—zippers, Velcro openers, large buttons
- Braille watches/talking clocks
- Adapted games
- Telephone adaptations for the visually impaired (e.g., giant push-button adapters or call makers)
- Braille or other coded markings at entrances to commonly used rooms

[a]Available from the Library of Congress; the National Federation of the Blind; or Books on Tape, Newport Beach, CA 92660.

SECTION D. VISION PATTERNS

1.	VISION	*(Ability to see in adequate light and with glasses if used)* 0. *ADEQUATE*—sees fine detail, including regular print in newspapers/books 1. *IMPAIRED*—sees large print, but not regular print in newspapers/books 2. *MODERATELY IMPAIRED*—limited vision; not able to see newspaper headlines, but can identify objects 3. *HIGHLY IMPAIRED*—object identification in question, but eyes appear to follow objects 4. *SEVERELY IMPAIRED*—no vision or sees only light, colors, or shapes; eyes do not appear to follow objects	
2.	VISUAL LIMITATIONS/ DIFFICULTIES	Side vision problems—decreased peripheral vision (e.g., leaves food on one side of tray, difficulty traveling, bumps into people and objects, misjudges placement of chair when seating self)	a.
		Experiences any of following: sees halos or rings around lights; sees flashes of light; sees "curtains" over eyes	b.
		NONE OF ABOVE	c.
3.	VISUAL APPLIANCES	Glasses; contact lenses; magnifying glass 0. No 1. Yes	

Figure 17-3 MDS assessment of vision patterns.

objective direct examinations by an eye care practitioner. Impairment with significant impact on functioning (e.g., mobility, reading, television viewing) should be further evaluated for existence of specific diagnoses that cause visual impairment (e.g., glaucoma, macular degeneration). **Table 17-11** summarizes the RAP for vision.

THE SKIN SENSES

Development of sensory neuropathies can decrease the individual's awareness of the environment. NH residents with neuropathies may benefit from utilizing highly textured objects. Rubber thimbles or rubber-tipped pencils may help these people to turn pages. Increased intensity of touch may be necessary when residents have lost deep touch. Vigorous massage may also restore a sense of adequate tactile sensation. The resident's response to a handclasp can identify the need for touch. The person who clings is clearly seeking increased touch. Touch can decrease anxiety, increase self-esteem, create a trusting relationship, and express caring and concern.

KINESTHESIS

Kinesthesis is the ability to recognize the position and movements of body parts without visual aid. Advancing age is associated with cerebellar dysfunction and a resultant failure to allow adequate discrimination of body movements. Passive movements for NH residents who are bed-bound or have had a stroke can help

Table 17-11 Key aspects of the vision resident assessment protocol (RAP)

Factors	Problems to be considered
Medications	Is resident receiving eye medication? IF YES, is resident experiencing any side effect?
Diagnosis	Does resident have: a. Cataracts? b. Glaucoma? c. Macular degeneration? d. Diabetes?
Neurological diagnosis or dementia	Is there a diagnosis related to perceptual vision problem? Are visual difficulties related to new environment?
Appropriate use of visual appliances	Does resident wear glasses? Are the lenses of glasses clean and free of scratches? Were glasses recently lost? Are glasses missing?
Functional need for eye exam/new glasses	Does resident have visual problems that impede his or her ability to: a. Eat? b. Walk on unit? c. Interact with other? Is resident's ability to recognize staff limited by visual problems? Does resident have problems with: a. Negotiating environment? b. Participating in self-care activities? Does resident: a. Report difficulty seeing TV/reading material of interest? b. Express interest in improved vision? Has resident refused to have eyes examined?
Environmental modifications	Does the resident's environment enable maximum visual function (e.g., glare on floors or table surfaces, lack of night lights)? Has the environment been adapted to resident's individual needs (e.g., large print signs marking room, color coded tape on dresser drawers, larger numbers on telephones) Could the resident be more independent with different: a. Visual cues (e.g., labeling items, task segmentation)? b. Other sensory cues (e.g., cane for locating objects in path)?
Other acute problems	Has the resident experienced: a. Eye pain? b. Blurry vision? c. Double vision? d. Sudden loss of vision?

to maintain kinesthetic sense. Upright posture using a tiltboard or waist support can also help to maintain the sense of equilibrium. Regular walking for chairbound residents or water exercises (where a pool is available) can serve a similar function.

SUGGESTED READINGS

Sensory Deprivation

Oster C: Sensory deprivation in geriatric patients. *J Am Geriatr Soc* 24:461, 1976.

Hearing

Jerger, J, Chmiel, R, Wilson, N, et al. Hearing impairment in older adults: New concepts. *J Am Geriatr Soc* 43:928–935, 1995.

Lichtenstein MJ, Bess FM, Logan SA: Validation of screening tools for identifying hearing-impaired elderly in primary care. *JAMA* 259:2875, 1988.

Mhoon E: Otology, in Cassel CK, Riesenberg DE, Sorensen LB, Walsh JR (eds): *Geriatric Medicine*, 2d ed. New York, Springer-Verlag, 1990, p 403.

Mulrow CD, Aguilar C, Endicott JE, et al: Association between hearing impairment and quality of life of elderly individuals. *J Am Geriatr Soc* 38:45, 1990.

Mulrow CD, Aguilar C, Endicott JE, et al: Quality-of-life changes and hearing impairment: A randomized trial. *Ann Intern Med* 113:188–194, 1990.

Mulrow, CD, Lichtenstein, MJ: Screening for hearing impairment in the elderly: Rationale and strategy. *J Gen Int Med* 6:249–258, 1991.

Nadol, Jr., JB: Hearing loss. *N Engl J Med* 329:1092–1102, 1993.

Uhlmann, RF, Larson EB, Rees TS, et al: Relationship of hearing impairment to dementia and cognitive dysfunction in older adults. *JAMA* 261:1916–1919, 1989.

Voeks SV, Gallagher CM, Langer EH, Drinka PJ: Hearing loss in the nursing home. *J Am Geriatr Soc* 38:141, 1990.

Vision

Hooyman NR, Lustbader W: *Taking Care of Your Aging Family Members*. New York, The Free Press, 1986.

Kollarits CR: The aging eye, in Calkins E, Davis PJ, Ford AB (eds): *The Practice of Geriatrics*. Philadelphia, Saunders, 1986, p 268.

Marx, MS, Werner, P, Cohen-Mansfield, J, et al: The relationship between low vision and performance of activities of daily living in nursing home residents. *J Am Geriatr Soc*, 40:1018–1020, 1992.

Mehelas TJ, Kliess RD, Kollarits CR, et al: Visual loss in geriatric residents of northwestern Ohio nursing homes. *Ohio State Med Assoc J* (March Issue):235, 1984.

Sturgess I, Rudd AG, Shilling J: Unrecognized visual problems amongst residents of Part III homes. *Age Ageing* 23:54–56, 1994.

CHAPTER
EIGHTEEN

ENDOCRINE AND METABOLIC PROBLEMS

Endocrine and metabolic problems are not rare among nursing home (NH) residents. This chapter will briefly discuss the practical considerations of managing these problems in the NH setting.

THYROID DISORDERS

A number of studies have demonstrated a fairly high prevalence of hypo- and hyperthyroidism in older individuals with medical illnesses. The prevalence of overt hypothyroidism ranges from 0.7 percent to 9.4 percent and of overt hyperthyroidism from 0.3 percent to 3.0 percent. Hypothyroidism has also been found to occur in up to 5 percent of patients with dementia. Based on these data, screening for thyroid disease would appear to be appropriate in all new admissions to a NH and thereafter on a yearly basis.

Clinical acumen plays no role in the diagnosis of hypo- or hyperthyroidism in the frail, older NH resident. Many NH residents suffer from the classical signs and symptoms of hypothyroidism due to the interaction of disease and aging processes rather than from true hypothyroidism. In addition, hyperthyroidism may present in an apathetic manner, with blepharoptosis instead of exophthalmos, anorexia instead of hyperphagia, depression instead of anxiety or agitation, weight loss, proximal muscle myopathy, heart failure, and atrial fibrillation. For these reasons we recommend regular biochemical screening for thyroid disease in the NH setting.

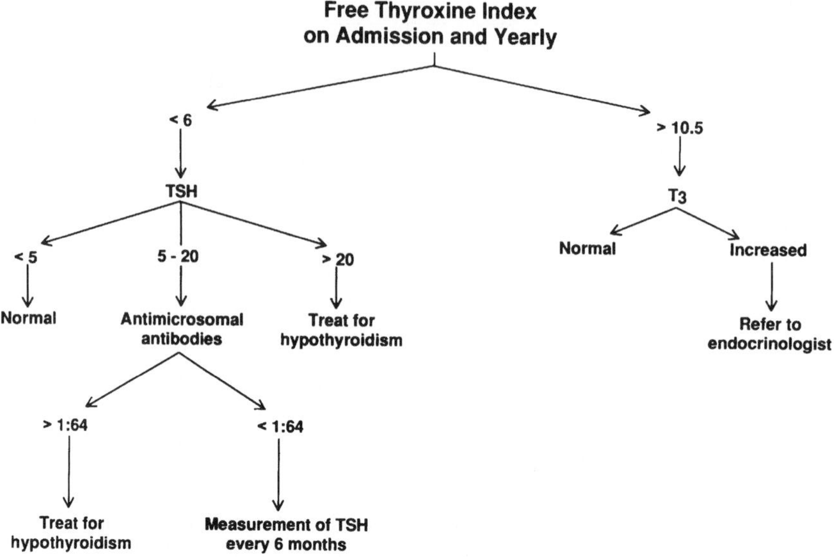

Figure 18-1 Approach to screening for thyroid dysfunction in the nursing home.

Figure 18-1 summarizes the approach to screening for thyroid dysfunction in the NH. Initial biochemical screening consists of thyroxine (T_4) and a triiodothyronine uptake (T_3U). When the T_3U uptake is normalized and multiplied by the T_4, a free thyroxine index is generated. For screening purposes, a narrower normal range than that reported by the laboratory is recommended (i.e., 6 to 10.5). When the value is greater than 10.5, a free triiodothyronine (T_3) level should be obtained to exclude T_3 toxicosis. When the value is below 6, a thyroid stimulating hormone (TSH) level should be obtained. If the TSH level is greater than 20 mIU/ml, the diagnosis of hypothyroidism is made and treatment should be instituted. Values between 5 and 20 mIU/ml are in a borderline zone and may revert to normal. In these cases antimicrosomal thyroid antibodies should be obtained. If the titer is 1:64 or less, the resident can be followed with TSH levels every 6 months. If the titer is greater than 1:64, the resident should be started on thyroid replacement, because individuals with the titer above this level have a higher probability of becoming hypothyroid. The supersensitive TSH assay is not recommended as a primary screen in NH residents, as illnesses and circulating antibodies decrease its sensitivity and specificity, making it less cost-effective for screening for thyroid dysfunction.

A major problem in the diagnosis of thyroid dysfunction in sick persons is the development of the "euthyroid sick syndrome." Illness can generate thyroid function tests similar to those seen in hypothyroidism. **Table 18-1** distinguishes between the euthyroid sick syndrome and hypothyroidism. Acute psychiatric illnesses can result in elevated thyroxine and/or triiodothyroxine levels.

Table 18-1 Comparison of thyroid function tests in the euthyroid sick syndrome, hypothyroidism, and the sick hypothyroid patient

	Euthyroid sick syndrome	Hypothyroid	Sick hypothyroid
Thyroxine (T_4)	Normal or decreased	Decreased	Decreased
Triiodothyronine (T_3)	Very low ($<$ng/dl)	Low normal	Very low
T_3 uptake (T_3U)	Increased	Decreased	Normal
Thyrotropin (TSH)	Normal, increased, or decreased	Increased	Increased or high normal

Depression may be associated with low thyroid hormone levels. A variety of drugs can also interfere with thyroid function tests. Beta blockers can produce an elevated free thyroxine index. Phenytoin, salicylates, and furosemide can result in a spuriously low free thyroxine index. Iodine-containing cough mixtures can result in suppressed thyroid function. Radioiodine contrast agents can result in an elevation in thyroxine and in an older person who is iodine-deficient, leading to iodine-induced thyrotoxicosis. The antiarrhythmic agent amiodarone (an iodine-containing drug) has both induced thyrotoxicosis and produced thyroid function tests consistent with hypothyroidism.

When thyroxine-binding globulin levels are abnormal, the free thyroxine index is usually normal because of the T_3 uptake value. A rare dysalbuminemia syndrome, which results in albumin with an abnormal avidity for binding thyroxine, may cause an elevated free thyroxine index in the presence of a normal triiodothyronine level.

Isolated T_4 toxicosis can occur in some older persons whose concomitant illness has suppressed their ability to convert T_4 to T_3. The TSH response at 30 minutes to 500 μmg of thyrotropin-releasing hormone (TRH) may be helpful in this situation. If the TSH is greater than 5 mIU/ml at 30 minutes, thyrotoxicosis is not present. A flat TSH response to TRH, however, does not necessarily indicate thyrotoxicosis, because aging, illness, and depression can all result in a flat response.

Treatment of hypothyroidism in the older individual involves slowly increasing L-thyroxine dosage from 25 μmg per day by 12.5 μmg every week to a dose between 50 and 100 μmg (0.05 to 0.10 mg) per day. Overreplacement of thyroid hormone may temporarily increase alertness but in the long run leads to an increased propensity for osteoporosis and muscle weakness. Older persons usually need a lower replacement dose of thyroid hormone as there is a decrease in plasma clearance rate of thyroxine with advancing age. Thyroid extract should not be used because of poor standardization from batch to batch. A TSH should be measured every 8 weeks until the TSH is below 5 mIU/ml. At this stage a thyroxine level should be checked and the resident should be maintained on 6 to 8 mg/dl.

Older individuals with hyperthyroidism should be treated with radioactive iodine. Beta blockers can be used to give temporary symptomatic relief. Some individuals with apathetic hyperthyroidism benefit symptomatically from treatment with an antidepressant. Goiter (an enlarged thyroid gland) is often seen in older individuals, particularly in those who were not exposed to sufficient iodine in the diet when they were growing up (i.e., those from some areas of the Midwest and Appalachian regions). If the individual is not biochemically hyperthyroid, the goiter is multinodular, and no symptoms of tracheal compression are present, the goiter should be ignored. With a large goiter and dyspnea, a computed tomography (CT) scan of the trachea to demonstrate narrowing or a ventilation flow-loop study may be useful.

Solitary thyroid nodules are at risk for being malignant. Approximately 5 percent of females over 50 years of age have a solitary nodule. The incidence of thyroid cancer falls rapidly after the age of 50 and most nodules are adenomas or cysts. Most thyroid cancers are of the follicular or papillary type and have a relatively benign course, though they tend to behave more aggressively in older individuals. Anaplastic thyroid carcinomas increase in prevalence with advancing age such that, by 80 years of age, half of the thyroid cancers are anaplastic.

Given these facts, how should one treat the solitary thyroid nodule in a NH resident? If, on admission to the NH, a solitary thyroid nodule is found, it should be observed at 3 and 6 months. If it is enlarging, the resident should be referred for a fine needle aspiration. If a new thyroid nodule is detected, fine needle biopsy is indicated because of the higher possibility of anaplastic cancer. It is, therefore, important that on admission to the NH the presence or absence of thyroid nodules be carefully documented.

DIABETES MELLITUS

Diabetes mellitus occurs commonly in older individuals. Approximately 20 percent to 30 percent of NH residents have diabetes mellitus. In addition, diabetes mellitus often leads to NH admission at a younger age. Major factors resulting in the increased admission of diabetics to NHs are blindness and amputations.

The increased propensity of older individuals to develop dehydration due to failure to perceive thirst puts the NH resident at particular risk of developing hyperosmolar coma. Minor infections (urinary tract, respiratory, sinuses) can often precipitate a rapid increase in blood glucose levels. For this reason, special attention must to be paid to the hydration of diabetic NH residents. The outcome for hyperosmolar coma is particularly poor among those hospitalized from NHs. Recently it has been recognized that many older persons with hyperosmolar coma have a mixed picture with some degree of ketoacidosis. Some older diabetics with type II diabetes mellitus develop pancreatic exhaustion and can develop diabetic ketoacidosis.

Hypoglycemia is an ever-present problem in NH residents receiving treatment for their diabetes. However, recent studies have suggested that if the physician aims generally to maintain the blood glucose between 100 to 200 mg/dl, hypoglycemia is rarely a problem in the NH. NH staff should be instructed to pay special attention to behavior changes (lethargy or agitation) in diabetic residents. Diabetic residents with abrupt behavioral changes should immediately receive sugar and the blood glucose level should be checked. Where possible, nursing staff should be allowed to administer 50 ml of 50 percent dextrose when starting an intravenous line on a diabetic resident suspected of being hypoglycemic. In addition, diabetic NH residents should have a standing order for 1 mg of glucagon intramuscularly in case of hypoglycemia associated with confusion and/or lethargy.

Table 18-2 lists the reasons for maintaining relatively good glucose control among diabetic NH residents. Blood glucose should be controlled before using pentoxifylline (Trental) to treat intermittent claudication in diabetics. It should be remembered that to see improvement in the symptoms of intermittent claudication, treatment for hyperglycemia must have been instituted for at least 120 days. Recent studies have suggested that depression may occur more commonly in older persons with diabetes mellitus, and the presence of depression may be directly related to poorer outcomes in diabetics. A number of studies have demonstrated that diabetics are more likely to complain of pain. This appears to be due to elevated glucose levels, which prevent a normal interaction of beta-endorphin with the opioid receptor.

Diabetics appear to be more likely to develop infections and, in particular, unusual infections. Tuberculosis should always be considered in the older diabetic with chest disease. Malignant otitis externa due to *Pseudomonas aeruginosa* is another example of an unusual infection seen in diabetics. All diabetics should have their pupils dilated and their fundi checked for retinopathy and glaucoma every 6 months. This is best done by the optometrist who visits the NH.

Diabetic amyotrophy is a progressive, painful proximal myopathy with minimal sensory changes. Diabetic neuropathic cachexia is a severe form of this

Table 18-2 Reasons for maintaining good glucose control in diabetic nursing home residents

Reduced incontinence due to diuretic effect of elevated glucose
Improved vision
Decreased platelet adhesiveness (reduces chance of myocardial infarction or stroke)
Improved outcome if a stroke should occur
Decrease in intermittent claudication
Improved cognitive function
Decreased pain perception
Decreased infection (possible)

disorder, which is associated with anorexia and extreme weight loss. Both of these conditions can lead to NH admission, and both often resolve spontaneously within 6 months to 2 years.

Diabetics often have hyperzincuria, which can lead to borderline zinc status. Zinc deficiency can lead to immune deficiency. All diabetic NH residents with ulcers related to peripheral vascular disease or pressure sores should receive zinc supplementation (220 mg three times a day with meals) to promote wound healing.

Table 18-3 outlines an approach to the management of diabetes mellitus in the NH. Chlorpropamide should never be used in the NH, because its long half-life can lead to prolonged hypoglycemia and it has a propensity to produce hyponatremia. The second-generation oral sulfonylureas examples are probably superior to the first-generation agents because of the decreased chances of drug–drug interactions. The choice of an oral agent should include consideration of the cost of the drug. When equal degrees of glucose control are obtained, glyburide and glysizide produce equal amounts of hypoglycemia. Especially higher doses of glysizide are needed to produce euglycemia and in a managed care situation switching from glypizide to glyburide resulted in substantial cost savings.

Table 18-3 Approach to management of diabetes mellitus in the nursing home

1. Diagnosis
   - Two fasting blood glucoses >140 mg/dl or
   - Two random blood glucoses >200 mg/dl
2. Initial management
   - Drug therapy
     - Low dose generation agent (e.g., glyburide 2.5 mg daily or glipizide 5 mg daily)
     - Increase dose twice weekly until glucoses are consistently 100–200 mg/dl
   - Diet
     - No added free sugar (ADA diabetic diet unneccessary unless resident has been on it long-term)
   - Exercise program compatible with resident's abilities
3. If inadequate response to maximal doses of oral agents (i.e., glyburide 10 mg daily or glipizide 20 mg daily)
   - Institute insulin therapy
     - NPH in the morning
     - Regular or NPH later in the day if necessary
4. Monitor glucose daily until stable with values >70 mg/dl and <200 mg/dl
5. Monitor glucose at least weekly by finger stick when resident is stable
6. Having standing orders for
   - Giving Glucoloa for glucose <50 mg/dl
   - Giving Glucagon 1 mg IM if glucose <30 mg/dl or if acute confusion or delirium occurs
7. When acute illness intervene, monitor glucose more frequently to detect stress-induced hyperglycemia

Glynase is a reformulated glyburide. Approximately 3 mg of glynase is equivalent to 5 mg of glyburide. The unique presstab formation makes it easier and more accurate to break in half when low doses are needed. Acarbose is an alpha-1-glucosidase inhibitor that slows the breakdown of carbohydrate in the gut resulting in slowed absorption of glucose and a smoothing out of the postprandial glycemic curve. Acarbose is particularly useful in persons who have large swings in glucose levels following a meal. The major side effect of acarbose is excessive gas formation. Occasional persons taking acarbose develop liver dysfunction and for this reason persons taking this drug need their liver function checked every 3 months.

Metformin is a biguanide that has recently become available for the treatment of diabetes in the United States but has been widely used in Europe for over 20 years. Metformin is an ideal drug for middle-aged and young-old obese type II diabetics. It increases insulin sensitivity and causes mild anorexia and weight loss. It cannot be given to persons with renal failure, liver disease, severe heart failure or those with chronic acidosis. Among NH residents with serum creatinine greater than 1.2 mg/dl, metformin should be avoided. It is also most probably better not to use it in persons over 80 years of age. Dosages should be reduced in older persons as metformin clearance is slowed. Metformin should be held if the resident develops cardiovascular collapse, severe infection or needs to have a radioiodine contrast study done. Metformin's major side effect is lactic acidosis, which presents with malaise and nonspecific complaints. This rarely occurs if the above prescribing conditions are carefully adhered to. Up to one-third of persons receiving metformin initially have some gastrointestinal disturbances and this persists in approximately 5 percent. Residents on metformin need to be carefully monitored for inappropriate weight loss, and if this occurs metformin should be stopped. Metformin can be given together with sulfonylureas when the sulfonylurea is no longer producing adequate glycemic control. Metformin may reduce the insulin requirement in obese diabetics.

Our preference is to use insulin twice a day in NH residents. One should use the human insulins whenever possible. The 70/30 combinations of NPH and regular have proved very satisfactory. There appears to be no real advantage of the 50/50 preparations over the 70/30 ones. New, ultrashort acting regular insulins are about to come available. Their rapid action may result in increased hypoglycemia in the NH where the resident often has to wait for food for unpredictable times following their insulin injection.

There appears to be little advantage to using American Diabetic Association (ADA) diabetic diets for NH residents. Most diabetic NH residents should be on a regular diet with no added free sugar. Diabetic NH residents need to be carefully observed for weight loss, as this may necessitate a reduction in the dose of insulin or of the oral sulfonylureas. All diabetics should receive a snack before going to sleep (the amount eaten recorded) and be on a regular exercise program (including those who are chair-bound).

When a diabetic NH resident is stabilized on an oral agent or insulin, measurement of a fasting glucose and at least two glucoses 2 to 3 h after meals by a finger-stick technique once a week should be sufficient. When diabetic residents are begun on a new treatment (insulin or oral agent), values should be monitored at least three times per week. Among residents who are difficult to control, a glucose between 2 and 3 a.m. should be measured to check for the Somogyi effect (hypoglycemia in the early hours of the morning, resulting in daytime hyperglycemia).

Adequate diabetic control can, in many cases, result in improved quality of life for NH residents. Glycosylated hemoglobin (MhA,C) and fructosamine measure diabetic control over the last few weeks to months. In the NH where similar information can be obtained by regularly obtaining accuchecks, their use is rarely necessary. However, for this to be a viable option, the medical director needs to carefully monitor the accuracy of the accucheck machines and nursing technique.

ADDISON'S DISEASE AND HYPOPITUITARISM

Addison's disease and hypopituitarism are rare but treatable conditions that are easily missed in the NH resident. Addison's disease should be suspected in the resident with postural hypotension, unexplained hyperkalemia and/or hyponatremia, fatigue, and in some cases difficulty in maintaining diabetic control because of hypoglycemia. The diagnosis of adrenal insufficiency is made by administering 250 μmg of synthetic 1–39 adrenocorticotrophic hormone (ACTH) (cosyntropin) intramuscularly after obtaining a basal cortisol level. Cortisol levels are then obtained at 30 and 60 min. Failure of cortisol levels to increase by at least 8 μmg/dl or to a level greater than 25 μmg/dl makes the diagnosis of adrenal insufficiency. Replacement treatment is with hydrocortisone 25 mg in the morning and 12.5 mg at lunchtime. Do not give steroids in the evening, as this may cause sleep disturbances. Doses should be doubled if the resident becomes infected.

Hypopituitarism should be suspected in the resident who is generally doing poorly and has borderline low thyroid function and in male residents with low testosterone levels. The diagnosis is often difficult to make, but an elevated prolactin level may be helpful. Computed tomography may demonstrate a pituitary tumor.

Low levels of dehydroepiandrosterone sulfate (DHEA-S) have been demonstrated in the male NH population. Very low levels seem to be correlated with poor functional status. Because DHEA-S has been shown to improve cognitive function in animals, it has been suggested that the low levels of DHEA-S may play a causative role in deteriorating functional status. One study has suggested a marked feeling of well being in persons taking DHEA. However, at present this is highly speculative, and DHEA replacement is not indicated to improve functional status. Recently testosterone has been shown to enhance muscle strength in older males. Its major side effect appears to be polycythemia and this may be particularly common in NH residents.

Low levels of somatomedin-C (insulin growth factor-I) are also seen in the NH population. The decrease in somatomedin-C appears to be greater than that normally seen with aging. The low levels of somatomedin-C in NH residents appear to be predominantly an indicator of protein-energy malnutrition. They also are predictive of death in the NH. Patients with low somatomedin-C levels may, in the future, be candidates for replacement with recombinant growth hormone.

Melatonin levels also decline with age and its use has been recently popularized in a variety of books for the lay public. There is little evidence that it has any major effects other than to promote sleep. It is not Food and Drug Administration (FDA) approved although widely available in health food stores.

VITAMIN D DEFICIENCY

Exposure of the skin to sunlight is necessary in order to obtain adequate amounts of vitamin D. Many NH residents have inadequate sunlight exposure and also ingest too few calories to obtain adequate amounts of vitamin D in the diet. In addition, with aging there is decreased conversion of 25(OH) vitamin D to 1,25(OH);12 vitamin D (the active form) and there is a decrease in the ability of vitamin D to activate its receptors in the gut. When older people go out of doors they often cover up sun-exposed areas, and those with skin cancer may use sunblock lotions to prevent exposure to ultraviolet light. This combination of factors causes many NH residents to develop borderline vitamin D status. Severe vitamin D deficiency (osteomalacia), while rare, presents with severe muscle pain and weakness.

Vitamin D deficiency should be suspected in any resident who has a low or low–normal calcium and elevated alkaline phosphatase. Vitamin D deficiency is present in up to 50 percent of individuals with hip fracture. Diagnosis can be made either by measuring 25(OH) vitamin D levels or giving a therapeutic trial of vitamin D. Treatment of vitamin D deficiency consists of giving 800 IU of vitamin D daily or 50,000 IU of vitamin D twice a year. Some older individuals develop vitamin resistance and require higher doses of vitamin D (e.g., 50,000 IU of vitamin D twice a week). When higher doses of vitamin D are given, calcium levels need to be closely monitored. Marie Chapuy and her colleagues in France have demonstrated that a combination of vitamin D (800 IU daily) and calcium (500 mg daily) given to elderly NH residents in France markedly decreased hip fractures for up to 4 years and decreased mortality by 15 percent. In our experience vitamin D replacement is appropriate in all NH residents whose calcium level is less that 9 mg/dl. These residents either have vitamin D deficiency or secondary hypoparathyroidism due to renal disease. Both of these conditions are treated with vitamin D.

OSTEOPOROSIS

Osteoporosis is a condition in which there is decreased bone mineral content. It is common in NHs and is associated with fractures of the vertebrae and hip. Vitamin D and calcium as alluded to above may be the most useful agents to prevent its progress. Alendronate has been shown to increase bone density and prevent hip fractures. Its major disadvantage is expense and the lack of long-term (5 or more years) safety trials. Nasal calcitonin can strengthen bone and may be particularly effective in decreasing pain associated with vertebral fracture. In older residents who have had a hysterectomy estrogen may be an acceptable therapy.

HYPONATREMIA

Hyponatremia is present in up to 20 percent of NH residents at any one time; up to 50 percent of all NH residents have a single episode of hyponatremia in a given year. In most cases the hyponatremia is mild and has no obvious symptomatic consequences. However, residents with mild hyponatremia are at increased risk of developing severe hyponatremia when they receive intravenous

Table 18-4 Cuases of hyponatremia in the nursing home

1. Tube feeding with inadequate salt
2. Syndrome of inappropriate antidiuresis (SIADH)
    - CNS disorders
    - Lung disease
    - Hypothyroidism
    - Drugs
        - Phenothiazines
        - Carbamazepine
    - Ectopic ADH production
        - Oat cell cancer of lung
        - Lymphoma
        - Pancreatic cancer
    - Idiopathic hyponatremia
3. Psychogenic polydipsia
    - Drugs, e.g., thioridazine (Mellaril)
    - Psychiatric disorders
4. ? Inappropriate atrionaturetic factor (ANF) release
5. Congestive heart failure
6. Liver disease

Note: ? = possible.

fluids. Limitation of fluids in residents with mild hyponatremia can prevent precipitation of severe hyponatremia (**Table 18-4**).

Two major causes of hyponatremia among NH residents have been identified. The first is tube feeding with inadequate salt loads. The majority of non-tube-fed residents with hyponatremia have the syndrome of inappropriate antidiuretic hormone secretion (SIADH). Major causes include phenothiazines, central nervous system disorders, pulmonary disease, hypothyroidism, and ectopic production of ADH by oat cell carcinoma of the lung. When a resident consistently has serum sodium levels less than 120 meq/liter, treatment with demeclocycline (600 to 1200 mg/dl) may be necessary. NH residents receiving the antipsychotic agent thioridazine (Mellaril) may develop psychogenic polydipsia, which can result in hyponatremia. The role of the newly identified atrionaturetic factor (ANF) in the hyponatremia seen among NH residents is uncertain.

SUGGESTED READINGS

Chapuy MC, Arlot ME, Duboeuf F, Brien J, et al: Vitamin D3 and calcium to prevent hip fractures in elderly women. *N Engl J Med* 327:1637–1642, 1992.

Drinka PJ, Sieben M, Vogel SK: Poor positive predictive value of low sensitive thyrotropin assay levels for hyperthyroidism in nursing home residents. *South Med J* 86:1004–1007, 1993.

Mooradian AD, Morley JE, Korenman SG: Endocrinology in aging. *Disease-a-Month* 34:395–461, 1988.

Mooradian AD, Osterweil D, Petrosek D, Morley JE: Diabetes mellitus in elderly nursing home patients: A survey of clinical characteristics and management. *J Am Geriatr Soc* 36:391–396, 1988.

Morley JE: Geriatric endocrinology, in Mendelsohn G (ed): *Diagnosis and Pathology of Endocrine Disorders*. Philadelphia, JB Lippincott Co, 1988, pp 603–617.

Morley JE, Perry HM: The management of diabetes in older individuals. *Drugs* 4:568–565, 1991.

CHAPTER
NINETEEN

INFECTIONS AND INFECTION CONTROL

Infections are among the most common medical conditions encountered in the nursing home (NH) setting, and in several studies, they have been the most common reason for the acute hospitalization of residents. The Centers for Disease Control estimate that close to 1.5 million infections occur annually in NHs, which averages out to almost one infection per year per resident. The monthly incidence of infections ranges from about 11–20 per 100 residents. With regard to nosocomial infections, point prevalence surveys (which overestimate chronic infections) have demonstrated a prevalence of 5 percent to 33 percent, which is comparable to the rate in acute care hospitals.

Several factors make NH residents susceptible to infections, including age-related changes in immunity, impaired functional status (especially urinary and fecal incontinence), and the high prevalence of chronic medical conditions, such as diabetes mellitus, chronic obstructive pulmonary disease, cancer, and peripheral vascular disease. All these conditions predispose NH residents to a variety of infections. A majority of infections in NHs are endemic, but many epidemics of respiratory infections (scabies, conjunctivitis), and gastroenteritis have been reported. The relatively closed environment of the NH in which regular interaction among residents and staff is encouraged, increases susceptibility to epidemic infections.

Three-quarters or more of all infections in the NH come from three sources: the urinary tract, the respiratory tract, and the skin and soft tissues. But infections among NH residents may be difficult to recognize and localize. Like other medical conditions, infections often present atypically in the frail, functionally impaired geriatric population. Fever and localizing signs of infection may be completely absent. Acute changes in functional status, decreased food and fluid intake, increased confusion or delirium, and falls may be the manifestations of an infectious process. **Table 19-1** lists symptoms and signs which may be the presenting manifestation of an infection in nursing home residents. When these conditions are reported, an infection should be considered. Although empiric antimicrobial therapy may be warranted in some situations, an attempt should be made to localize an infection by means of appropriate diagnostic studies. The overuse of empiric antimicrobial therapy can lead to the development of a variety of resistant organisms within the facility.

Despite the prevalence, morbidity, and costs associated with NH infections, several surveys have suggested that infection control policies and procedures are poorly developed in many NHs. In addition, many unnecessary cultures are probably performed, and antimicrobials are often administered inappropriately. The purpose of this chapter is twofold: to provide a perspective on the management of common infections in the NH and to provide an overview of appropriate infection control practices for the NH setting.

Table 19-1 Symptoms and signs which may be the presenting manifestation of infection among nursing home residents

- Changes in vital signs
  - Change in temperature
    - Fever $\geq 100°F$
    - Change from baseline $\geq 2.4°F$
  - Hypothermia T $< 96.5°F$
  - Tachypnea
  - Orthostatic hypotension
- Acute mental status change
  - New or worsened confusion
  - Lethargy
  - Delirium
  - Agitation
- Unexplained change in functional status
- Loss of appetite
- Weakness
- Falls
- New or worsened urinary incontinence

After Yoshikawa, TT and Norman DC: Approach to fever in the nursing home. *J Amer Geriatr Soc* 44:74–82, 1996.

Table 19-2 Common infections in the nursing home

A. Urinary tract
   1. Noncatheterized residents
      (a) Asymptomatic bacteriuria (with or without pyuria)
      (b) Symptomatic infection/urosepsis
   2. Catheterized residents
      (a) Asymptomatic bacteriuria (with or without pyuria)
      (b) Symptomatic infection/urosepsis

B. Respiratory tract
   1. Upper respiratory tract infections
   2. Bronchitis
   3. Influenza, respiratory syncytial virus, other viruses
   4. Pneumonia
   5. Tuberculosis

C. Skin and soft tissues
   1. Conjunctivitis
   2. Cellulitis
   3. Infected pressure sores
   4. Herpes zoster

D. Gastrointestinal tract
   1. Gastroenteritis/infectious diarrhea
   2. Antibiotic-associated enterocolitis (*C. difficile*)
   3. Other
      (a) Appendicitis
      (b) Diverticulitis
      (c) Cholecystitis

MANAGEMENT OF COMMON INFECTIONS IN THE NH

In general, the approach to treating infections in the NH depends on three factors:

1. Characteristics of the resident (underlying diseases, functional status, quality of life, goals for care and preferred intensity of treatment)
2. Nature and severity of the infection
3. Resources available within the NH

Table 19-2 lists infections that occur commonly in the NH. Each of these will be discussed briefly, emphasizing what is important in the NH setting. Readers should refer to textbooks of medicine and infectious disease for more detailed information on these conditions.

Urinary Tract Infections

The approach to managing urinary tract infections (UTI) in the NH setting should take into account two fundamental considerations:

1. Residents with indwelling bladder catheters should be considered separately from those without them.
2. There is a high prevalence of "asymptomatic" bacteriuria. If it is truly asymptomatic, it should not be treated, even if it is accompanied by pyuria.

Table 19-3 lists key principles of managing UTI in noncatheterized NH residents. In most NHs, the prevalence of bacteriuria, defined as growth of more than 100,000 colony forming units per milliliter of urine, is between 30 percent and 50 percent in women and slightly lower in men. Epidemiological studies have clearly shown that this bacteriuria comes and goes without treatment. Several studies have demonstrated that attempts to eradicate asymptomatic bacteriuria do not have a prominent influence on morbidity and mortality and can lead to the development of resistant organisms. Thus, it is clear that true asymptomatic bacteriuria should not be treated in the NH. An important caveat, however, lies in the definition of asymptomatic. Because symptoms and signs of infection may be nonspecific, there should be a high index of suspicion for infection when acute or subacute changes in status occur.

If infection is suspected, a good clean catch specimen of urine for urinalysis and culture is necessary. It is possible to collect specimens that accurately reflect bladder urine without catheterizing NH residents. For women, the procedure involves cleaning the urethra and perivaginal area with a disinfectant such as betadine, and having the resident void into a disinfected fracture pan or toilet insert. Among functionally capable men, especially those who are circumcised, an accurate specimen can often be obtained from an uncleansed, freshly voided specimen. In functionally or cognitively impaired men, an accurate bladder specimen can be obtained by cleaning the penis with an antiseptic solution, applying an external catheter, and rapidly processing the first voided specimen. Some residents may need to be catheterized because a specimen cannot be collected by the above methods in a practical or timely manner. Other laboratory studies should also be done to determine the severity of illness (**Table 19-3**).

NH residents who appear clinically unstable and possibly septic should be transferred to an acute care hospital (or "subacute" unit if available and appropriate) for parenteral antimicrobial therapy, intravenous hydration, and close monitoring. If such residents are clinically stable and taking oral fluids, oral antimicrobial therapy can be initiated. The selection of an antimicrobial should take into account resistance patterns noted at the facility. In the absence of a history of recurrent UTI or recent antimicrobial therapy, trimethoprim–sulfamethoxazole or norfloxacin would be adequate initial therapy. If the resident has a history of recurrent UTI or was recently treated with an antimicrobial, a different drug should be prescribed until sensitivity data become available. Older men should be treated initially with ampicillin (or another drug if allergic) to cover *Enterococcus*. Nitrofurantoin should generally be avoided because its effectiveness is dependent upon a creatine clearance of at least 40 ml/min, which is often not present in frail NH residents.

empiric antimicrobial coverage should include Group D enterococci as well as gram-negative organisms. If symptomatic UTI recurs frequently, a urological evaluation is indicated to identify genitourinary abnormalities, such as periurethral abscess or bladder calculi—which may predispose to recurrent episodes.

Respiratory Tract Infections

Three types of respiratory tract infections will be discussed in some detail because of their prevalence and associated morbidity and mortality: influenza, bacterial pneumonia, and tuberculosis. Upper respiratory infections—including viral nasopharyngitis, bacterial sinusitis, and acute viral and bacterial tracheobronchitis are also common in the NH—but the principles of managing these conditions do not differ substantially from those for the community-dwelling geriatric population. Overprescription of antimicrobials for what are predominantly viral illnesses should be avoided so as not to promote the development of resistant organisms and side effects from the medications. On the other hand, NH residents with significant chronic lung disease are susceptible to decompensation from acute bronchitis; antimicrobial therapy is appropriate for these residents when they become symptomatic, producing purulent sputum in the absence of signs of pneumonia.

Epidemics of influenza can be devastating in the NH setting. **Table 19-5** lists some general principles regarding influenza in the NH. A vigorous attempt should be made to vaccinate all residents as well as direct-care staff annually, between late October and early December. There should be a high index of suspicion for an outbreak in the NH if there is an outbreak in the community or if residents and/or staff begin to develop symptoms (**Table 19-5**). If this occurs, throat cultures should be obtained to determine if the outbreak represents type A influenza, because prophylaxis with ramantidine (or amantadine) may be useful in preventing infection due to this virus (but not to type B influenza). Serological testing is not necessary unless an epidemic is being investigated. If amantadine prophylaxis is used, the dose must be adjusted for age and renal function. The standard dose of 200 mg/day should be reduced to 100 mg/day or less in NH residents because of their reduced renal excretion and propensity to develop side effects, especially delirium. Recurrent fever or signs of respiratory distress suggest superimposed bacterial pneumonia.

Pneumonia, known as the "old person's friend," is one of the most common causes of hospitalization and death among NH residents. Pneumonia should be at the top of the differential diagnosis list for any NH resident who has an acute or subacute change in mental or functional status or a decrease in food or fluid intake. Typical symptoms are frequently absent, although tachypnea is an especially important sign and is easily missed by nursing staff. **Table 19-6** lists several key principles of managing pneumonia in the NH, and **Table 19-7** lists antimicrobials that are appropriate for the therapy of NH-acquired pneumonia. In general, NH residents should be treated in an acute care hospital or subacute unit

Table 19-5 Influenza in the nursing home

1. Influenza, especially Type A, is a major cause of preventable morbidity and mortality in the NH setting.
2. All residents and staff providing direct care should be immunized annually between late October and early December.
3. A high index of suspicion for an influenza outbreak is necessary during winter months when:
   a. An outbreak occurs in the community
   b. Staff are absent with respiratory illnesses
   c. Residents begin to develop clinical manifestations:
      (1) Fever
      (2) Headache, malaise, myalgias, arthralgias
      (3) Rhinorrhea, nasal congestion, cough
4. Symptomatic residents and staff should have throat cultures early in the course of a suspected outbreak of Influenza A.
   a. Once a case is confirmed by culture, all similar illnesses should be considered influenza
   b. Serologic testing is not necessary unless an epidemic is under investigation
5. Ramantadine (or amantadine) is useful for prophylaxis for Influenza A. (Not Type B.)
   a. If given within 24–48 hours of onset of illness, it may reduce the severity of symptoms
   b. Should be given to vaccinated residents and staff only if outbreak occurs within two weeks of vaccination (antibody protection takes about two weeks to develop)
   c. May be given to asymptomatic unvaccinated residents and staff as prophylaxis throughout the duration of a severe outbreak
   d. The usual dose of 200 mg per day must be reduced to 100 mg or less in residents over age 65, and reduced further if renal function is impaired
   e. NH residents are susceptible to side effects of amantadine, especially delirium
6. Recurrent fever, tachypnea or other signs of respiratory distress may indicate superimposed bacterial pneumonia.

where adequate staff and diagnostic capabilities are present because of the high incidence of concomitant conditions such as hypoxia, dehydration, metabolic disturbances, and cardiac decompensation. Antimicrobial therapy should generally be administered parenterally for at least 7 days. In carefully selected cases in which the resident is mildly ill, alert and taking in adequate fluids and nutrition, oral therapy may be appropriate. Because adequate sputum specimens are difficult to obtain from NH residents, antimicrobial therapy is most often empiric. It should cover organisms that are known to cause NH-acquired pneumonia, including gram-negative rods (especially *Klebsiella*), *Streptococcus pneumoniae*, *Haemophilus influenzae*, and *Staphylococcus aureus*. Anerobic coverage should be provided if aspiration is suspected. Excellent supportive care is also essential for the successful treatment of pneumonia and the prevention of iatrogenic complications (**Table 19-6**).

Tuberculosis, though relatively uncommon, is very important in the NH population for several reasons. First, NH residents are especially susceptible to the reactivation of *Mycobacterium tuberculosis*. Second, like bacterial pneumo-

Table 19-6 Management of pneumonia in nursing home residents

1. Fever and pulmonary symptoms are often absent in nursing home residents with pneumonia (see **Table 19-1**)
2. Initial diagnostic evaluation should include:
   a. Complete blood count
   b. Glucose, electrolytes, BUN, creatinine
   c. Blood cultures (if very ill)
   d. Chest X-ray
   e. Oximetry or arterial blood gas or oximetry (if indicated)
   f. Gram stain and culture of sputum (if obtainable; respiratory therapist may be helpful if available)
3. Most nursing home residents with pneumonia should be hospitalized (or transferred to a "subacute" unit if available) for parenteral antimicrobial and fluid administration
4. In carefully selected cases in which the resident is mildly ill, alert and taking in adequate fluid and nutrition, oral therapy may be appropriate
5. Aspiration should be suspected if any of following are present:
   a. Nasogastric tube
   b. Gastrostomy tube with high gastric residuals
   c. Decreased level of consciousness
   d. Dysphagia and/or a neurological deficit which predisposes to swallowing disorder and aspiration
6. Antimicrobials should generally be administered parenterally for at least 7 days or more, depending on the clinical condition.
   a. Antimicrobial therapy should cover organisms frequently isolated in nursing home acquired pneumonia (see **Table 19-7**):
      (1) *Streptococcus pneumoniae*
      (2) Gram-negatives (especially *Klebsiella*)
      (3) *Haemophilus influenzae*
      (4) *Staphylococcus aureus*
      (5) Anaerobes (especially with aspiration)
   b. When clinically stable, oral antimicrobial therapy can be initiated and continued for a total treatment course of 14 days
7. Excellent supportive care is essential.
   a. Proper hydration
   b. Adequate nutrition
   c. Adequate oxygenation
   d. Pulmonary care
   e. Management of other medical illnesses
   f. Skin care
   g. Early and frequent mobilization to prevent complications from immobility

After Yoshikawa TT: *Geriatrics* 44(10) pp 32–43, 1989.

nia, pulmonary tuberculosis is difficult to recognize but curable if appropriate treatment is instituted. Third, unrecognized tuberculosis can result not only in the death of the resident but also in an epidemic within the facility. Finally, in many areas of the country a substantial proportion of the staff are immigrants who may have an increased susceptibility to tuberculosis.

Table 19-7 Antimicrobial therapy for nursing home acquired pneumonia

Empiric parenteral therapy	
Drug	**Dose**[a]
General	
Second generation cephalosporins	
Cefuroxime	750 mg–1.5 g every 8–12 hours
Cefoxitin	2 g every 6 hours
Cefotetan	1–2 g every 12 hours
Third generation cephalosporins	
Cefotetan	1 g every 12 hours
Ceftriaxone	1–2 g every 12–24 hours
Cefotaxime	1 g every 8 hours
Cefoperazone	1–2 g every 12 hours
Ceftazidine	1 g every 8 hours
Ticarcillin (3 g)–clavulanate (0.1 g)	2.0–3.1 g every 4–8 hours
Ampicillin (1 g)–sulbactam (0.5 g)	1.5 g every 8 hours
Oxacillin plus Aztreonam	2 g every 6 hours (oxacillin) 1 g every 12 hours (Aztreonam)
Cefazolin plus Aminoglycoside[b]	1 g every 8 hours (Cefazolin) 1.5 mg/kg every 8–12 hours (gentamicin)
Aspiration suspected[c]	
Coverage for anerobic organisms should be added with either:	
Ampicillin-sulbactam	
Metronidazole	
Ticarcillin–clavulanate	
Pseudomonas suspected	
Coverage should include one of the following:	
Aztreonam	
Cefoperazone	
Ceftazidime	
Ticarcillin–clavulanate	
For empiric coverage with penicillin allergy	
Reasonable regimens include:	
Clindamycin plus Aztreonam	
Clindamycin plus ciprofloxacin	
Oral therapy[b]	
Known organism	Treat based on susceptibility
Unknown organism	Amoxacillin–Clavulanic–acid Cefuroxime–axetil Ciprofloxacin (with or without penicillin G or ampicillin) Trimethoprim–sulfamethoxazole (with clindamycin or another agent)

After Yoshikawa TT: *Geriatrics* 44(10) pp 32–43, 1989.

[a]Doses are based on absence of significant renal dysfunction.

[b]In general aminoglycoside use for longer than 3 days should be avoided in the elderly.

[c]Initiate after 7 or more days of parenteral therapy when clinically stable; total duration of therapy should be 14–21 days.

Table 19-8 Principles of managing tuberculosis in the nursing home setting

1. All staff should have tuberculin skin testing at the time of employment and annually with intermediate strength (5 tuberculin units) of purified protein derivative (PPD) antigen
2. All new admissions to the facility should have an intermediate strength PPD placed, *unless* they have had a well documented and evaluated positive skin test in the past
   a. If the initial test is negative (less than 10 mm of induration at 48 hours), they should be *retested* within 2 weeks
   b. Dermal control antigens (*Candida*, *Trichophyton*, mumps) may be used in order to detect cutaneous anergy
3. All residents with a positive PPD (including booster) should have a chest X-ray and careful evaluation to determine if active disease may be present
4. Although not mandatory, annual skin testing of all residents is recommended
5. *Chemoprophylaxis* should be considered for residents with either of the following:
   a. >5 mm PPD reactivity
      (1) Close contact with active case
      (2) Known or suspected HIV infection
      (3) Abnormal chest X-ray with fibrosis consistent with old healed tuberculosis
   b. >10mm PPD reactivity on initial or second test, or >6 mm more induration on second test compared with first, and either:
      (1) Silicosis or other chronic lung disease
      (2) Undernutrition
      (3) Diabetes mellitus
      (4) End-stage renal disease
      (5) Immunosuppression (e.g., 15 mg or more of prednisone daily)
      (6) Hematologic malignancy (lymphoma, leukemia)
      (7) Gastrectomy or jejunoileal bypass
      (8) Intravenous drug use
   c. >15 mm PPD reactivity (suspected new conversion)
6. *Chemoprophylaxis* includes:
   a. Isoniazid (INH) 300 mg daily or 900 mg twice per week and pyridoxine (B_6) 50 mg daily for a minimum of 6 months if chest X-ray is normal
   b. If chest X-ray is abnormal (stable lesion, negative mycobacteriology), or if resident has HIV infection, 12 months of therapy is recommended
7. For *active* pulmonary tuberculosis:[a]
   a. 9 months of therapy
      (1) INH 300 mg per day
      (2) Rifampin 600 mg per day
      (3) Pyridoxine (B_6) 50 mg per day
8. All residents treated with INH should have liver function tests *every 3 months*.
   a. If the SGOT increases greater than 3-fold, therapy should be stopped
   b. If indicated, after normalization of liver function tests, rechallenge with 50 mg per day, increasing by 50 mg at weekly intervals (up to 300 mg) may be attempted, following liver function tests carefully
      (1) If liver function tests deteriorate again, do not rechallenge
      (2) If prophylaxis absolutely necessary, ethambutol plus rifampin may be tried

[a]In some areas four drug treatment is necessary because of the prevalence of multi-drug resistant strains.

Table 19-8 provides a detailed outline of the principles of managing tuberculosis in the NH. These recommendations are straightforward and consistent with recommendations published elsewhere. Although it is not mandatory in all areas, we recommend that residents and staff have a tuberculin skin test annually. Further details on the management of tuberculosis can be found in some of the suggested readings, and an example of a policy for NHs is included in the Appendix.

Infections of Skin and Soft Tissues

A wide variety of infections of the skin and soft tissues occur among NH residents, including conjunctivitis, cellulitis, scabies, herpes zoster (shingles), and infected ulcers and pressure sores. In addition colonization of the skin and nares with methicillin resistant staphylococcal aureus (MRSA) is common and a source of considerable confusion and anxiety among NH staff. Although it is very rare, tetanus is always a concern, because many NH residents have not had adequate immunization.

Conjunctivitis In some point prevalence surveys, conjunctivitis is among the most common infections identified in the NH setting. The predominant symptoms and signs are conjunctival erythema and a purulent discharge. Most conjunctivitis is bacterial; it should be treated with a topical antimicrobial solution and warm compresses (the latter if significant discomfort is present). Cultures are not necessary. When conjunctivitis is recurrent, regular attention should be given to the cleanliness of the eyelids in order to help prevent recurrences. This is best done with lid scrubs utilizing baby shampoo.

Cellulitis Bacterial cellulitis most commonly affects the lower extremities. An obvious source of the cellulitis, such as an ulcer or abrasion, is found in only half or less of cases. Cultures are generally not indicated; attempts to get cultures by needle aspiration do not generally yield clinically useful information. The most common pathogens involved are *S. aureus* and beta-hemolytic streptococci, except in cellulitis related to infected pressure sores and diabetic ulcers in which gram negative and anaerobic organisms are also found. Culture results may be helpful if there is a poor response to initial therapy, or if there is an outbreak of skin infections in the facility. Cellulitis of the lower or upper extremities is often treatable in the NH. An oral semisynthetic penicillin, first generation cephalosporin, or amoxicillin–clavulanic acid are reasonable initial therapy. Penicillin allergic residents can be treated with clindamycin orally. If parenteral therapy is necessary, cefazolin, or nafcillin/oxacillin can be given intramuscularly. The affected area should be observed carefully for the first 24 to 48 hours; if there is no improvement or the condition becomes worse, hospitalization for parenteral therapy should be considered. It is helpful to mark the borders of the cellulitis to document improvement or progression. Cellulitis involving the face or neck should generally be treated with parenteral therapy in an acute care setting.

Bacterial cellulitis should be differentiated from two other skin infections in the NH: candidiasis and scabies. NH residents, especially diabetics and those who have been on broad-spectrum antibiotics, are susceptible to mucocutaneous candidiasis. The most common manifestation is acute intertriginous infection of the perianal skin, perineum, and genitalia and macerated skin surfaces under breasts or skin folds. The diagnosis can be confirmed by observing the fungus microscopically in a skin scraping exposed to potassium hydroxide. Treatment includes good hygiene and a topical antifungal agent.

Scabies Scabies is caused by a mite (*Sarcoptes scabiei*) that burrows under the skin. It can become epidemic in the NH if not diagnosed and managed properly. Residents with excoriated pruritic papules should be suspected of having scabies. The excoriations can become severe and be complicated by cellulitis. The diagnosis is made by observing the mite microscopically in a skin scraping. All affected residents and their contacts should be treated with an antiscabetic solution and antipruritic agents as needed. Effective treatment can be achieved with 1 percent lindane solution or 5 percent permethrin cream. These agents must be applied to all skin surfaces from the neck down, including toe webs and beneath the fingernails and removed 8–12 hours later by bathing. All clothing and linens should be thoroughly laundered, and residents should be reevaluated in 3 to 6 weeks if pruritus persists.

Herpes zoster (shingles) Herpes zoster, generally known as shingles, results from a reactivation of latent varicella-zoster virus. This virus is also responsible for chickenpox, and 95 percent of adults have had a primary infection. The incidence of shingles increases with advancing age. A prodrome of fever, malaise, or pain (which may be severe and can mimic many conditions) may precede the eruption of skin lesions by a few days. Early skin lesions are grouped vesicles on a red base in a specific dermatome, which does not cross the midline. The most commonly affected dermatomes are the ophthalmic division of the trigeminal nerve and T_3 to L_3 The lesions become pustular in 3 to 4 days, crust within 7 to 10 days, and generally disappear within 2 to 3 weeks. The management of shingles involves the prevention of complications, the relief of acute symptoms, and the treatment of chronic complications. The major complications of herpes zoster are local infection, dissemination and chronic pain or postherpetic neuralgia. Antiviral therapy is beneficial in reducing the acute pain and shortening the duration of postherpetic pain if begun within 48 hours. The recommended oral therapy is acyclovir 800 mg 5 times per day for 7 days or famciclovir 500 mg 3 times per day for 7 days. Doses should be adjusted for renal dysfunction. Routine use of steroids to reduce the frequency of postherpetic neuralgia is not recommended. Dissemination is extremely rare in people who are not immunosuppressed. In the presence of significant immunosuppression (hematological or reticuloendothelial malignancy, cancer chemotherapy, chronic steroid treatment), intravenous acyclovir 500 mg/m^2 of body surface area should be administered every 8 h for 7 days in order to prevent dissemination (pneumonia, myelitis, paralysis, ocular complications).

The pain during the acute phase of shingles may be severe and often requires narcotic analgesics, even among those with a high tolerance for pain. Postherpetic neuralgia, defined as pain lasting longer than a month, is the most common complication of shingles and can last months or even years. Management of postherpetic neuralgia is difficult. A wide variety of measures have been used with variable and limited success including amitriptyline, carbamazepine, transcutaneous electrical stimulation, nerve blocks, and capsaicin topical cream.

During the acute phase of shingles, the skin vesicles contain infectious material. Staff, children, and other individuals who have not had chickenpox, as well as possibly pregnant females, should not come in contact with the affected resident until all the lesions are crusted and dry. Although gowns, gloves, and masks are not necessary, proper handwashing techniques should be used after contact with an affected resident. Residents with shingles do not have to be isolated but should not be in the same room with residents who are immunosuppressed.

Infected pressure ulcers The basic principles of managing infected pressure ulcers are outlined in **Table 19-9**. The approach to infected ulcers and other skin wounds are basically the same. Several points should be emphasized. As in the case of urine in residents with chronic indwelling catheters, bacterial colonization without evidence of infection is the rule. Growth of organisms on a culture is not in itself an indication for antimicrobial therapy. Topical antimicrobial therapy may occasionally be helpful when ulcers are not healing in the presence or absence of purulent drainage. Systemic antimicrobial therapy should be reserved for specific indications, including cellulitis, osteomyelitis, or signs of sepsis without another source. When systemic antimicrobial therapy is indicated, it should be based on properly collected cultures. Surface swabs of pressure ulcers and other skin wounds are of no value and may be misleading. Cultures should be taken by injecting 1 ml of nonbacteriostatic saline through uninfected skin surrounding the infected. Site and aspirating from a nearby site for culture material. Cultures can also be taken from debrided necrotic tissue or bone biopsy. Anaerobic cultures should be done in addition to standard aerobic cultures because of the prevalence of anaerobic pathogens in deep tissue infections. When such infection is present, antimicrobial therapy should be parenteral and should include adequate anaerobic coverage. **Table 19-9** contains a list of antimicrobials that would be appropriate in this situation.

Methicillin resistant *Staphylococcus aureus* (MRSA) A considerable degree of confusion and anxiety generally accompany discussions of MRSA in NHs. **Table 19-10** outlines several key points about MRSA. While colonization is common, clinical infection is infrequent and is generally no more severe than

Table 19-9 Principles of managing infected pressure ulcers in the nursing home

1. Bacterial colonization without clinical evidence of infection is common—analogous to catheter related bacteriuria.
   a. Growth of organisms on culture is not in itself an indication for treatment
2. Cultures must be done properly in order to determine the cause of deep tissue infection.
   a. Surface swabs are of no value and may be misleading
   b. Cultures of needle aspirates of injected saline and/or tissue biopsy are more predictive of causative organisms
   c. If osteomyelitis is suspected based on X-ray and/or bone scan, a bone biopsy for culture is necessary to identify the pathogen(s)
   d. If systemic infection is suspected, blood cultures should be obtained
   e. Anaerobic as well as aerobic cultures should be done
3. Pathogens in deep tissue infections are generally polymicrobial
   a. In stage 1 and 2 ulcers, gram positive cocci and aerobic gram negative rods are common
   b. In stage 3 and 4 ulcers, a mixture of aerobic gram negative rods and anaerobes is common
4. Antimicrobial therapy should be reserved for specific indications
   a. Cellulitis (not just erythema of healing tissue)
   b. Osteomyelitis
   c. Clinical signs of sepsis in the absence of another source
5. Antimicrobial therapy should be based on culture results whenever possible.
   a. Unless a superficial cellulitis is being treated, initial antimicrobial therapy should generally be parenteral
   b. Anaerobic coverage should be included for deep tissue infections

Appropriate antimicrobials include (not in order of preference):

Ampicillin sulbactam	Cefotetan
Cefoxitin	Metronidazole
Clindamycin	Ticarcillin–clavulanate

infections caused by other organisms. Transmission can generally be prevented by good handwashing and universal precautions. Isolation is not generally indicated, but immunocompromised residents and those with open skin lesions should not be roomed with residents with known MRSA. In facilities with high colonization or infection rates it is reasonable to cohort residents with MRSA in specific rooms. Treatment of colonized residents or staff is not indicated, and such treatment commonly results in rapid re-colonization and the development of resistant organisms.

Vancomycin resistant *enterococcus* (VRE) Vancomycin-resistant enterococcus (VRE) is increasingly being recognized as a common problem. VRE is most commonly isolated from stool samples and from wounds. It tends to be more common in persons who have been treated for anerobes with metronidazole, intrabdominal surgical procedures, and preexposure to vancomycin. VRE tends to last for hours on surfaces in residents' rooms. Transmission has occurred by

Table 19-10 Key points about methicillin-resistant *Staphylococcus* (MRSA) in the nursing home

1. 10–25 percent of NH residents may be colonized with MRSA
   a. Colonization rates are higher among those with poorer functional status, have feeding tubes or urinary catheters, or have wounds
2. Active infection with MRSA is relatively infrequent
   a. Less than 5 percent of residents develop active infection
3. Roommate-to-roommate transmission is relatively uncommon
   a. When MRSA is spread it is by direct transmission from the hands of staff members
4. Handwashing is the most important measure to prevent spread
   a. There is no evidence that barriers (e.g., gowns, masks) are necessary
   b. Gloves should be used when treating colonized wounds or handling MRSA infected specimens (e.g., urine)
5. Isolation is generally not necessary for colonized or infected residents
   a. Except for residents with an active MRSA respiratory infection, isolation is not necessary
      (1) Infected wounds should be properly covered
      (2) Handwashing and universal precautions will prevent spread
   b. Immunocompromised residents or those with open skin wounds should not be roomed with a resident with known MRSA
   c. In facilities with high colonization rates, it is reasonable to attempt to cohort (i.e., place in the same room) colonized residents
6. Antibiotic treatment of colonized residents or staff is not indicated
   a. Re-colonization occurs quickly, and antibiotic resistance develops
7. Residents with active MRSA infection require parenteral vancomycin therapy

use of electronic thermometers. Management of residents with VRE requires continuous use of universal precautions and body substance isolation. VRE represents a challenge in the nursing home. There is little point in screening for VRE carriage in noninfected individuals. In locally incontinent persons with VRE isolation may be necessary.

Tetanus Tetanus is a rare disease, but it is serious and preventable. Most elderly people except those who served in the armed forces, have either never had a primary series of immunizations or have not had a booster shot in many years, which may make a single booster at the time of injury ineffective in achieving sufficient protection from subsequent wounds. The method of immunization depends on the nature of the wound and the immunization status of the resident. The cost-effectiveness of tetanus immunization in the NH setting is not known. If the resident has had three or more doses of tetanus diphtheria toxoid (Td) with the last being within the previous 5 years, no immunization is necessary. For clean, minor wounds, Td may be administered. Consideration should be given to giving a primary series of three Td injections (at the time of injury, 4 to 6 weeks later, and 6 to 12 months after the second dose) to residents with deep or contaminated lesions who have never been immunized or had their last dose many years earlier. Tetanus immune globulin, 250 to 500 units, can be administered (by a separate syringe at a different site) in addition to Td to residents with contaminated or gangrenous deep lesions.

Gastrointestinal Tract Infections

Though not as prevalent as the infections already discussed, infections in the gastrointestinal tract are relatively common and are an important source of morbidity and mortality in the NH population. In addition, some of these infections can cause serious epidemics in an institutional setting.

With the exception of diarrhea caused by *Clostridium difficile*, which is increasingly common in NHs, and salmonella, a pathogen is not identified and the illness is generally attributed to a virus among residents with an acute diarrheal illness or gastroenteritis. Residents with the new onset of diarrhea who have not had a recent course of systemic antimicrobial (which predisposes to *C. difficile* colitis) should have a stool specimen collected and sent for examination for leukocytes. The absence of fecal leukocytes suggests a viral etiology or a toxin-induced illness (e.g., staphylococcal or clostridial food poisoning). Fecal leukocytes are present when there is tissue invasion or inflammation of the intestinal mucosa, as can be seen in bacterial or parasitic infection, toxin-induced illness, or inflammatory bowel disease (i.e., Crohn's). Residents who have fecal leukocytes should have a specimen sent for culture and *C. difficile* toxin assay. Infectious agents can come from a human reservoir (e.g., *Salmonella typhi*, *Shigella*, *Giardia*) or from food or water (e.g., nontyphoid *Salmonella*, *Yersinia* spp., *Campylobacter*, *Eschesichia coli* 0157:H7). *E. coli* 0157:H7 has been responsible for epidemics associated with the eating of undercooked beef.

Treatment of acute gastroenteritis with antimicrobials should be limited to residents with severe bacterial dysentery, systemic infection, or parasitic infection. NH residents with profuse diarrhea should be hospitalized for management of fluid and electrolyte balance. Enteric precautions should be instituted for all residents with an acute gastroenteritis and prolonged diarrhea.

Diarrhea occurs commonly during or just after antibiotic therapy. This is generally due to changes in intestinal flora, and is often mild and self-limited. In many cases, however, diarrhea can lead to intestinal inflammation and damage. This entity is generally termed "antibiotic-associated enterocolitis". Its signs and symptoms usually develop within a week after a course of antibiotics is initiated but may occur as long as 6 weeks later. A high index of suspicion for this disorder is necessary for any NH resident who develops diarrhea and/or other gastrointestinal symptoms within a month after a course of antibiotics. Diarrhea in this situation should not automatically be attributed to other factors common in this population, such as enteral feedings, nutritional supplements, or laxatives. Most antibiotic-associated enterocolitis is caused by *Clostridium difficile*. NH residents may be colonized with *C. difficile* without symptoms, however presence of the toxin suggests active infection. The *C. difficile* toxin assay is highly sensitive and specific. However, this assay may need to be repeated several times if initially negative and there is a high suspicion of *C. difficile* infection. Many cases of antibiotic-associated enterocolitis are severe enough to cause pseudomembranous colitis, which can be diagnosed by characteristic intestinal mucosal changes will be seen on endoscopy. Consideration should be given to sigmoidoscopy to diagnose this condition based on the severity of symptoms. If the clinical picture is consistent with antibiotic-associated enterocolitis, all NH residents with positive stool assays for *C. difficile* toxin should have antibiotics discontinued and be treated with oral metronidazole (250 mg three times per day) for 10 days. If the resident fails to respond, then oral vancomycin, 125 mg 4 times per day for 10 days should be prescribed. Enteric precautions should be instituted for all residents with antibiotic-associated enterocolitis.

Other infections of the gastrointestinal tract also occur in the NH population. Acute appendicitis, cholecystitis, and diverticulitis should always be considered in the differential diagnosis of an infection and abdominal pain in a NH resident. As with other infections, the clinical manifestations may be minimal, nonspecific, or deceiving. A careful abdominal examination is essential in any NH resident with a fever or unexplained gastrointestinal symptoms, no matter how vague. Although leukocytosis may be absent, a white blood cell count and differential should be ordered. Unexplained leukocytosis or a left shift should make an intra-abdominal infection a strong consideration, even in the absence of localizing signs or symptoms. Surgical consultation should be obtained early in the course of any suspected intra-abdominal infection.

Hepatitis is an important infection in the NH, not so much because of its prevalence but because of its potential to cause an epidemic in an institutional setting. Any NH resident or staff suspected of having hepatitis should have appropriate blood studies performed. If hepatitis is diagnosed, it is imperative to identify a source whenever possible in order to prevent a potential epidemic within the institution. Norwalk (or small round) virus is commonly associated with episodes of severe vomiting in the NH. The incubation period is 24 to 48 hours. Spread can be inhibited by isolating resident (and their roommates) with new onset vomiting from the dining room for 72 hours. Diagnosis can be made by submitting specimens of vomit and blood from 6 infected residents to the IDC.

AIDS

Acquired immunodeficiency syndrome (AIDS) is of increasing importance to providers of NH care. With the increasing prevalence of this disorder and the potential for those afflicted with AIDS to develop dementia and other functional disabilities, there will be an increasing need for institutional care for this population. NHs should develop educational programs and policies and procedures about AIDS, so that these individuals can be properly cared for if they require institutional care.

INFECTION CONTROL

All NHs are required to have an infection control program. This requirement has been reinforced by the OBRA 1987 legislation. The broad goals of such a program are to provide a sanitary and comfortable environment and to prevent the development and transmission of infection whenever possible. Infection control activities range from the development of policies and procedures to

Table 19-11 Key aspects of an infection control program in a nursing home

1. The goal of an infection control program is to provide a safe and comfortable environment, and to prevent the development and transmission of infections whenever possible
2. The facility should have an Infection Control Committee (ICC)
   a. Members should include representatives of multiple departments, including nursing, medical, dietary, pharmacy, housekeeping, maintenance, and laundry
   b. Meetings should be quarterly with minutes kept for each meeting
3. Written policies and procedures should be developed for the prevention and control of infections and the maintenance of a sanitary environment (See examples in "Appendix")
   a. Definitions of various infections
   b. Reporting procedures
   c. Universal precautions
   d. Handwashing and aseptic techniques
   e. Isolation and disposal procedures
   f. Immunizations
      (1) Influenza
      (2) Pneumococcal
      (3) Tetanus
   g. Tuberculosis
      (1) Skin testing of residents and staff
      (2) Prophylaxis
   h. Employee health
      (1) Pre-employment immunizations and infectious disease history
      (2) Tuberculosis skin testing
      (3) Screening of dietary personnel
   i. Processing laundry
   j. Pest control
   k. Cleaning and care of equipment
4. Surveillance should be ongoing
   a. Regular reporting of all infections
   b. Collation of culture results
   c. Review of antimicrobial susceptibility patterns
   d. Review of antibiotic usage
   e. Quarterly summary to identify trends
   f. Potential epidemics should be continuously considered
      (1) Respiratory illness
      (2) Gastroenteritis
      (3) Skin and soft tissue infections

screening and preventive activities for residents and staff to ongoing surveillance to determine the incidence of infection and identify outbreaks.

Table 19-11 lists several key aspects of an infection control program for the NH setting. The program is best overseen by a multidisciplinary infection control committee that should meet at least quarterly. In addition to reviewing surveillance data, this committee should be involved in the development of policies and procedures that are relevant to infection control (see **Table 19-11**). The committee should be chaired by a physician or nurse with a special interest and experience in infectious diseases. In addition, a staff person, usually a nurse, should be designated as the infection control practitioner. A defined proportion of this individual's time (the amount depending on the size of the facility) should be dedicated to surveillance and other infection control activities. Surveillance can be simplified by regularly entering data into a computerized database and reviewing appropriate reports.

It is beyond the scope of this chapter to discuss all aspects of infection control. "Suggested Readings" contain sources of more detailed information

Table 19-12 Estimated risk of infective endocarditis associated with selected preexisting cardiac disorders

Relatively high risk
Prosthetic heart values
Previous infective endocarditis
Aortic regurgitation
Aortic stenosis
Mitral regurgitation
Mitral stenosis with regurgitation
Surgically repaired intracardiac lesions with residual hemodynamic abnormality
Intermediate risk
Mitral valve prolapse with regurgitation
Pure mitral stenosis
Asymmetric septal hypertrophy
Bicuspid aortic value or calcific aortic stenosis with minimal hemodynamic abnormality
Degenerative valve disease in the elderly
Surgically repaired intracardiac lesions with minimal or no hemodynamic abnormality, <6 months after surgery
Very low or negligible risk
Mitral valve prolapse without regurgitation
Trivial valvular regurgitation (on echocardiography) with no structural abnormality
Arteriosclerotic plaque
Coronary artery disease
Cardiac pacemaker
Surgically repaired intracardiac lesions, with minimal or no hemodynamic abnormality >6 months after surgery

After Durack, DT: *N Engl J Med* 332:38–44, 1995.

about infection control for NHs. In addition, the "Appendix" contains some examples of specific definitions, forms, policies, and procedures relevant to infections in the NH setting. A few points are worthy of emphasis. Because of the nature of documentation in NH records, the laboratory resources available, and the clinical presentation of infectious diseases already discussed, it is generally not possible to apply standard definitions of infections used in hospitals. Standard definitions recommended by the Centers for Disease Control should be modified for surveillance procedures (see "Appendix" for examples). Proper techniques to prevent the spread of infections in an institutional setting are critical. In addition to universal precautions, these techniques include handwashing, aseptic techniques for handling sterile equipment (such as catheters), proper care and cleaning of equipment (such as respiratory equipment and whirlpools), explicit procedures for isolation and waste disposal when contagious diseases are identified (e.g., infectious diarrhea, herpes zoster, hepatitis, tuberculosis), thorough laundering of bed linens soiled by incontinent urine or stool, and proper pest control whenever this is a problem.

Screening and preventive activities are essential components of any infection control program. These activities should extend to staff as well as residents. As noted earlier in this chapter, NH residents should receive proper immunizations to help prevent influenza, pneumococcal pneumonia, and tetanus.

Table 19-13 Examples of procedures for which antimicrobial prophylaxis is and is not recommended

Prophylaxis recommended
- Dental procedures which induce gingival bleeding (including cleaning and scaling)
- Surgery involving gastrointestinal or respiratory mucosa
- Bronchoscopy with rigid bronchoscope
- Esophageal dilatation
- Gall bladder surgery
- Genitourinary procedures
  - Urinary tract surgery (including prostate)
  - Cystoscopy
  - Urethral dilation
  - Urethral catheterization if urinary infection present

Prophylaxis not recommended
- Dental procedures not likely to cause bleeding (e.g., adjustment of appliances, fillings above the gum line)
- Bronchoscopy with flexible bronchoscope (with or without biopsy)
- Cardiac catheterization
- Gastrointestinal endoscopy (with or without biopsy)
- Genitourinary procedures in the absence of infection
  - Urethral catheterization
  - Dilatation and curettage

After Durack, DT: *N Engl J Med* 332:38–44, 1995.

Table 19-14 Basic recommendations for antimicrobial prophylaxis

For dental, oral and upper respiratory tract procedures

1. Standard regimen in patients at risk
   a. Amoxicillin, 3 g orally 1 hour before procedure and 1.5 g 6 hours after initial dose
2. If allergic to amoxicillin or penicillin:
   a. Erythromycin ethylsuccinate, 800 mg, or erythromycin stearate, 1 g orally 2 hours before procedure and ½ the dose 6 hours after initial dose **or**
   b. Clindamycin, 300 mg orally 1 hours before procedure and 150 mg 6 hours after initial dose
3. Alternative prophylactic regimens for patients at risk
   a. Standard:
      Ampicillin, 2 g intravenously or intramuscularly 30 minutes before procedure, followed by 1 g intravenously or intramuscularly, or amoxicillin, 1.5 g orally 6 hours after initial dose
   b. If allergic to amoxicillin or penicillin:
      Clindamycin, 300 mg intravenously 30 minutes before procedure and 150 mg intravenously or orally 6 hours after initial dose
   c. Alternative regimen for high-risk patients who are not candidates for the standard regimen:
      Ampicillin, 2 g intravenously or intramuscularly, plus gentamicin, 1.5 mg/kg intravenously or intramuscularly not to exceed 80 mg 30 minutes before procedure, followed by amoxicillin, 1.5 g orally 6 hours after initial dose, or repeat the parenteral regimen 8 hours after initial dose
   d. For high-risk patients allergic to amoxicillin, ampicillin, or penicillin:
      Vancomycin, 1 g intravenously administered during a 1-hour period, beginning 1 hour before procedure. No repeat dose is necessary

For genitourinary and gastrointestinal procedures

1. Standard regimen:
   Ampicillin, 2 g intravenously or intramuscularly, plus gentamicin, 1.5 mg/kg intravenously or intramuscularly not to exceed 80 mg 30 minutes before procedure, followed by amoxicillin, 1.5 g orally 6 hours after initial dose. Alternatively, the parenteral regimen may be repeated once 8 hours after initial dose
2. If allergic to amoxicillin, ampicillin, or penicillin:
   Vancomycin, 1 g intravenously administered during a 1-hour period, plus gentamicin, 1.5 mg/kg intravenously or intramuscularly not to exceed 80 mg 1 hour before procedure. May be repeated once 8 hour after initial dose
3. Alternative oral regimen for low-risk patients:
   Amoxicillin, 3 g orally 1 hour before procedure and then 1.5 g 6 hours after initial dose

All residents should be tested for tuberculosis and an appropriate policy of prophylaxis for skin-test converters should be developed (see "Appendix" for an example). Employees should also be screened for tuberculosis, and their immunization and infectious disease histories should be recorded at the time of employment. Proper screening of dietary personnel is especially important because of their potential to spread contagious diseases. Employees should also be encouraged to receive influenza vaccine and to report any potentially contagious conditions, such as diarrhea and respiratory illness, and not to report to work during such episodes.

NH residents have a high prevalence of conditions which require antimicrobial prophylaxis. Since NH residents commonly undergo a variety of procedures which are associated with a relatively high risk of endocarditis and for which prophylaxis is recommended, it is important for NH providers to identify residents in need of prophylaxis. **Tables 19-12**, **19-13**, and **19-14** summarize risk factors for endocarditis, procedures for which prophylaxis is recommended, and prophylactic regimens for common procedures.

Although standard software packages are available for infection control, any spreadsheet program can be utilized to enter and analyze the incidence of various infections. An example of a reporting format is included in the "Appendix". In addition to the incidence of infections, ongoing surveillance should include examination of culture results, sensitivity patterns of cultured organisms, and antibiotic usage. In many areas, clinical laboratories and pharmacies can provide valuable assistance in accumulating these data. Surveillance results are generally examined quarterly to identify trends and potential problem areas; it is extremely important, however, to identify potential outbreaks early in their course so that appropriate measures can be instituted to manage the outbreak and prevent an epidemic in the facility.

SUGGESTED READINGS

General

Beck-Sague C, Banerjee S, Jarvis WR: Infectious diseases and mortality among US nursing home residents. *Am J Pub Health* 83:1739–1742, 1993.

Degelau J, Guay D, Straub K, Luxenberg MG: Effectiveness of oral antibiotic treatment in nursing home-acquired pneumonia. *J Am Geriatr Soc* 43:245–251, 1995.

Magaziner J, Tenney JH, DeForge B, Hebel R, Muncie Jr. HL, Warren JW: Prevalence and characteristics of nursing home-acquired infections in the aged. *J Am Geriatr Soc* 39:1071–1078, 1991.

Orr PH, Lidnsay NE, Duckworth H, Brunka J, et al: Febrile urinary infection in the institutionalized elderly. *Am J Med* 100:71–77, 1996.

Verghese A and Berk LS (eds): *Infections in Nursing Homes and Long Term Care Facilities*. Karger, New York, 1990.

Yoshikawa TT, Norman DC: Approach to fever and infection in the nursing home. *J Am Geriatr Soc* 44:74–82, 1996.

Yoshikawa TT: Pneumonia, UTI, and decubiti in the nursing home: Optimal management. *Geriatrics* 44:32–43, 1989.

Yoshikawa TT, Norman DC: *Aging and Clinical Practices: Infectious Diseases, Diagnosis and Treatment*. New York, Igaku-Shoin, 1987.

Infection Control and Antibiotic Use

Centers for Disease Control: Recommendations of the Immunization Practices Advisory Committee, Centers for Disease Control: Prevention and control of influenza. *J Am Geriatr Soc* 36:963–968, 1988.

Crossley K, Henry K, Irvine P, Willenbring K: Antibiotic use in nursing homes: Prevalence, cost and utilization review. *Bull NY Acad Med* 63:510–518, 1987.

Crossley KB, Irvine P, Kaszar DJ, Loewenson RB: Infection control practices in Minnesota nursing homes. *JAMA* 254:2918–2921, 1985.

John JF, and Ribner BS: Antibiotic resistance in long-term care facilities. *Infect Control Hosp Epidemiol* 12:245–250, 1991.

McGeer A, Campbell B, Emori TG, et al: Definitions of infection for surveillance in long-term care facilities. *Am J Infect Control* 19:1–7, 1991.

Patriarca PA, Arden NH, Koplan JP, Goodman RA: Prevention and control of type A influenza infections in nursing homes. *Ann Intern Med* 107:732–740, 1987.

Smith PW (ed): *Infection Control in Long Term Care Facilities.* New York, Wiley, 1984.

Smith PW, Daly PB, Roccaforte JS: Current status of nosocomial infection control in extended care facilities. *Am J Med* 91:3B–281S–285S, 1991.

Zimmer JG, Bentley DW, Valenti WM, Watson NM: Systemic antibiotic use in nursing homes: A quality assessment. *J Am Geriatr Soc* 34:703–710, 1986.

Methicillin-Resistant *Staphylococcus aureus*

Boyce JM: Methicillin-resistant *Staphylococcus aureus* in hospitals and long-term care facilities: Microbiology, epidemiology, and preventive measures. *Infect Control Hosp Epidemiol* 13:725–737, 1992.

Bradley SF, Terpenning MS, Ramsey MA, et al: Methicillin-resistant *Staphylococcus aureus*: Colonization and infection in a long-term care facility. *Ann Intern Med* 115:417–422, 1991.

Muder RR, Brennen C, Wagener MM, et al: Methicillin-resistant *Staphylococcus* colonization and infection in a long-term care facility. *Ann Intern Med* 114:107–112, 1991.

Strausbaugh LJ, Jacobson C, Sewell DL, Potter S, Ward TT: Antimicrobial therapy for methicillin-resistant *Staphylococcus aureus* colonization in residents and staff of a veterans affairs nursing home care unit. *Infect Control Hosp Epidemiol* 13:151–159, 1992.

Clostridium difficile

Anaud A, Bashey B, Mir T, et al: Epidemiology, clinical manifestation, and outcome of *Clostridium difficile*-associated diarrhea. *Am J Gastroenterol* 89:519–523, 1994.

Bentley DW (ed): *Clostridium difficile*-associated disease in long-term care facilities. *Infect Control Hosp Epidemiol* 11:434–438, 1990.

Fedety R, Shah AB: Diagnosis and treatment of *Clostridium difficile* colitis. *JAMA* 269:71–75, 1993.

Kelly CP, Pothoulakis C, La Mont JT: *Clostridium difficile* colitis. *N Engl J Med* 330:257–262, 1994.

Thomas DR, Bennett RG, Laughon BE, et al: Postantibiotic colonization with *Clostridium difficile* in nursing home patients. *J Am Geriatr Soc* 38:415–420, 1990.

Tuberculosis

Finucane T: The American Geriatrics Society statement of two-step PPD testing for nursing home patients on admission. *J Am Geriatr Soc* 33:77–78, 1988.

Stead WW, To T: The significance of the tuberculin skin test in elderly persons. *Ann Intern Med* 107:837–842, 1987.

Stead WW, To T, Harrison RW, Abraham JH: Benefit-risk considerations in preventive treatment for tuberculosis in elderly persons. *Ann Intern Med* 107:843–845, 1987.

Yoshikawa TT: Tuberculosis in aging adults. *J Am Geriatr Soc* 40:178–187, 1992.

Endocarditis Prophylaxis

Durack DT: Prevention of infective endocarditis. *N Engl J Med* 332:38–44, 1995.

Van Scoy RE, Wilkowske CJ: Prophylactic use of antimicrobial agents in adult patients. *Mayo Clin Proc* 67:288–292, 1992.

CHAPTER

TWENTY

CHRONIC NEUROLOGICAL CONDITIONS

STROKE

The most common chronic neurological condition in nursing homes (NHs) is cerebrovascular accident or stroke. Stroke often results in major impairment of quality of life. Stroke can result not only in impaired ability to walk and to utilize an upper limb but also in the inabilities to communicate, think, or see adequately. The different causes of stroke are outlined in **Table 20-1**. Recognition of these is important to allow both the diagnosis of treatable causes of stroke and intervention to prevent a recurrence of stroke.

When a stroke victim is admitted to the NH, the physician should make sure that the resident has had a platelet count, Westergren sedimentation rate (looking for vasculitis), CT scan (to distinguish hemorrhage from ischemia), and electrocardiogram. Where embolus is suspected, echocardiography can be performed. A two-dimensional echocardiogram is, however, only 50 percent sensitive for mural thrombi in individuals with atrial fibrillation, and it provides poor images of mechanical prosthetic valves. It should be recognized that the presence of mural thrombi does not predict embolic risk in dilated cardiomyopathy. The presence of cardiolipin antibodies may indicate vasculitis, but aging per se may also increase titers of these antibodies.

Up to 25 percent of residents will have another stroke within a year of their first one. The risk of another stroke is increased in residents with any of the conditions outlined in **Table 20-2**. Control of blood glucose levels to under 150 mg/dl in residents with diabetes mellitus may not only prevent the recurrence of stroke but also result in improved rehabilitation potential. Diastolic blood

Table 20-1 Causes of stroke

Ischemic (82%)
- Thrombosis
- Embolus
  - cardiac
  - cartoid
- Hypotension
  - myocardial infarction
  - other
- Vasculitis

Hemorrhage (18%)
- Intercerebral
  - hypertension
  - A-V malformations
  - metastatic tumors
  - iatrogenic coagulopathy
  - congophilic angiopathy
- Subarachnoid
  - Berry anuerysms
  - A-V malformations
  - coagulopathies
  - infectious endocarditis
  - vasculitis
  - idiopathic hemorrhage

pressure should be kept to between 90 to 95 mmHg to prevent recurrence of stroke.

The use of anticoagulation or antiplatelet therapy in ischemic stroke depends on the general health status of the resident and the history of previous bleeds. In the short-term stayer admitted for acute rehabilitation, low-dose aspirin should be used on a daily basis. Anticoagulation with coumadin, making sure that the prothrombin time is maintained at an INR of 1.8 to 2.5 should be used for cardiogenic embolism and possibly also for artery-to-artery thromboembolism. This appears to give maximum protection with minimum bleeding. Our experience has suggested that in the very frail resident, anticoagulation greatly

Tab!e 20-2 Factors predisposing to stroke

- Cardiac disease
- Hypertension
- Diabetes mellitus
- Diabetes vascular disease
- Cervical bruit
- Transient ischemic attacks

increases the potential of gastrointestinal bleeding. Thus, decisions on the use of aspirin or anticoagulation must be individualized. The combination of low-dose aspirin and a nonsteroidal anti-inflammatory agent makes little sense and may potentiate bleeding. Some of the general principles of rehabilitation are discussed in Chapter 24. The success of rehabilitation in residents with stroke is improved by early intervention (within 48 h). In addition, it is important to ensure that there is no hiatus in rehabilitation when transfer to the NH occurs. Range-of-motion exercises are extremely important, and each affected extremity should be moved through the complete range of motion with five repetitions twice daily. Stretching should be done with care and overstretching avoided. Foot boards and splints for wrists and fingers can help to maintain these parts of the extremities in a functional position. Flaccid extremities should be kept in the neutral position and the shoulder should be abducted for some period each day. Hands should be elevated if edema is present. Subluxation of the shoulder can occur, and use of a sling, pillow, or wheelchair board may be necessary in order to prevent its occurrence in a flaccid limb. A painful shoulder may respond to hot packs or ultrasound, though local or systemic corticosteroids may be necessary. Spasticity can be treated by diazepam (though with careful dosing in older individuals) or by baclofen. Biofeedback may also help. Judicious use of adaptive devices may result in major functional improvement. Residents should be taught how to use paralyzed extremities in order to passively assist in activities of daily living.

For mobility, the resident must regain balance. Standing in parallel bars is helpful in this regard. Most residents with stroke will require a hemiwalker or quad cane to allow mobility in the early phase after a stroke. Braces too can play an important part in allowing full mobility. Therapy focusing on completing tasks necessary for dressing and grooming is also critical. In many NHs, the failure of nursing staff to be prepared to wait a sufficient period of time for the resident to complete a task is a major hindrance to rehabilitation. It can take a resident with a stroke up to 2 h to complete bathing, brushing teeth, combing hair, shaving, and dressing. With patience, this time can be reduced within 1 to 2 months to less than a half hour.

Dysphagia occurs in 39 percent of all residents following stroke. With good speech therapy intervention and altered diet texture aspiration is rare. All NH residents following stroke should have a screening assessment for swallowing dysfunction following a stroke. Among those with dysfunction fully intact swallowing will be recovered in about one in five residents.

Residents with nondominant frontoparietal infarcts often have hemineglect. This can cause them to bump into objects on the neglected side and fail to be able to read half of a page. Such residents often have problems not only in dressing but also in shaving on the affected side. **Figure 20-1** shows an example of a drawing made by a resident with hemineglect.

Problems with speech are common following stroke. Dysarthria (difficulty in pronouncing words) can be due to involvement of either the peripheral or central nervous system. Involvement of Wernicke's area (anterior lesions) leads

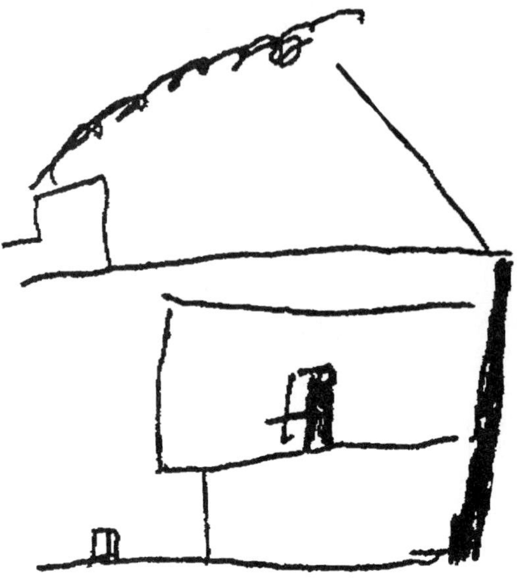

Figure 20-1 Picture of a house drawn by a man with a severe left hemineglect.

to a fluent speech defect that often includes "nonsense" words. These residents also tend to find word or sentence substitutions for the word they wish to use and can have impaired understanding of verbal commands. Involvement of Broca's area, on the other hand, leads to a "nonfluent" speech (expressive aphasia). The resident may be able to pronounce the nouns and verbs but leaves out the in-between words. Aphasia following stroke can take up to a year to resolve maximally. All residents with speech problems can benefit from a consultation with a speech pathologist. Residents with speech defects should be formed into groups to facilitate communication and social support.

Residents with lesions in the supplementary motor area supplied by the anterior cerebral artery may develop impairment of carrying out automatic movements such as those used for brushing their teeth, despite having the necessary motor function to carry out the task. Such residents require painstaking retraining to reestablish the necessary motor patterns.

Approximately one-third of residents will develop a major depressive episode within 2 years of a stroke. Untreated depression is associated with worse rehabilitation outcomes. Residents should be screened for depression at 3-monthly intervals following a stroke. The management of depression is discussed in detail in Chapter 12. Stroke may also result in a reduced attention span and cognitive dysfunction. Emotional lability and inappropriate emotional responses are also seen in residents who have had strokes.

The resident who has had a stroke requires special attention to a number of syndromes. Lack of awareness of the syndromes associated with stroke can cause frustration for both NH residents and staff. **Table 20-3** summarizes the common

Table 20-3 Common syndromes associated with stroke and approaches to their management

Syndrome	Management
Painful shoulder	Hot packs or ultrasound
Hemineglect	Occupational therapy concentrating on neglected side
Speech problems dysarthria aphasia	Speech pathologist Communication groups
Impairment of automatic movements	Recognition and retraining
Dysphagia	Speech pathologist Special foods Enteral tube feeding if necessary
Spasticity/cramping	Baclofen Diazepam (low dose) Biofeedback
Depression	Low-dose antidepressant Group therapy
Reduced attention span	Limited activity sessions
Cognitive problems	Memory aids Memory retraining
Emotional lability	Staff awareness that this is related to stroke
Incontinence	Frequent toileting Exclude unrinary retention, urinary tract infection Consider pharmacologic treatment for urge incontinence (see Chap. 13)
Shoulder sublaxation	Sling may help

conditions associated with stroke and some of the available management approaches. It is important to involve the resident's family members in the understanding of the various syndromes associated with stroke. Involvement in family counseling may be necessary to allow family members to deal with their own psychological stress associated with a stroke occurring in a family member.

PARKINSON'S DISEASE

Parkinson's disease occurs in 1 percent of persons over the age of 65. Parkinson's disease is characterized by tremor, difficulty in initiating movement (akinesia), and slowness in movement (bradykinesia). Cognitive impairment can occur in up to 20 percent of residents with Parkinson's disease, and depression can be present in up to 40 percent. Visual hallucinations and illusions can also occur, sometimes as a result of antiparkinsonian medication.

Several complications of immobility are common in residents with Parkinson's disease. Gait and balance difficulties are common in Parkinson's patients and predispose them to falls and consequent decreases in mobility (see Chapter 16). Ankle and pedal edema can be limited by increased exercise of the lower extremities. Incontinence, usually of the urge type, can be managed behaviorally and/or pharmacologically (see Chapter 15). Constipation is related to decreased movement, inability to develop adequate abdominal pressure when straining at stool, and decreased bowel mobility (due to both the disease and its therapy). Thus, residents with parkinsonism should be on some type of bowel regimen that includes stool softeners and regular toileting after breakfast in order to "train" the bowel habit and prevent fecal impaction. Orthostatic hypotension can be particularly troublesome in residents with Parkinson's disease (see Chapter 21).

Weight loss is common in Parkinson's residents. This may be associated with difficulties in swallowing, particularly when the head can no longer be maintained in an erect position. It is often associated with sialorrhea. The major cause of weight loss in many parkinsonian residents, however, is the energy expended by the incessant tremors at rest.

Residents with Parkinson's disease often show poor motivation to maintain an exercise program. Group sessions may help provide peer pressure to keep residents in such a program. Exercise sessions for these residents should be limited to 10 min at a time and repeated three to four times per day. Full range-of-motion exercises for those muscle groups necessary for activities of daily living should be carried out at each session. Exercises to prevent stooped posture and leaning to one side are important. Leg-raising exercises may reduce the accumulation of edema. Placing objects on the ground and making the resident step over them can improve gait speed and possibly help prevent tripping due to the typical shuffling gait. The availability of virtual reality glasses that project objects in front of the person with Parkinson's has enhanced the mobility of these persons. The resident with Parkinson's disease and poor balance requires a wheeled walker. Nonwheeled walkers can cause these residents to fall backwards when they lift the walker off the ground.

The drug therapy of choice for Parkinson's disease is a combination of L-dopa and carbidopa (Sinemet). Sinemet should be taken 30 to 60 min before meals to enhance absorption. However, if nausea develops, it may have to given with meals. Excessive protein intake should be avoided in residents with Parkinson's disease because it may interfere with the brain's uptake of L-dopa. Some residents develop abnormal movements 3 h after taking Sinemet. They may benefit from the addition of a direct dopamine agonist such as bromocriptine (Parlodel) or pergolide (Permax) or of the long acting Sinemet CR. Sellegine, a monoamine B oxidase inhibitor, may enhance the effect of Sinemet by 20 percent to 30 percent, perhaps improves the longevity of residents with Parkinson's

Table 20-4 Modalities useful to manage residents with Parkinson's disease

1. Leg exercises four times per day for 3 to 5 min at a time if edema is present.
2. Range-of-motion exercises three to four times per day for 5 min at a time. Usually better compliance if carried out in groups.
3. Exercises to correct stooped posture and leaning to one side.
4. Regular walking using a wheeled walker.
5. Training to step over real or imaginary objects to help initiate gait.
6. Support the neck muscles with exercise, a soft cervical collar may be helpful.
7. Limit protein intake to 40 g per 70 kg of body weight in diet. (Resident may need increased calories because of energy expenditure due to tremors.)
8. Adequate fluid intake.
9. Train resident to push on abdomen when straining at stool. (For this purpose a soft cushion pushed into the abdomen may help.)
10. Screen regularly for depression and treat when present.
11. Assess and treat incontinence when present.
12. Medications
    - Avoid anticholinergics in the older NH resident.
    - Sinemet (L-dopa and carbidopa)
    - Dopamine agonists: bromocriptine, pergolide
    - Deprenyl (monamine oxidase B inhibitor)—expensive, but may improve mental function
    - Amantadine, low-dose (100–200 mg/day)

disease, and enhance mental functioning. Anticholinergic drugs are usually not useful in NH residents because of side effects. Anticholinergic drugs should be tapered slowly, as they may otherwise result in a withdrawal syndrome consisting of 2 to 3 days of worsening parkinsonian symptoms. Amantadine at 200 mg/day or less may result in some improvement. Side effects include hallucinations, purple mottling of the skin, and ankle swelling. In residents with end-stage Parkinson's disease, tapering of drugs can be tried, but this needs careful monitoring for increased rigidity and immobility, which can, in turn, lead to complications such as pressure sores and aspiration. Depression is common early in Parkinson's disease and should be vigorously treated. Hallucinations are relatively common in endstage Parkinson's disease sufferers, and may be a side effect of antiparkinsonian medications (especially L-dopa). When a Parkinson resident needs a neuroleptic, clozapine is the drug of choice because it does not have the extrapyramidal effects of haloperidol and thiothixene.

Table 20-4 summarizes the major modalities useful for management of the resident with Parkinson's disease.

TREMORS

A number of drugs may cause tremors in NH residents. These include anticholinergic drugs, neuroleptics, lithium, adrenergic agonists, theophylline, corticosteroids, and thyroid hormone (given in excessive amounts for replacement). Pathological causes of tremor include anxiety, hyperthyroidism, cerebellar disease, Parkinson's disease, alcoholism, and alcohol withdrawal. Essential tremor is extremely common with advancing age. Beta blockers (e.g., propranolol 240 mg/day) are partially effective at controlling tremors, but in older individuals they may cause serious side effects (e.g., heart failure, bronchospasm, fatigue, limb "heaviness"). Primidone (start at 62.5 mg and increase to 250 mg three times per day over 3 weeks) has been suggested, but its severe side effects, including vomiting, ataxia, and headache, make it a poor choice for NH residents. Methoxolamide, a carbonic anhydrase inhibitor, has also been effective in some persons. Drug therapy of essential tremor in NH residents is justified only when the tremor interferes substantially with the resident's ability to carry out activities of daily living.

EPILEPTIC SEIZURES

By 70 years of age, 2 to 3 percent of the older population will suffer from epilepsy. There is little information on the management of epileptic seizures in NH residents. New-onset seizures in any person over age 60 should be investigated to rule out the possibility of tumor or subdural hematoma. Older persons with petit mal, temporal lobe epilepsy or prolonged post-ictal states may present with delirium. The major complications of epilepsy in older persons are listed in **Table 20-5**. Many residents are placed on antiepileptic therapy at the time of a single seizure associated with a stroke, hypoxia, or neurosurgery. Many of these residents do not need this treatment long-term and the medication can be discontinued 6 weeks following the event with no adverse consequences. There are also many NH residents who are on anticonvulsant medication for unclear reasons. In view of the severity of side effects of these medications, these residents are deserving of a trial off medication. This is also true of residents who have had a single seizure at some time in the past. Of individuals with a single

Table 20-5 Complications of epilepsy in nursing home residents

Traumatic
Tongue bites producing anorexia
Fractures
Head injury
Subdural hematoma
Delirium
Aspiration pneumonia
Cognitive dysfunction
Decreased functional status
Status epilepticus
Medication side effects

Table 20-6 Side effects of antiepileptic medications

Phenytoin	Carbamazepine	Sodium valproate	Gabapentine
Drowsiness	Dizziness	Tremor	Drowsiness
Ataxia	Ataxia	Agitation	Ataxia
Gingival hypertrophy	Nausea	Weight gain	Dizziness
Folate deficiency	Hyponatremia	Hair loss	Nystagmus
Neuropathy	Aplastic anemia	Liver dysfunction	Status epilepticus when drug stopped
Hirsutism	Dyslalia	Delirium	
Vitamin D deficiency	Delirium	Thrombocytopenia	
Pseudolymphona		Nausea	
Delirium			
Nystagmus			

seizure, 60 percent will not have a repeat seizure within 5 years. Phenytoin is protein bound and the upper limit of safety for serum levels needs to be adjusted downwards when the person has low albumin level is low. Recent studies have suggested that sodium valproate has high efficacy and tolerability as first line therapy. The side effects of antiepileptic medications are listed in **Table 20-6**.

MULTIPLE SCLEROSIS

Multiple sclerosis is a common cause of institutionalization, especially among those suffering from the chronic progressive form. Institutionalized residents with multiple sclerosis are often much younger than the majority of residents in a NH. Symptoms are commonly worse in the afternoon and when the temperature increases. Keeping the temperature low, use of swimming therapy and vigorous therapy of elevated temperatures with acetaminophen and external cooling may all play a useful role in limiting symptomatology.

Infections may trigger an exacerbation of the underlying disease. Even in young persons with multiple sclerosis, infections often present atypically either with delirium or a failure to see the expected fever normally associated with infection. Any NH resident with multiple sclerosis who has a change in functional mental status, even if it is subtle, should be evaluated to exclude a treatable infection.

Spasticity is a common problem in advanced multiple sclerosis and may respond to baclofen or diazepam in addition to range-of-motion exercises. Incontinence is also very common and is generally associated with detrusor hyperreflexia. Individuals with multiple sclerosis can, however, develop a wide variety of lower urinary tract dysfunctions, including detrusor-sphincter dyssynergy and acontractile bladder. For these reasons, residents with multiple sclerosis who develop new or worsened incontinence should have a careful urodynamic evaluation (see Chapter 15).

Many residents with multiple sclerosis also develop some degree of cognitive dysfunction. Depression is very common and requires active therapy. Sexual dysfunction may be a major concern among younger males with multiple sclerosis. Vacuum tumescence devices or penile prostheses may be a reasonable therapy for some of these residents. Physicians should be supportive of residents with multiple sclerosis and be optimistic concerning the possibility of improved treatments. The length of exacerbations may be shortened by treatment with methylprednisone or adrenocorticotrophic hormone (ACTH). Interferon-beta (Betaseron) can reduce the frequency of relapses. Immunosuppressive agents such as azathioprine and cyclophosphamide have also been used for treatment of chronic progression.

HUNTINGTON'S CHOREA

Huntington's chorea is a dominant disorder associated with a gene on chromosome four. It involves degeneration of the caudate nucleus and the putamen of the basal ganglia and is associated with a selective loss of γ-aminobutyric acid.

Huntington's chorea presents in the fourth or fifth decades of life, and those afflicted generally develop disabilities severe enough to need NH care at a young age. Residents with this disorder will typically survive 10 to 20 years in the NH. These residents have a cognitive disturbance predominantly involving the ability to carry out complex processes and to maintain good judgment. The ability to maintain long-term memory and speech functions often remains intact until late in the disorder. The major debilitating feature is the abnormal choreiform movements that involve both upper and lower limbs, the face, and the trunk. These movements often respond well to baclofen. However, as the disease progresses, extremely high doses of neuroleptics may be necessary to maintain the abnormal movements at an acceptable level—one that allows the staff to care for the resident. Abnormal movements are worse when the resident is disturbed and flailing motions can injure staff. Staff need to be warned that the resident understands what is being said. It is important to provide support for the resident's family and provide sensory stimulation for the resident.

MEIGS SYNDROME (BLEPHAROSPASM AND OROFACIAL CERVICAL DYSTONIA)

This disorder usually presents after the age of 60. It consists of blepharospasm, abnormal movements of the mouth, clenching of the jaw, lip smacking, and occasionally spasms of cervical muscles. Dysarthria and swallowing difficulties may also be associated with this syndrome. Meigs syndrome may be confused with tardive kinesia secondary to neuroleptic use. When blepharospasm interferes with function, it may be controlled by injecting botulinum toxin into the eyelid muscle or by surgery.

SUGGESTED READINGS

Stroke

Diamond PT, Halroyd S, Macciocche SN, Felsenthal A: Prevalence of depression and outcome on the geriatric rehabilitation unit. *Am J Phys Med Rehab* 76:216–217, 1995.

Kelly JF, Winograd CH: A functional approach to stroke management in elderly patients. *J Am Geriatr Soc* 33:48–60, 1985.

Nadeau SE: Stroke. *Med Clin North Am* 73:1351, 1989.

Odderson IR, Keaton JC, McKenna BS: Swallow management in patients on an acute stroke pathway: Quality is cost-effective. *Arch Phys Med Rehab* 76:1130–1133, 1995.

Sarno MT: Communication disorders in the elderly, in T. Franklin Williams (ed): *Rehabilitation in the Aging*. New York, Raven Press, 1984, p. 161.

Yibson CJ, Caplan BM: Rehabilitation of the patient with stroke, in T. Franklin Williams (ed): *Rehabilitation in the Aging*. New York, Raven Press, 1984, p. 165.

Parkinson's Disease

Cote LJ, Henly M: Parkinson's disease, in Hazzard WR, Andres R, Bresman EL, Blass JP (eds): *Principles of Geriatric Medicine and Gerontology*. New York, McGraw-Hill, 1990, p. 954.

Rich SS, Friedman JM, Ott BR: Resperidone versus clozepine in the treatment of psychosis in six patients with Parkinson's disease and other akinetic-rigid syndromes. *J Clin Psychiat* 56:556–559, 1995.

Sweeny PJ: Parkinson's disease: Managing symptoms and preserving function. *Geriatrics* 50:26–31, 1995.

Tremor

Cleaves L, Findley LJ: Tremors. *Med Clin North Am* 73:1307, 1989.

Purushothaman R, Morley JE: Differential diagnosis and management of tremors in the elderly. *Clin Geriatr* 3:44–56, 1995.

Multiple Sclerosis

Rosenthal MJ: Chronic care issues in multiple sclerosis. *Geriatric Med Today* 7(4):73, 1988.

Lynch SG, Rose JW: Multiple sclerosis. *Disease-a-Month* 42:1–55, 1996.

Epilepsy

Wilson M-MG: Epilepsy in older persons: Part I: Pathophysiology, classification, etiology and clinical evaluation. *Clin Geriatr* 3:18–30, 1995.

Wilson M-MG: Epilepsy in older persons. Part II: Approaches to Management. *Clin Geriatr* 3:33–51, 1995.

CHAPTER
TWENTY-ONE

SELECTED MEDICAL CONDITIONS

The purpose of this chapter is to briefly review the management of several common clinical disorders in nursing home (NH) residents that are not covered in other chapters of this text. We do not mean to imply that conditions discussed are unimportant; we have tried to focus on conditions that are most common and treatable in the NH population.

ANEMIA

Anemia (a hemoglobin below 12 g/dl) is present in 30 to 50 percent of institutionalized older persons. In approximately 30 percent of these individuals, the anemia will be unrecognized; in another 30 percent, it will be recognized but not treated. The causes of anemia are outlined in **Fig. 21-1**. In a NH population, the major cause of a hemoglobin between 10 and 12 g/dl will be an anemia of chronic disease and/or malnutrition. It is important, however, to distinguish the treatable anemias from the anemia of chronic disease. It is also critical to recognize that NH residents with acute blood loss or dehydration may have anemia in the presence of a normal hemoglobin.

The first step in diagnosing the cause of an anemia is to obtain a reticulocyte count and calculate the reticulocyte index (**Table 21-1**). If the reticulocyte index is greater than 3 percent, the anemia is due either to hemorrhage or hemolysis. In these residents the stool should be checked for blood and medication lists reviewed to exclude drugs (e.g., methyldopa) that may cause an autoimmune

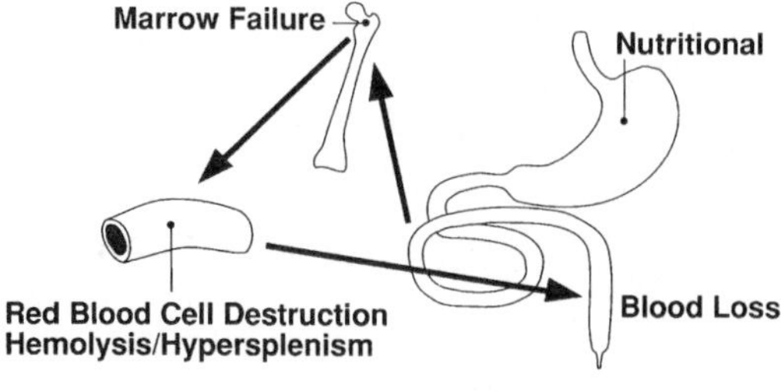

Figure 21-1 Basic causes of anemia in the nursing home population.

Table 21-1 Reticulocyte index (RI)

$$RI = \text{reticulyte count} \times \frac{\text{resident's HCT}}{\text{normal HCT}} \times \frac{1}{\text{maturation time}}$$

Maturation time	HCT, %
1.0	45
1.5	35
2.0	25
2.5	15

Note: HCT = Hematocrit. Normal RI is 73 percent.

hemolytic anemia or gastrointestinal bleeding (e.g., nonsteroidal anti-inflammatory agents). If blood loss cannot be identified, the next step is to obtain a Coombs test to rule out the presence of autoimmune hemolytic anemia, which is the most common cause of hemolysis in older persons. **Table 21-2** lists the most common causes and the treatment options for autoimmune hemolytic anemia. Microangiopathic hemolytic anemias associated with neoplasms or severe infection are not uncommon in older individuals. Diagnosis is made by finding decreased platelet levels, a prolonged partial thromboplastin time, hemosiderin in the urine, and red cell fragments on the smear.

When the reticulocyte index is less than 3 percent, the next step is to determine whether the red cell indices are micro-, normo-, or macrocytic. Normocytic indices may suggest a combination of vitamin B_{12} and iron deficiency. Currently it is recommended that these residents undergo further investigation only when the hemoglobin is below 11 g/dl. Multiple myeloma can occur in this population. If it is suspected, a serum and urine protein electrophoresis should be obtained. Residents with microcytic anemia should undergo iron studies, including iron transferrin saturation, total iron binding capacity, and ferritin (**Table 21-3**). This should allow the diagnosis of either iron-deficiency anemia or the anemia of chronic disease to be made. When the results are equivocal, a bone marrow biopsy may be necessary to make the final diagnosis. Iron-deficiency anemia is often overtreated. To correct an iron-

Table 21-2 Common causes and treatment of hemolytic anemias in nursing home residents

Causes
- Mycoplasma infections (bilateral infiltrate on chest X-ray)
- Chronic lymphocytic leukemia
- Non-Hodgkin's lymphoma
- Collagen vascular disorders

Drugs
- Methyldopa
- Quinine
- Quinidine
- Salicylates
- Penicillins

Treatment
- Ig/G red cell antibodies: steroids and possibly splenetomy
- Ig/M red cell antibodies: refractory to treatment

Table 21-3 Differential diagnosis of iron-associated anemias

	Iron deficiency	Anemia of chronic disease	Sideroblastic anemia
Iron	Low	Low	High
Transferrin saturation	<20%	<20%	High
Ferritin	<20 ng/dl	<100 ng/dl	20–100 ng/dl
Total iron-binding capacity	>375	<250	250–375
Bone marrow	Absent iron stores	Normal or increased iron stores	Ringed siderblasts

deficiency anemia, approximately 20 mg of iron per day for 7 weeks is needed, and 300 mg of iron sulfate contains 60 mg of iron (325 mg of iron gluconate contains 37 mg of iron). Thus one tablet of iron a day is sufficient to correct the anemia. A reticulocyte count should be obtained after 1 week of therapy with iron to check for an adequate response. Residents with a normal transferrin saturation (>20 percent) should be worked up for hypothyroidism, Addison's disease, protein–energy malnutrition, or a hemoglobinopathy. When iron deficiency is diagnosed, the resident should have at least three stools collected for occult blood. If any of these stools contains blood, both a lower and upper GI endoscopy should be performed (**Table 21-4**).

Sideroblastic anemia is a disorder of older persons. Iron is deposited in the mitochondria of normoblasts, resulting in the presence of ringed sideroblasts in the marrow. The peripheral smear is dimorphic, with both macrocytes and normocytes being present and approximately 50 percent of them showing

Table 21-4 Causes of anemias associated with low serum iron in older subjects

Blood loss
- Gastrointestinal
  - Gastritis
  - Esophagitis
  - Ulcers
  - Neoplasia
  - Angiodysplasia
  - Diverticular disease
  - Aspirin and nonsteroidal anti-inflammatory drugs
  - Alcohol
- Epistaxis
- Hemoptysis
- Hematuria
- Hematoma (especially after hip fracture)
- Coagulation disorders
- Coumadin

Anemia or chronic disease
- Infections
- Neoplasia
- Pressure sores
- Collagen vascular disorders
- Rheumatoid arthritis
- Polymyaglia rheumatica

hypochromia. The reticulocyte count may be normal or increased and there is often a mild neutropenia. Clinically, in addition to symptoms of anemia, residents may have a lemon-yellow hue to their skin, hepatosplenomegaly, and anorexia. Sideroblastic anemia occurs more commonly in residents with diabetes mellitus or congestive heart failure. Residents with sideroblastic anemia have an increase in serum iron and transferrin saturation, normal total iron binding capacity and ferritin, and an increased free erythrocyte protoporphyrin. Most sideroblastic anemias are idiopathic, and approximately 10 percent of these will respond to 200 mg of pyridoxine three times per day. Sideroblastic anemias are occasionally associated with drug administration (e.g., isoniazid, pyrazinamide, chloramphenicol) or with lead toxicity or chronic neoplastic or inflammatory disease. Drug-associated sideroblastic anemia may also respond to pyridoxine. Residents with sideroblastic anemias are at increased risk for developing acute myelogenous leukemia.

Macrocytic anemias are due either to vitamin B_{12} or folate deficiency. Pernicious anemia occurs in 3 percent of females and 1 percent of males over the age of 60. It is associated with a lack of intrinsic factor, which binds the vitamin B_{12} to allow its absorption in the small intestine. A blood smear demonstrates macrocytosis, pancytopenia, and hypersegmented polymorphonuclear leukocytes. The resident may have increased indirect circulating bilirubin levels and an increased lactic dehydrogenase. Besides anemia, residents with pernicious anemia may have dementia, ataxia, posterior column abnormalities (loss of position sense), and glossitis. Residents with pernicious anemia have increased risk of developing hypothyroidism, diabetes mellitus, Addison's disease, and nontropical sprue. Vitamin B_{12} deficiency may also be due to ileal disease or to protein–energy malnutrition. Serum vitamin B_{12} levels below 200 pg/ml are considered low. Residents with values between 200 to 400 pg/ml should have their serum B_{12} level measured at 6-monthly intervals. If a macrocytic anemia is present serum levels of methylmalonic acid and homocysteine should be measured. If both are elevated the resident has vitamin B_{12} deficiency, if only homocysteine is elevated the diagnosis is folate deficiency. The Schilling test is now rarely used in the diagnosis of pernicious anemia. Treatment of vitamin B_{12} deficiency is by biweekly injection of 100 μg of vitamin B_{12} until the anemia corrects and then monthly injections.

Some elderly NH residents develop severe anemia due to bone marrow failure. This is generally associated with one or more chronic diseases. In some cases, the marrow contains an increased number of blast cells, but not enough to make the diagnosis of leukemia. These residents may require repeated blood transfusions to maintain their hemoglobin values above the range of 7 to 8 g/dl. We have now seen a number of patients like this whose anemia has responded to erythropoietin injections. Although expensive, this option should be considered as it can markedly enhance quality of life.

CARDIOVASCULAR DISORDERS

Cardiovascular disease is the major cause of death in older persons, accounting for nearly half the deaths in those over age 75. Digoxin, diuretics, beta blockers, calcium channel blockers, nitrates, and angiotensin converting enzyme inhibitors are among the most common drugs utilized in the NH. A full discussion of cardiovascular disease is beyond the scope of this chapter. Only a few points of special importance to NH residents will be highlighted.

Myocardial Infarction

In older persons, myocardial infarction often presents without chest pain. The new onset of dyspnea is the most common presentation of myocardial infarction in institutionalized elderly individuals. Myocardial infarction should also be suspected in any NH resident who has acute onset of confusion. The incidence of syncope as a presentation of myocardial infarction doubles in institutionalized individuals. Syncopal episodes should, therefore, arouse suspicion of an acute myocardial infarction in a NH resident.

Cardiac Amyloidosis

Cardiac amyloidosis is a disease of older persons. It may cause heart failure and angina (when the coronary arteries are involved). Diagnosis should be considered when the resident has a restrictive cardiomyopathy with an electrocardiogram demonstrating low-voltage left axis deviation and a pseudoinfarct pattern (decreased R waves in the precordium and Q waves anteriorly). An echocardiogram demonstrates "granular speckling." Residents with amyloidosis may be especially likely to develop digoxin toxicity.

Congestive Heart Failure

Congestive heart failure (CHF) occurs in approximately 10 percent of persons in their eighties. Heart failure can be due to inadequate contraction of the ventricle (systolic dysfunction) or the failure of the heart to relax adequately during diastole (diastolic dysfunction). Up to 40 percent of older residents with heart failure have diastolic dysfunction. Residents with ischemia in combination with diastolic dysfunction have a particularly poor prognosis. The major factors distinguishing between systolic and diastolic dysfunction are outlined in **Table 21-5**. In residents with diastolic dysfunction and heart failure digoxin and arterial vasodilators should be avoided. Regulation of tachycardia in diastolic dysfunction is key and is best obtained with beta-blockers. Diuretics should be utilized in low doses in diastolic dysfunction in combination with angiotensin converting enzyme inhibitors. Calcium channel blockers are also used for this condition.

Table 21-5 Diagnosis of heart failure: differentiation and treatment of diastolic compared to systolic dysfunction

	Diastolic dysfunction	Systolic dysfunction
Age	Over 65 years	Less than 65 years
Presentation	Acute dyspnea	Progressive dyspnea
Examination	S_4 heart sound	S_3 heart sound
Chest X-ray	No cardiomegaly	Cardiomegaly
EKG	Left ventricular hypertrophy	Q waves
Echocardiogram	Normal ejection fraction	Decreased ejection fraction
Treatment	Slow heart rate Avoid digoxin and arterial vasodilators	Diuretics Digoxin ACE inhibitors

Digoxin Use and Arrhythmia Treatment

Digoxin is a dangerous drug in older persons and it is greatly overused in NHs. Many residents receive digoxin because of lower extremity edema, which is due to stasis, varicose veins, and decreased serum albumin rather than heart failure. Digoxin can cause protein-energy malnutrition in as many as 25 percent of older residents receiving this drug, because it causes anorexia. Digoxin can also produce dementia and depression in a substantial number of residents. In NH residents, digoxin use should probably be limited to those with atrial fibrillation and a ventricular response greater than 100 beats per minute or a history of other recurrent symptomatic supraventricular arrhythmias. Digoxin can, however, precipitate heart block in individuals with sick sinus syndrome, and 24-h monitoring should be used to exclude this diagnosis. Contraindications to digoxin include idiopathic hypertrophic subaortic stenosis and ventricular diastolic dysfunction, which are being increasingly recognized in the geriatric population. These conditions are better treated with calcium channel blockers.

Management of ventricular arrhythmias should initially ensure that potassium and magnesium values are normal. The incidence of ventricular arrhythmias, even among elderly individuals without symptomatic cardiac disease, is high. No studies have documented improved outcomes resulting from treatment of these arrhythmias, and antiarrhythmic drugs have numerous serious side effects. In most cases, the advantages of drug therapy for ventricular arrhythmias is offset by these side effects. Therefore, we rarely use antiarrhythmics in NH residents unless a resident is bothered by palpitations or treatment is strongly recommended by a cardiologist. Automatic implantable defibrillation systems are available for recurrent ventricular tachycardia or fibrillation.

Hypertrophic Obstructive Cardiomyopathy

The diagnosis of hypertrophic obstructive cardiomyopathy should be considered in residents with heart failure, angina, and syncope or in residents who had hypertension that is no longer present and are not malnourished. Echocardiography demonstrates septal hypertrophy. Like heart failure associated with ventricular diastolic dysfunction, this disorder responds specifically to beta blockers and calcium channel blockers. Digoxin is not indicated for congestive heart failure associated with hypertrophic obstructive cardiomyopathy and may exacerbate this condition.

Aortic Stenosis

Aortic stenosis is common in the very old and may progress to cause syncope, heart failure, and angina. NH residents who are suspected of having aortic stenosis and who are candidates for surgical interventions should be followed with periodic (6 to 12 months) echocardiography with Doppler flow to detect progression. Clinically, aortic stenosis of increasing severity presents with dyspnea. This worsening dyspnea must be distinguished from that due to coexistent chronic obstructive pulmonary disease. Properly timed valve replacement surgery can preserve several years of life. For some residents who are too ill to undergo valve replacement, balloon valvuloplasty may provide at least temporary relief of disabling symptoms. Residents with aortic stenosis are also at greater risk of having gastrointestinal bleeds from angiodysplasia.

Hypertension

Hypertension is present in approximately 40 percent of individuals over age 65. The European multicenter study has demonstrated that there is a U-shaped mortality curve associated with diastolic blood pressure, with blood pressures below 90 mmHg being as liable to result in death as those over 100 mmHg. For this reason, it is recommended that blood pressure control in NH residents aims at a diastolic blood pressure between 90 and 95 mmHg. The Systolic Hypertension in the Elderly Program (SHEP) demonstrated that reducing isolated systolic blood pressure greater than 160 mmHg was associated with a reduced stroke risk. Where possible, monotherapy should be attempted. Costs suggest that thiazide diuretics are the drugs of choice to treat hypertension in this population. The dose should be limited to 25 mg daily of hydrochlorothiazide. Only when potassium depletion is demonstrated should potassium supplementation or triamterene be added. Hyperkalemia is more likely than hypokalemia to cause sudden death without prior symptoms. Triamterene can be associated with triamterene kidney stones, particularly in dehydrated residents. If a thiazide diuretic fails, an angiotensin converting enzyme (ACE) inhibitor as monotherapy can be tried. Many NH residents have concomitant disorders that may guide drug therapy (e.g., a calcium channel blocker may be appropriate in residents with angina and hypertension, and ACE inhibitors may be appropriate in those with concomitant heart failure or in persons with diabetes). Classical step therapy can be tried if these approaches fail. Weight loss in NHs often results in improvement in the resident's blood pressure; hence the need for antihypertensive medications should be regularly reevaluated. In addition, the possibility that the resident is suffering from side effects of antihypertensive therapy should regularly be reviewed. While hypertension is often responsive to low-salt diets in NH residents, we do not recommend this approach routinely because it may unnecessarily interfere with the resident's dietary satisfaction and result in the potential for producing protein-energy malnutrition through dietary manipulation.

Pseudohypertension

A small percentage of older persons (less than 5 percent) have "pseudohypertension" due to rigidity of the arteries. This should be suspected when the radial artery (not the pulse) is palpable while the blood pressure cuff is inflated above the systolic blood pressure. This is called Osler's sign and has debatable sensitivity and specificity. Care should be taken not to overtreat if such an individual is to be considered for antihypertensive therapy.

Meal-Associated Hypotension

A number of older NH residents have been found to have declines in mean blood pressure of between 5 to 20 mmHg following ingestion of a meal and the release of a vasodilatory peptide hormone, calcitonin gene related peptide. The blood pressure drop may last for 2 to 3 h. This drop in blood pressure has been correlated with an increased prevalence of falls following a meal in the NH population. The fall in blood pressure is predominantly related to the carbohydrate content of the meal. It can be ameliorated by giving meals with a higher fat content or by giving multiple small meals. A somatostatin analog has been shown experimentally to prevent the meal associated fall in blood pressure and is available in the United States for treatment of acromegaly.

Orthostatic Hypotension

Postural hypotension (a drop of 10 mmHg in systolic blood pressure or 5 mmHg in diastolic blood pressure within 2 min after arising from the recumbent position) has been reported to be present in 8 percent to 11 percent of NH residents. Old age alone is not a sufficient reason for postural hypotension, and

Table 21-6 Causes of postural hypotension

Medications	Autonomic neuropathy
Diuretics	Diabetes mellitus
Antidepressants	Amyloidosis
Neuroleptics	Alcoholism
Antihypertensives	Central nervous system
Antianginals	Parkinson's disease
Antiparkinsonians	Stroke
Anticholinergics	Peripheral nervous
Hypovolemia	Guillain-Barré
Dehydration	Familial dysautonomia (Riley-Day)
Blood loss/anemia	Cardiovascular
Malnutrition	Hypertrophic cardiomyopathy
Prolonged recumbency	Venous insufficiency (varicose veins)
Endocrine	Baroreceptor destruction/dysfunction
Adrenal insufficiency	Idiopathic
Hypoaldosteronism	Multisystem atrophy (Shy-Drager)
Pheochromocytoma	Idiopathic orthostatic hypotension

the cause of postural hypotension should be documented in all NH residents in whom it is present. The major causes of postural hypotension are outlined in **Table 21-6**. When a full-blown autonomic neuropathy is suspected, the diagnosis can be confirmed by demonstrating the presence of one or more of the following:

1. Failure of the diastolic blood pressure to increase by 10 mmHg during isometric hand grip
2. The absence of sinus arrhythmia
3. Demonstration that, during Valsalva maneuver, the ratio of the R-R interval during the bradycardia phase to the R-R interval during the tachycardia phase is less than 1.3.

The first approach to the management of orthostatic hypotension should be nonpharmacological (**Table 21-7**). The use of support hose is controversial. If they are to be of any use, support hose must extend to the level of the groin and be put on before the resident gets out of bed. The major pharmacological treatment of postural hypotension is the mineralocorticoid 9-alpha fludrocorticosterone. The

Table 21-7 Nonpharmacological management of postrual hypotension

1. Teach patient to get up slowly
2. Teach prestanding exercises
3. Supply bedisde urinal/bedpan
4. Have walker or rail next to bed
5. Raise head of bed
6. Ensure adequate fluid intake
7. Ensure adequate salt intake
8. Provide support hose (thigh high)
9. Stop or decrease medication dose of implicated medicines
10. Treat electrolyte disturbances

Table 21-8 Drugs used to treat postural hypotension

- Fludrocortisone (0.1 to 1 mg/day)
- Prostaglandin synthetase inhibitors
- Somatostatin analog (experimental)
- Xamoterol (better than prindol)
- Alpha-adrenergic agonists
- Vasopressin
- Dehydroergotamine
- Caffeine
- Dopamine antagonists
- Desmopressin

starting dose should be 0.1 mg a day, and the maximum dosage should be 1 mg/day. This agent can precipitate hypokalemia, supine hypertension, and congestive heart failure and thus must be used cautiously in residents with cardiovascular disease. Other drugs that may be helpful in treating postural hypotension are listed in **Table 21-8**. In those residents with central nervous system (CNS) involvement, desmopression and/or the somatostatin analog (now experimental) may prove to be useful. **Fig. 21-2** outlines an approach to the management of orthostatic hypotension.

Hypotension

Most American physicians pay little attention to low blood pressures. However low blood pressures often interfere with quality of life in NH residents and may be associated with increased depression and mortality. The common treatable causes of low blood pressure are excessive antihypertensive medications, malnutrition, hypertrophic obstructive cardiomyopathy, low salt diets, anemia, and Addison's disease. These conditions should be excluded in any NH with a systolic blood pressure below 110 mmHg.

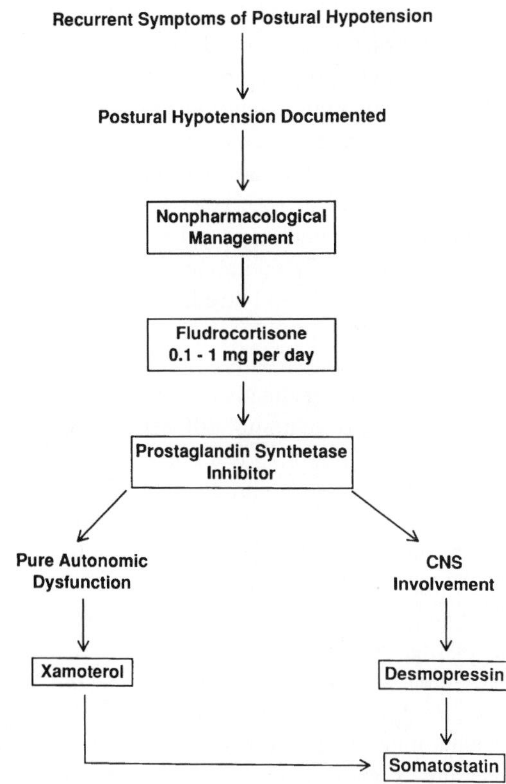

Figure 21-2 Basic approaches to the management of postural hypotension.

RHEUMATOLOGICAL CONDITIONS

Table 21-9 lists the major diagnostic criteria for different rheumatological conditions seen in NH residents.

Arthritis is the most prevalent chronic disorder, afflicting almost half the population over 75 years of age. The most common form of arthritis in older individuals is osteoarthritis. The approach to management of this disorder is outlined in **Table 21-10**. Recent studies have suggested that the more potent nonsteroidal anti-inflammatory agents may accelerate the progression of the disease. For this reason the lowest dose that gives adequate pain relief should be prescribed. While the prostaglandin analog misoprostol has been shown to be protective against nonsteroidal anti-inflammatory drug-induced bleeding, NH residents can rarely tolerate the dosages needed for cytoprotection. The common side effects of anti-inflammatory agents are listed in **Table 21-11**. Systemic steroids have no place in the management of osteoarthritis. Enteric-coated aspirin and ibuprofen are the cheapest anti-inflammatory agents available and are a reasonable choice for initial therapy. The newly available Tylenol extended relief has provided another alternative when given every 6 to 7 hours. We have seen dramatic responses to this drug formulation in persons in whom regular Tylenol was ineffective. Tramadol has proven to be an excellent drug for the treatment of severe arthritis. In those residents with severe arthritis pain unresponsive to these measures, oral morphine or other narcotic preparations should be considered. This is an important quality of life issue.

Polymyalgia rheumatica is not rare in older females. Muscle aching, muscle weakness and fatigue are the common features. The Westergren erythrocyte sedimentation rate is greater than 40 mm/h. Treatment is with steroids. Polymyalgia rheumatica may be associated with temporal arteritis, which can cause blindness. Temporal arteritis should be suspected when the resident complains of unilateral headache or visual changes. Diagnosis is made by temporal artery biopsy. If temporal arthritis is suspected, this should be treated as a medical emergency with high-dose steroids.

Soft tissue rheumatism (fibrositis) is associated with aching, stiffness (especially early morning stiffness), fatigue, anorexia, and sleep disturbances. Passive range of motion is usually not restricted. There are usually tender areas which, when pressed, reproduce the pain (trigger points). Laboratory tests are all normal. Treatment includes antidepressants, local heat, direct pressure to trigger points, and local anesthetic or steroid injections.

Inflammation of a bursal sac is a common problem in NH residents. **Figure 21-3** shows locations of bursal sacs that commonly become inflamed. Bursitis involving the anserine or one of the peripatellar bursae is a common cause of knee pain, which responds to local injection of lidocaine into the bursa. One to four local injections with corticosteroids is generally curative. Trochanteric bursitis may mimic hip pain. The diagnosis is made by eliciting the pain when pressure is applied over the bursa. Again, local injection of lidocaine and a

Table 21-9 Common manifestations of rheumatological conditions in nursing home residents

	Osteoarthritis	Rheumatoid arthritis	Polymyalgia	Gout	Pseudogout
Onset	Gradual	Gradual	Gradual	Acute	Acute
Early morning symptoms	0	+	±	0	±
Joint pain	+++	+++	+	+++	+++
Joint swelling	++	+++	+	+++	+++
Muscle pain	±	±	+++	0	0
Westegren sedimentation rate	Normal	Elevated	Elevated	Normal	Normal
Rheumatoid factors	0	Positive	Positive	0	0
Synovial fluid crystals	0	0	0	Yellow, needle-shaped, negatively birefringent (monosodium urate)	Weakly positive birefringent rhomboid crystals (calcium pyrophosphate dihydrate crystals)

Note: 0 = none; varying numbers of + related to greater frequency of event.

Table 21-10 Approach to the management of osteoarthritis in nursing home residents

1. Provide adequate analgesia
   - Enteric-coated aspirin
   - Nonsteroidal anti-inflammatory agents
   - Acetaminophen
   - Codeine
2. Weight reduction if greater than 130% of average body weight
3. Regular exercise programs
4. Application of heat to joints, particularly prior to exercise
5. Use of cane or other walking aides to relieve weight bearing
6. Consider prosthetic joint replacement
7. Screen for and treat depression when present

Table 21-11 Potential side effects of nonsteroidal anti-inflammatory agents

Gastrointestinal bleeding
Platelet inhibition
Cognitive problems
Depression
Dizziness
Water retention
Hyperkalemia
Acute renal failure
Nausea and vomiting
Hepatoxicity

corticosteroid may provide dramatic relief. NH residents are also prone to other disorders, such as bicipital tendinitis (which can occur as a result of pushing the wheels of a wheelchair). It may respond well to local injections.

Another disorder that is relatively common in the NH population is carpal tunnel syndrome. This generally presents as pain and/or paresthesias in the hands and should not be confused with more typical degenerative joint disease. Symptoms often begin with paresthesias at night and a feeling of clumsiness of the hand. The diagnosis can be made clinically by reproducing the symptoms by compressing the median nerve (this can be done by flexing the wrist for a prolonged period) and by documenting neurological deficits in the first four digits. The primary therapy is immobilization with a splint. If this fails and symptoms are disabling and/or weakness develops, surgical relief of pressure on the nerve should be considered.

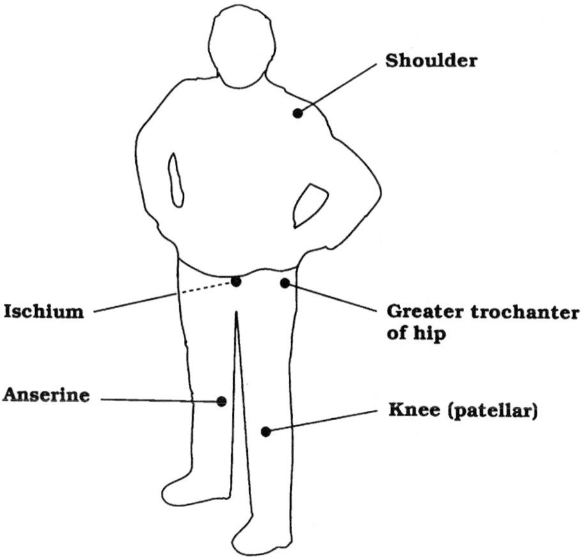

Figure 21-3 Common sites of bursal inflammation. Bursitis in these areas can mimic other conditions and often responds to local injections (see text).

Low back pain is an important condition in the NH, not only because of complaints from residents but also because of employees and the toll it can take on the worker's compensation system. The major causes of low back pain are listed in **Table 21-12**. In most persons low back pain is not due to a severe underlying condition and can be managed conservatively with 90 percent of persons recovering within 4 weeks. The history and examination should be

Table 21-12 Causes of low back pain

Musculoskeletal injuries
Arthritic changes of facets
Spinal stenosis
Compression fractures
Ankylosing spondylitis
Cancer
Infection
Herniated disc
Cauda equina
Visceral disease:
Kidney
Aorta
Pancreas
Pelvic disorders
Gastrointestinal disease

sufficient to elucidate which persons need work-up before 4 weeks. A history of trauma in an older person suggests vertebral fracture. Incontinence and saddle anesthesia suggest severe compromise of the lumbar spine. Weight loss, night pain or fever and a history of cancer, recent infection or intravenous drug abuse suggest cancer or infection. Neuroclaudication presents with failure of pain to resolve without bending the back (i.e., either sitting or bending forward). Muscle atrophy, decreased strength (particularly lack of strength in spontaneous movements) or a patulous oral sphincter suggest cord compression. Sciatica is elicited by straight leg raining and dorsiflexion and/or internal rotation of the foot when discomfort is felt. Other foot movements do not elicit sciatic pain.

The approach to low back pain is to use the history and physical to exclude possible cancer, injection, trauma or cord compression syndromes. For all others, activity and pain management to support activity are the key to recovery. Nonsteroidal antiinflammatory agents and long acting acetominophen seem to be the best pain medications. These need to be given continuously and not just when pain develops. In most cases opioid use should be limited to 4 days or less. Education concerning prevention of back strain and appropriate lifting exercises should be carried out. Physical therapy manipulation of the back may help continuity of normal activity and appears to produce better outcomes than rest or passive exercise. If pain persists beyond 4 weeks without improvement a CT scan and discussion of possible surgical options is appropriate. Bone scans and needle electromyography (EMG) may be useful in some cases. There is no evidence that back belts protect nursing staff when lifting residents.

SUGGESTED READINGS

Anemia

Kushner JP, Lee GR, Wintrobe MM, Cartwright GE: Idiopathic refractory sideroblastic anemia: Clinical and laboratory investigation of 17 patients and review of the literature. *Medicine* 50:139, 1971.

Lipshitz DA, Mitchell CO, Thompson C: The anemia of senescence. *Am J Hematol* 11:47, 1981.

McLennan WJ, Andrews GR, Macleod C, Caird FI: Anemia in the elderly. *Q J Med* 52:1, 1973.

Cardiovascular Disorders

Ahmad RAS, Watson RDS: Treatment of postural hypotension. *Drugs* 39:74, 1990.

Aronow WS: Management of congestive heart failure in the elderly patient. *Comprehensive Therapy* 21:329–338, 1995.

Jansen RW, Lipsitz LA: Postprandial hypotension: Epidemiology, pathophysiology and clinical management. *Ann Intern Med* 122:286–295, 1995.

Mamivaara A, Hoklunen U: The treatment of acute low back pain-bed rest, exercises or ordinary activity. *N Engl J Med* 332:352–355, 1995.

Morley JE, Reese SS: Clinical implications of the aging heart. *Am J Med* 80:77, 1989.

Tresh DD, McGough MF: Heart failure with normal systolic function: A common disorder in older persons. *J Am Geriatr Soc* 63:1035–1062, 1995.

Rheumatological Disorders

Baum J: Rehabilitation aspects of arthritis in the elderly, in Williams TF (ed): *Rehabilitation in the Aging*. New York, Raven Press, 1984, p 177.

Kantrowitz FG, Munoz G, Roberts N, et al: Rheumatology in geriatrics, in Gambert SR (ed): *Contemporary Geriatric Medicine* (Vol. 2). New York, Plenum Press, 1986, p 183.

Nesher G, Moore TL: Clinical presentation and treatment of arthritis in the elderly. *Clinics in Geriatr Med* 10:659–675, 1994.

CHAPTER
TWENTY-TWO

GASTROINTESTINAL DISORDERS

The major gastrointestinal (GI) problems in nursing home (NH) residents are dysphagia, gastrointestinal bleeding, and constipation. These conditions will be discussed in some detail in the sections that follow. In addition, a number of other GI disorders can interfere with quality of life in NH residents. These conditions will also be discussed briefly in this chapter.

XEROSTOMIA

Xerostomia, or dry mouth, is present in 40 percent to 50 percent of NH residents. Classical presentations of xerostomia include difficulty in swallowing, inability to speak clearly, difficulty in maintaining dentures in the mouth, hypogeusia, lips sticking to teeth, and dental caries. The major causes of xerostomia are listed in **Table 22-1**. Management of xerostomia includes, whenever possible, discontinuing drugs that may be contributing, ensuring adequate hydration, and providing artificial saliva, such as carboxymethylcellulose. If the resident still has teeth, the synthetic saliva chosen should contain fluoride. Squeeze bottles which the resident can use to squirt saliva into the mouth are the cheapest delivery system. In some residents, ease of delivery may be improved by a pump spray bottle or aerosol spray. Care should be taken to see that the resident maintains a good hydration status. Residents with teeth should brush with toothpaste before going to bed, and, after rinsing the mouth, apply 0.4 percent stannous fluoride by brushing again with a toothbrush. They should then spit the fluoride out without further rinsing to obtain full protection throughout the night.

Table 22-1 Causes of xerostomia

Drugs
Antidepressants
Other psychotropic drugs
Anticholinergics
Calcium channel blockers
Radiation therapy
Sjögren's syndrome
Dehydration
Systemic illness

ORAL MUCOSAL DISORDERS

Approximately 60 percent of NH residents have oral mucosal lesions. Hyperplasia and stomatitis of the tongue are the commonest lesions. Ulcerations are usually associated with dentures. Other oral conditions seen in the NH population include hyperkeratotic lesions, fistulas, and angular cheilitis. Pain associated with these lesions is present in approximately 12 percent. Leukoplakia and carcinoma are rare oral lesions. Regular examination of the oral cavity, inquiry concerning oral pain, and periodic evaluation by a dentist experienced with the geriatric population are an important part of the care of NH residents.

DYSPHAGIA

Dysphagia is a relatively common and potentially life-threatening condition in the NH. It is associated with aspiration pneumonia, excessive expectoration of saliva, weight loss, heartburn, laryngeal irritation, and Zenker's diverticulum. In persons over the age of 80, there are decreased esophageal peristaltic waves, increased nonperistaltic waves, and delayed relaxation of the esophageal sphincter, all of which, physiologically, can lead to mild dysphagia and/or aspiration. Residents with achalasia can have nocturnal aspiration, with coughing spasms that wake them. The major causes of dysphagia in NH residents are listed in **Table 22-2**. Severe dysphagia is almost always due to an organic cause, and the cause should be documented in all NH residents. The evaluation should include an assessment by a speech therapist trained to evaluate swallowing disorders and a barium swallow under observation of an experienced radiologist and/or speech therapist. NH residents with dysphagia should have such an evaluation before a permanent or temporary enteral feeding tube is placed. It is necessary to re-evaluate the appropriateness of the dietary level of NH residents with dysphagia at regular intervals.

Up to one-third of older persons have some degree of cricopharyngeal dysfunction, making this a potentially important cause of dysphagia in the NH.

Table 22-2 Causes of dysphagia in nursing home residents

Preesophageal	**Esophageal**
Neuromuscular	Neuromuscular
Pseudobulbar palsy	Cricopharyngeal muscle dysfunction
Myasthenia gravis	Achalasia
Parkinson's disease	Diffuse esophageal spasm
Multiple sclerosis	Diabetes mellitus
Amytrophic lateral sclerosis	Structural—intrinsic
Diabetes mellitus	Esophageal ring
Structural—intrinsic	Peptic stricture
Pharyngitis due to moniliasis	Candidal esophagitis
Structural—extrinsic	Herpes simplex esophagitis
Oropharyngeal abcess	Carcinoma
Neoplasm	Structural—extrinsic
Diverticulum	Aortic aneurysm
	Peritracheal lymph node enlargement
	Bronchogenic carcinoma
	Enlarged left atrium

Cricopharyngeal muscle dysfunction leads either to failure to swallow food or to the trapping of food at the entrance of the esophagus. Solids are easier than liquids for residents with this disorder to swallow. The treatment is cricopharyngeal myotomy.

Not only does esophageal spasm cause dysphagia, but it can also produce chest pain, which is often confused with angina. Treatment consists of nitroglycerin before meals, isosorbide dinitrate, or calcium channel blockers. Occasionally, dilatation of the esophagus may be necessary.

GASTROESOPHAGEAL REFLUX DISEASE

Gastroesophageal reflux disease (GERD) is a common disease with up to 7 percent of the adult population having daily symptoms. GERD can present as atypical chest pain and be misdiagnosed as angina. Anticholinergic drugs should be discontinued in residents with symptoms of GERD. Endoscopy and biopsy may be necessary to rule out Barrett's esophagitis if there is no response to treatment. GERD can also result in nocturnal asthma. Optimal treatment of GERD includes the use of proton pump inhibitors (i.e., omperazole). H_2 blockers are often used for symptoms of GERD (in fact in 1995 ranitidine was the most commonly prescribed drug for NH residents). However, they are often used for too long a period of time, and may cause side effects and adverse drug interactions. In selected persons addition of prokinetic agents (e.g., cisapride) and surgical therapy may be utilized. Metoclopramide should be avoided because it can cause parkinsonian side effects.

UPPER GASTROINTESTINAL HEMORRHAGE

Upper GI hemorrhage is a major problem in NH residents. The most common causes of upper GI bleeding in older persons are duodenal ulcer, gastric erosions, gastric ulcer, hiatal hernia associated esophagitis, and carcinoma of the stomach. Mallory–Weiss tears can also be seen in older persons after repeated retching or vomiting. Drugs are a common precipitating factor in GI bleeding. Drugs associated with bleeding include aspirin, nonsteroidal anti-inflammatory drugs, steroids, warfarin, and alcohol. Enteric-coated drugs reduce the possibility of bleeding. While misoprostol, a prostaglandin analog, can reduce the possibility of bleeding associated with the use of nonsteroidal anti-inflammatory drugs, diarrhea often limits its effectiveness in the NH resident. NH residents on any of these drugs should have their hemoglobin levels checked periodically (e.g., every 1 to 2 months). Coffee ground emesis and occult GI bleeding in NH residents is often associated with systemic infection or respiratory failure. Endoscopy has limited usefulness in the work-up of NH residents. Most residents will respond to conservative therapy and the discontinuation of ulcerogenic drugs which is similar for gastritis and ulcers. If bleeding continues after this therapy endoscopy would be indicated.

Peptic ulcer disease increases in prevalence in older persons despite the age-related decrease in the secretion of gastric acid. Recently, the bacterium *Helicobacter pylori* has been demonstrated to play a role in the pathogenesis of ulcers and gastritis. This organism increases in frequency with advancing age due

Table 22-3 Side effects of H_2-receptor antagonists

Mental confusion[a]
Diarrhea
Myalgias
Rashes
Hypotension
Bradycardia
Impotence
Neutropenia
Renal dysfunction
Drug interactions[b]
Diazepam
Warfarin
Theophylline
Phenytoin
Propranolol
Metronidazole

[a]Worse in presence of renal or hepatic disease.
[b]Cimetidine reduces the hepatic metabolism of these drugs.

to achlorhydria and mucosal damage. All older persons with a gastrointestinal bleed due to ulcers or gastritis may benefit from 14 days of treatment with amoxycillin, metronidazole and pepto-bismol in an attempt to eradicate this bacterium. All older persons with indigestion should be given pepto-bismol.

Management of acute or chronic gastrointestinal bleeding in older persons involves a choice of H_2 blockers (cimetidine or ranitidine) or sucralfate. Antacids often cause diarrhea, are difficult to administer regularly at 3-h intervals (which is necessary for optimum effects), alter absorption of drugs, and may cause magnesium or aluminum toxicity in the presence of renal disease. Omperazole is an inhibitor of gastric acid that is associated with an increased colonization of *Helicobacter pylori*. The side effects of H_2 blockers are listed in **Table 22-3**. The ideal dose of cimetidine in a 90-year-old is 100 mg daily and in an 80-year-old 200 mg twice daily. This reduced dosage decreases the risk of toxicity. Sucralfate has virtually no systemic side effects but needs more frequent administration than H_2-receptor antagonists. H_2-receptor antagonists are often misused in NH residents when they are given chronically in an attempt to prevent bleeding. There is little evidence that this practice is useful, and it increases the possibility of side effects, as well as drug–drug interactions.

HEPATOBILIARY DISORDERS

Gallstones are common in older persons, particularly females. Emergency surgery carries a 10 percent mortality rate, compared to less than 2 percent for elective surgery. The availability of extracorporeal shock-wave lithotripsy has further enhanced the safety of gallstone treatment. Abdominal pain is present in most NH residents with acute cholecystitis, but fever and peritoneal signs are absent in half or more. Jaundice, which may be painless, occurs in one-third. Gallbladder disease may mimic myocardial infarction, with referred chest pain and Q waves on electrocardiography. Chronic gallbladder disease can produce early satiation and severe weight loss. Cholecystectomy results in weight gain. Complications of acute cholecystitis that occur commonly in older persons are perforation, empyema, emphysematous cholecystitis, and ischemic necrosis of the gallbladder with gangrene. NH residents with symptoms or signs consistent with gallbladder disease should undergo abdominal ultrasonography as a first diagnostic step.

Hepatitis (especially hepatitis C) is not rare in older persons. It is often transient, presenting with right-upper-quadrant pain, fever, mild jaundice, and changes in liver function tests. It may mimic gallbladder disease. Treatment is observation. Acetaminophen should be avoided in these residents. All NH residents suspected of having hepatitis should have serologic studies because of the risks of spread throughout the NH and the need for proper infection control precautions (see Chapter 19). In one study the prevalence of hepatitis B surface antigen and anti MCV were 0.6 percent and 1.4 percent, supporting the use of hepatitis B vaccine for nursing staff and the implementation of universal precautions on long-term care facilities.

MESENTERIC VASCULAR OCCLUSION

Acute intestinal infarction is a life-threatening condition in older persons. Surgery may be lifesaving. This condition may present with relatively few signs or may be manifested by periumbilical pain or symptoms suggestive of intestinal obstruction. Approximately 30 percent of NH residents may have an acute confusional episode associated with this disorder. Mesenteric occlusion is often accompanied by severe acidosis, elevated white blood cell count, and fever. Any NH resident with a sudden mental status change, leukocytosis, and acidosis should be suspected of having acute intestinal infarction even in the absence of GI signs or symptoms.

Chronic intestinal ischemia or "abdominal angina" is often missed in older NH residents. This condition may present with midabdominal pain that is often worse after eating or with early satiation. Diarrhea and chronic weight loss are also common. Treatment is with nitrates or calcium channel antagonists.

APPENDICITIS

Older persons who have appendicitis have a high mortality rate. On admission to the NH, previous appendectomy should be documented. If the appendix is still intact, the physician should always include appendicitis in the potential diagnosis of abdominal disease. As in most other intra-abdominal conditions, localizing symptoms and signs may be absent, requiring a high index of suspicion. This is especially important, because perforation occurs in approximately 50 percent of older persons with appendicitis and early diagnosis can be lifesaving. When appendicitis is suspected, modern ultrasound techniques are usually diagnostic.

DIVERTICULAR DISEASE

Diverticula are present in 50 percent of persons over 80 years of age. While diverticula are generally asymptomatic, approximately one-fourth of NH residents who have them are at risk for diverticulitis, intestinal obstruction, perforation, or gastrointestinal bleeding. Older persons are more likely than younger individuals to have more extensive colonic involvement, including both left and right sides of the colon. In younger persons, fever, leukocytosis, and rebound tenderness are commonly associated with acute diverticular disease. However, these findings are much less common in older persons. The signs and symptoms of diverticular disease are outlined in **Table 22-4**. Residents with any

Table 22-4 Signs and symptoms of diverticular disease

Symptoms	Signs
Abdominal pain	Bleeding
Constipation	Left ileal fossa mass
Rectal bleeding	Abcess
Flatulence	Perforation
Vomiting	Fistula
Diarrhea	Peritonitis
Urinary complaints	Obstruction

of the symptoms listed and unexplained fever and/or leukocytosis should arouse suspicion for diverticulitis even in the absence of suggestive abdominal signs.

DIARRHEA

Diarrhea in NH residents can be either acute or chronic. Acute diarrheas are usually associated with an infectious process, dietary change, ingestion of milk by those with lactase deficiency, or tube feeding. Infectious diarrheas are discussed in some detail in Chapter 19. Chronic diarrheas are either secretory or nonsecretory. Secretory diarrheas continue after a 24-h fast, whereas non-secretory diarrheas are dependent on food to stimulate the process. The most common causes of chronic diarrhea are fecal impaction, malabsorption syndromes, chronic intestinal ischemia, laxative abuse, neoplasms, and anorectal incontinence. All NH residents with diarrhea should be checked for fecal impaction, which is probably the most common cause of diarrhea in this population. Fecal impaction can also cause fecal incontinence. (The causes and management of fecal incontinence are discussed in Chapter 15.) If diarrhea persists for more than 2 or 3 days or if it occurs in several residents simultaneously, an infectious cause should be considered. Stool should be sent for a culture for pathogens as well as for Clostridium difficile toxin. Antibiotic-associated diarrhea or enterocolitis should be suspected in residents who develop diarrhea while on or within 2 to 4 weeks of treatment with antibiotics (see Chapter 19).

CONSTIPATION

Constipation, either real or imagined, is a major problem in NH residents. It should be remembered that normal bowel function ranges from three times per day to three times per week. With advancing age and immobility, there is a

Table 22-5 Causes of constipation in nursing home residents

1. Immobility (the terminal reservoir syndrome)
2. Poor hydration
3. Fecal impaction
4. Depression (tricyclics may make constipation worse)
5. Drugs (Table 22-6)
6. Organic causes
    - Hypothyroidism
    - Hypercalcemia
    - Intestinal obstruction
    - Hypomagnesemia
    - Other electrolyte disorders
    - Parkinsonism
7. Laxative abuse (Table 22-9)
8. High-fiber diet in immobile resident

tendency for stools to occur less often. A major cause of constipation in NH residents is the "terminal reservoir syndrome." This syndrome occurs because the gastrocolic reflex needs physical activity for its initiation. In addition, in NH residents who require help with toileting, there is often failure to respond to the gastrocolic reflex at the appropriate time. The major causes of constipation in older NH residents are listed in **Table 22-5**. The new onset of constipation should prompt a search for treatable causes. Several drugs commonly prescribed for NH residents can also cause or aggravate constipation. In particular a strong association exists between anticholinergic drug use and constipation (**Table 22-6**). It should be noted that fiber, often used to treat constipation, may actually cause constipation in residents who are immobile, because the gastrocolic reflex is necessary to move fiber through the gastrointestinal tract. A high tea intake

Table 22-6 Drugs commonly associated with constipation

Antacids
Anticholinergics
Calcium
Iron
Opiates
Calcium channel antagonists
Antidepressants
Antiparkinsonian drugs
Ephedrine
Terbutaline
Nonsteroidal anti-inflammatory drugs
Neuroleptics

Table 22-7 Complications of constipation

Megacolon
Sigmoid volvulus
Fecal impaction
Fecal incontinence
Rectal prolapse
Refactory straining
- Syncope
- Arrhythmias
- Transient ischemic attacks

may also aggravate constipation. Major complications of constipation include megacolon, volvulus, and fecal incontinence (**Table 22-7**).

An overview of the approach to the management of constipation in the NH is illustrated in **Fig. 22-1**. The first step is to make sure that the resident is adequately hydrated. A BUN-to-creatinine (BUN, blood urea nitrogen) ratio of 20:1 or greater is suggestive of poor hydration. Treatment is four to 8 glasses (1 to 2 liters) of fluid daily unless contraindicated by severe heart or renal failure or hyponatremia. The second step is to use fiber in the mobile resident. Psyllium (in

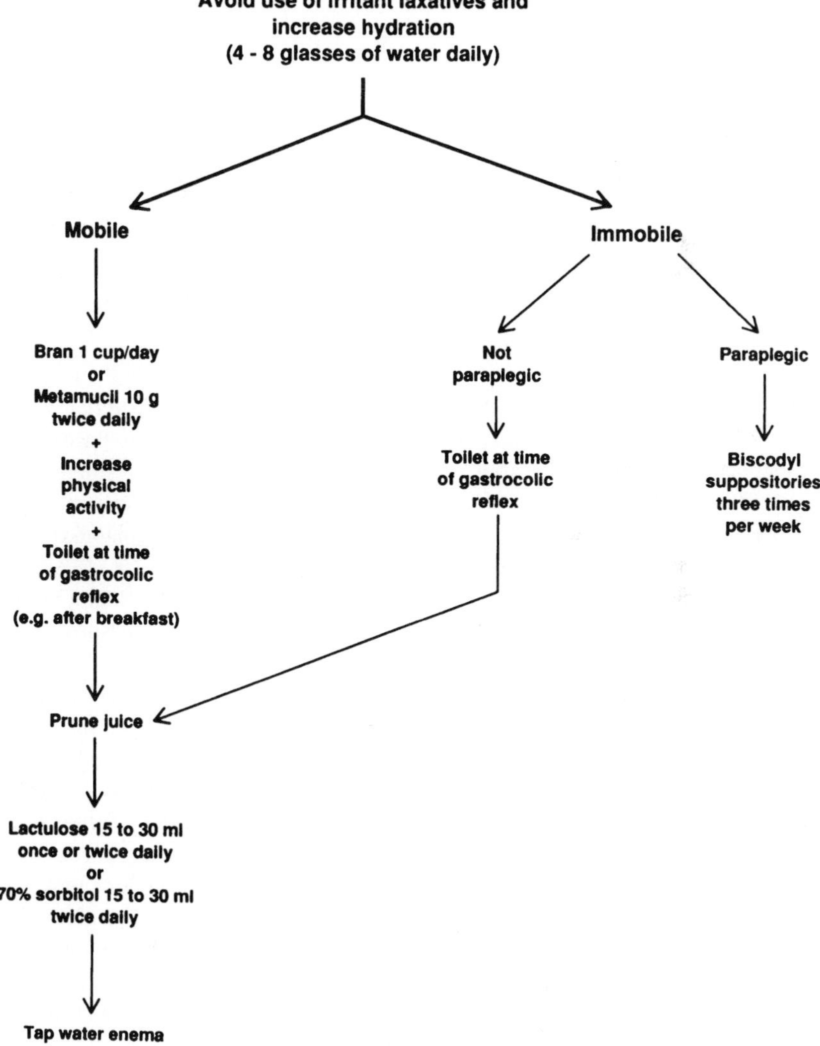

Figure 22-1 Approach to chronic constipation in nursing home residents.

Table 22-8 Causes of fecal incontinence

Fecal impaction with overflow
Altered reservoir capacity
Irradiation
Surgery
Neuronal damage
Local
Laxative abuse
Diabetes mellitus neuropathy
Spinal cord
Autonomous or reflex colon
Surgery
Functional impairment
Dementia
Delirium
Depression
Immobility
Poor access to toilet facility
Diarrhea

Metamucil) at 20 g/day (10 g twice daily) generally works well. Alternatively, a cup of bran will give approximately the same amount of fiber. The third step is to increase physical activity after meals and attempt to toilet the resident at the time of the gastrocolic reflex. We do not use stool softeners in the majority of residents. Many are marketed with irritant laxatives, may be hepatotoxic, and may be aspirated in those residents with swallowing problems.

Discontinuation of stool softeners coupled with adequate hydration has produced no complaints in our NH residents. When the above measures fail, a subgroup of residents may need osmotic diuretic therapy (e.g., lactulose 15 to 30 ml once or twice per day or 70 percent sorbitol 15 to 30 ml twice a day). Prune juice is cheap and may be an excellent agent in some residents who insist on a laxative. Sorbitol is cheaper when it is prepared in bulk quantities in the institution. Tap water enemas distend the rectum and colon and produce reflex evacuation. Regular enema use can lead to fecal incontinence (**Table 22-8**). Biscodyl suppositories (Dulcolax) 10 mg three times per week are necessary in some residents with paraplegia or significant immobility who cannot take advantage of the gastrocolic reflex. In addition, residents with lax abdominal muscles may benefit from pushing with their hands on the lower abdomen at the time of toileting.

Irritant laxatives and stool softeners (**Table 22-9**) are overprescribed for NH residents. Up to three-quarters of NH residents are prescribed a laxative "as needed," and 50 percent receive daily scheduled laxatives. The prescribing of

Table 22-9 Irritant laxatives and stool softeners[a]

Generic name	Trade name	Side effects
Bisacodyl	Dulcolax Carter's Little Pills	Gastric irritation
Anthraquinone (senna)	Senokot Perdiem (with psyllium) Fletcher's Castoria (with alcohol)	Degeneration of Meisner's and Auerbach's plexus
Phenolphthalein	Correctol[b] Ex-Lax Doxidan[b] Feen-A-Mint[b] Laxative mints[b]	Rashes
Casanthrol	Dialose Plus[b] Peri-Colace	Rashes
Magnesium hydroxide	Milk of magnesia Haley's MO (with mineral oil)	Magnesium toxicity
Docusate sodium	Colace Dialose DOSS	Rashes

[a]These drugs should be avoided in most NH residents (see text).
[b]Also contains docusate.

multiple laxatives for the same resident is also very common. Although prune juice can often be substituted for irritant laxatives, nurses tend to strongly prefer the use of the latter—especially Dulcolax suppositories and milk of magnesia with cascara. Chronic use of irritant laxatives can lead to severe constipation (so-called laxative colon). There is much mythology concerning laxatives among NH staff, and physicians need to be aware that many residents will not need irritant laxatives if they are managed by the strategy outlined above.

SUGGESTED READINGS

Altman DF: Gastrointestinal diseases in the elderly. *Med Clin North Am* 67:433, 1983.

Bennett RG, Greenough WB III: Approach to acute diarrhea in the elderly. *Gastroenterol Clin N A* 22:517–533, 1993.

Bennett RG: Diarrhea among residents of long-term care facilities. *Infect Contr Hosp Epidemiol* 14:397–404, 1993.

Castle SC: Constipation: Endemic in the elderly. *Med Clin North Am* 73:1497, 1990.

DeVault KR, Castell DO: Current diagnosis and treatment of gastroesophageal reflux disease. *Mayo Clin Proc* 69:867–876, 1996.

Ekelund R: Oral mucosal disorders in institutionalized elderly people. *Age Ageing* 17:193, 1988.

Finucane PM, Arunachalum T, O'Dourd J, Pathy MSJ: Acute mesenteric infarction in elderly patients. *J Am Geriatr Soc* 37:355, 1989.

Goldstein MK, Brown EM, Holt P, et al: Fecal incontinence in an elderly man. *J Am Geriatr Soc* 37:991, 1989.

Groher ME, McKaig TN: Dysphagia and dietary levels in a skilled nursing facility. *J Am Geriatr Soc* 43:528–532, 1995.

Harari D, Gurwitz JH, Minakes KL: Constipation in the elderly. *J Am Geriatr Soc* 41:1130–1140, 1993.

Heading RC: Long term management of gastroesophageal reflux disease. *Scand J Gastroenterol* Suppl 213:25–30, 1995.

Monane M, Avorn J, Beers MM, Everett DE: Anticholinergic drug use and bowel function in nursing home patients. *Arch Int Med* 153:633–638, 1994.

Navazesh M: Salivary gland hypofunction in elderly patients. *J Calif Dental Assn* 22:62–68, 1994.

Sautengco R, Posner GL, Marsh F, Jr: The significance and work-up of minor gastrointestinal bleeding in hospitalized nursing home patients. *J Natl Med Assn* 87:745–750, 1995.

Shamburek RD, Farrar JT: Disorders of the digestive system in the elderly. *N Engl J Med* 322:438, 1990.

Simon AE, Gordon M, Bishai FR: Prevalence of hepatitis B surface antigen, hepatitis C antibody and HIV-1 antibody among residents of a long-term care facility. *J Am Geriatr Soc* 40:218–220, 1992.

Wald A: Constipation and fecal incontinence in the elderly. *Gastroenterol Clin North Am* 19:605, 1990.

PART THREE

GENERAL MANAGEMENT ISSUES

Quality of Life

To live or not to live, that is the question.
Whether 'Tis nobler to suffer slings and
Arrows of old age, or being warehoused in a nursing home,
Opposing the years and praying not to end up on a peripad.

To sleep a drugged sleep, to awake confused,
And end the thousand thoughts the mind is heir to.
"Mama, where is my doll? What happened to my quality of life?"
'Tis a consummation devoutly to be avoided.

To feed oneself, to bathe, to walk perchance
To fall and break a hip, Ay there's the rub.
For in those simple skills, what peace of mind may come,
To avoid the calamity of so long a life.

For who can bear the whips and scorns of bureaucrats
Who have never suffered the burning of an N/G tube.
They mean full well—they want us all to die in good health.
May they be spared the torture of such assaults.

Nature calls at last, so please don't let them
  Subject my tired body to a gastrostomy tube.
Oh, here they come with enemas and catheters.
  My bed sores scream in stench and pain.

Look! The Pearly Gates have come into view.
  Relief is finally within my grasp.
The bitter battle has been won.
  Nature will give me rest at last.

I hear a siren. An ambulance is on its way!
  Oh no! My doctor forgot to document my plea for no heroics.
I struggle to escape. A needle is my reward.
  Even the ambulance ride I can't enjoy.

In the E.R., the interns and nurses grunt and sweat.
  They start IVs and respirators and even intubate.
The Pearly Gates soon fade from view.
  Have I no right to decide my fate?

But I am not made of immortal stuff,
  My worn out body can't even cry.
They have wasted their priceless resources,
  And plans of great pitch and moment go awry.

The Health Department has new rules which no one knows thereof
Soon the ECF will not have to bear the inspector's wrong.
They don't have to hydrate, just let us go in peace.
Soft you now—my final sleep cometh.

The late Phillip L. Rossman, MD
Los Angeles, California

CHAPTER

TWENTY-THREE

DRUG USE

DRUG USE

Numerous studies and reviews have highlighted the excessive number of drugs that many nursing home (NH) residents receive, the inappropriateness of many drugs and/or dosage regimens ordered in NHs, the susceptibility of NH residents to adverse drug reactions, and the relatively high incidence of bothersome as well as potentially serious adverse drug reactions that occur in the frail geriatric NH population. Because of the seriousness and pressing nature of the problems created by this excessive and inappropriate prescription of drugs in NHs, the federal government has gotten into the act. The 1987 Omnibus Reconciliation Act (OBRA), which establishes many new rules and regulations for NH care, focuses on drug use in general as well as antipsychotic drugs in particular.

Several surveys indicate that on average, NH residents are prescribed six to eight drugs and that some are prescribed over 20 different medications simultaneously. Close to half of these prescriptions are for prn drugs, many of which are rarely used. Drugs are clearly necessary for many residents in order to manage chronic medical conditions. Pressure from residents, families, and NH staff to prescribe drugs often plays an important role as well. However, drug prescribing in the NH, unlike the ambulatory care unit or acute care hospital, is frequently done without direct assessment of the resident and is based on information provided by NH staff. In some situations, the prescription of a drug is a substitute for a careful assessment of the resident leading to a precise diagnosis and management plan. Primary care physicians and medical directors must take appropriate steps to improve their prescribing habits in the NH setting.

The purpose of this chapter is not to provide primary care physicians with a compendium of specifics on the prescription of various drugs for NH residents. Selected aspects of drug therapy for specific conditions common among NH residents are included in several other chapters throughout this text, and more detailed information is available in general textbooks of medicine and geriatrics. The objective of this chapter is to give primary care physicians and medical directors some general guidelines for drug use in the NH. Because of the prevalence of psychiatric conditions and behavioral disturbances in this population, the commonplace prescription of inappropriate psychotropic drugs for NH residents, and the specific focus of OBRA on antipsychotics, a separate section of this chapter discusses psychotropic drug use.

GENERAL PRINCIPLES OF DRUG PRESCRIBING

Because the involvement of consultant pharmacists is a federally mandated requirement, most NHs have a consultant pharmacist who regularly reviews drug regimens. The American Society of Consultant Pharmacists (based in Arlington, Virginia), a national organization of pharmacists, provides services to NHs. Many state and local organizations of pharmacists also include groups whose practice focuses on the NH setting. Medical directors and primary care physicians should work collaboratively with consultant pharmacists and nursing staff in order to maximize the appropriateness of drug regimens for individual NH residents as well as to develop appropriate policies and procedures for the prescription, administration, and monitoring of drug therapy. The latter activities should be accomplished in conjunction with a pharmacy and/or quality assurance committee.

Table 23-1 lists several general principles of drug prescribing for NH residents. These can be divided into two basic sets of recommendations: one focusing on general principles of drug therapy for the frail geriatric population and the other on practical considerations in writing drug orders in the NH. As in prescribing for geriatric patients who are not in NHs, drug treatment should be ordered only when a specific indication exists and the risk/benefit considerations favor drug therapy. Any time a drug is ordered, a corresponding diagnosis or specific indications should be documented in the medical record—on a problem list, in a progress note, and in the order itself if appropriate (especially for p.r.n. orders). Age- and disease-related changes in the pharmacology of various drugs are well documented. Drug doses should therefore take into account the route of elimination of the drug and the resident's ability to eliminate the drug by that route. Renal function, liver function, cardiac output, body mass, and hydration are critical factors to consider in adjusting drug dosages and dosage intervals. "Start low and go slow" is a general rule of thumb that is particularly appropriate for NH residents. Several criteria have been published for inappropriate drug prescriptions for NH residents which are based on expert consensus (**Table 23-2**).

Table 23-1 General principles of drug prescribing in the nursing home

1. Make sure that a drug is necessary to treat the resident's condition.
2. An appropriate diagnosis should be recorded for each drug prescribed.
3. When a drug is ordered:
   a. The dose should be appropriate for the resident's condition and ability to eliminate the drug
   b. "Start low and go slow" is an appropriate guideline for most drugs in the NH population
   c. Avoid significant drug–drug interactions (see **Table 23-3**)
   d. Avoid potential drug–condition interactions (see **Table 23-4**)
   e. Pay attention to the practical aspects of drug orders:
      (1) Order the minimum number of doses necessary
      (2) Avoid timed orders (e.g., "every 8 hours") unless absolutely necessary based on the kinetics of the drug
      (3) Write time limited orders (e.g., "for 7 days") whenever possible
      (4) Include a specific indication for all prn orders
   f. Pay attention to the cost of the drug:
      (1) For residents on medical assistance programs (i.e., Medicaid), use drugs reimbursed by the program whenever possible
4. Write appropriate orders for drug monitoring (see **Table 23-5**)
   a. Avoid unnecessary "hold if" orders which increase nursing time necessary for drug administration
      (1) Most "hold if" orders can be discontinued after the resident's condition is stable on the drug
   b. Follow drug blood levels periodically for drugs with a narrow therapeutic index, and when clinical efficacy correlates with blood levels
5. Review each drug order monthly.
6. Discontinue all unnecessary drugs.
7. Work collaboratively with consultant pharmacists to ensure the appropriateness of drug orders and drug monitoring.
8. Regularly review drug prescribing, administration and monitoring through a Pharmacy and/or Quality Assurance Committees.

Because multiple drugs are often prescribed for NH residents, the chance of adverse drug interactions is high. Many software programs are available to detect potential drug–drug interactions. However, a caveat about these programs is that they tend to spew out all possible interactions rather than just the clinically important ones. Many programs do have the capability to identify only potentially serious interactions. **Table 23-3** lists some examples of potential drug–drug interactions that are important clinically. This is an area where consultant pharmacists can provide valuable assistance in identifying the interactions, determining their clinical importance, and helping to identify an alternative drug regimen if necessary. "Drug–condition" interactions may be just as important if not more so than drug–drug interactions. Most NH residents have at least one or more chronic conditions that can influence the response to drugs prescribed for other conditions. **Table 23-4** lists several examples of such drug–condition interactions. Primary care physicians should therefore document each

Table 23-2 Criteria for inappropriate drug prescribing in nursing home residents based on expert consensus

Drug name or class	Statement
Sedative/hypnotics	
Long-acting benzodiazepines; chlordiazepoxide, diazepam, flurazepam	All use should be avoided; use short-acting benzodiazepines if needed
Meprobamate	All use should be avoided, except in those already addicted
Oxazepam	Any single dose >30 mg should be avoided
Short-acting benzodiazepines; oxazepam, triazolam, alprazolam	Nightly use for >4 weeks should be avoided
Short-duration barbituates: pentobarbital, secobarbital	All use should be avoided, except in those already addicted; safer sedative/hypnotics are available
Triazolam	Any single dose >0.25 mg should be avoided
Antidepressants	
Amitriptyline	All use should be avoided; use less anticholinergic antidepressant if needed
Combination antidepressants–antipsychotics, e.g., amitriptyline–perphenazine (Triavil)	All use should be avoided; if needed, prescribe individual components at proper geriatric doses; avoid amitriptyline
Antipsychotics	
Haloperidol	Doses >3 mg/d should be avoided; patients with known psychotic disorders may require higher doses
Thioridazine	Doses >30 mg/d should avoided; patients with known psychotic disorders may require higher doses
Antihypertensives	
Hydrochlorothiazide	Doses >50 mg/d should be avoided
Methoyldopa	Use should be avoided; safer antihypertensives are available
Propranolol	All use should be avoided except if used to control violet behaviors; other beta blockers offer less CNS penetration or more beta selectivity
Reserpine	Use should be avoided; safer antihypertensives are available
NSAIDs	
Indomethacin	All use should be avoided; other NSAIDs cause less CNS toxic reaction
Phenylbutazone	All use should be avoided; other NSAIDs are less toxic

Table 23-2 (*Continued*)

Drug name or class	Statement
Oral hypoglycemics	
Chlorpropamide	All use should be avoided; other oral hypoglycemics have shorter half-lives and do not cause syndrome of inappropriate antidiuretic hormone (SIADH)
Analgesics	
Propoxyphene	All use should be avoided; other analgesics are safer and more effective
Pentazocine	All use should be avoided; other narcotics are more effective and safer
Dementia treatments	
Cyclandelate	All use should be avoided; effectiveness is in doubt
Isoxsuprine	All use should be avoided; effectiveness is in doubt
Platelet inhibitors	
Dipyridamole	All use should be avoided; effectiveness at low doses is in doubt; toxic reaction is high at higher doses; aspirin is safer alternative
Histamine$_2$ blockers	
Cimetidine	Doses >900 mg/d and therapy beyond 12 weeks should be avoided
Ranitidine	Doses >300 mg/d and therapy beyond 12 weeks should be avoided
Antibiotics	
Oral antibiotics	Therapy >4 weeks should be avoided except when treating osteomyelitis, prostatitis, tuberculosis, or endocarditis
Decongestants	
Oxymetazoline, phenylephrine, psuedophedrine	Daily use for >2 weeks should be avoided
Iron	Doses >325 mg/d should be avoided; they do not substantially increase iron absorption and increase side effects
Muscle relaxants/antispasmodics	
Cyclobenzaprine, orphenidrate, methocarbamol, carisoprodol	All use should be avoided; potential for toxic reaction is greater than potential benefit
GI antispasmodics	All long-term use should be avoided; potential for toxic reaction is greater than potential benefit
Antiemetics	
Trimethobenzamide	All use should be avoided

Table 23-3 Examples of potentially clinically important drug–drug interactions

Mechanism	Example	Potential effects
Interference with drug absorption	Antacids interacting with digoxin, INH antipsychotics, histamine-2 blockers	Diminished drug effectiveness
Displacement from binding proteins	Warfarin, oral hypoglycemics, dilantin, aspirin and other nonsteroidals, sertraline and paroxetine	Enhanced effects and increased risk of toxicity
Altered distribution	Digoxin and quinidine	Increased risk of toxicity
Altered metabolism	Cimetidine interacting with propranolol, theophylline, dilantin	Decreased drug clearance, enhanced effects, increased risk of toxicity
	Tricyclic antidepressants and phenothiazine antipsychotics	Increased blood levels and increased risk for toxicity
	Serotonin reuptake inhibitors and tricyclic antidepressants, phenothiazines and quinidine	Decreased metabolism and increased risk of toxicity
Altered excretion	Lithium and diuretics	Increased risk of toxicity and electrolyte imbalance
Pharmacological antagonism	L-dopa and clonidine	Decreased anti-parkinsonian effects
Pharmacological synergism	Tricyclic antidepressants and antihypertensives	Increased risk of hypotension
	Narcotic analgesics and psychotropics	Increased risk of delirium, sedation, falls

resident's chronic conditions and be aware of how the efficacy of drug therapy may be influenced by these conditions, as well as whether a newly prescribed drug may adversely affect another underlying condition.

Several practical aspects of drug orders for NH residents are important in reducing the nursing time necessary to administer and monitor the drugs (thus lowering the cost and also allowing nursing staff to spend time in other areas) as well as in minimizing disruption to the residents' routines. The lowest possible number of drug doses should be prescribed. Many drugs that are prescribed three or four times a day may be needed only once or twice. Long-acting and slow-release preparations are becoming increasingly available and should be prescribed when appropriate. Long-acting psychotropic drugs should, however, generally be avoided (see discussion under "Psychotropic Drugs" below). When multiple doses of drugs are necessary, timed orders (e.g., every 8 h) should be avoided unless they are essential in view of the kinetics of the drug and the

Table 23-4 Examples of potentially clinically important drug–condition interactions

Drug	Conditions	Clinical implications
Diuretics	Diabetes	Decreased glucose tolerance, especially with hypokalemia
	Poor nutritional status	Increased risk of dehydration and electrolyte imbalance
	Urinary frequency, urgency	Precipitate incontinence
Beta blockers	Diabetes	Sympathetic response to hypoglycemia masked
	Chronic obstructive lung disease	Increased bronchospasm
	Congestive heart failure	Decreased myocardial contractility
	Peripheral vascular disease	Increased claudication
Narcotic analgesics	Chronic constipation	Worsening symptoms, fecal impaction
Tricyclic antidepressants	Congestive heart failure, angina	Tachycardia, decreased myocardial contractility, postural hypotension exacerbating cardiovascular conditions
Tricyclic antidepressants, antihistamines, and other drugs with anticholingeric effects	Constipation, glaucoma and other visual impairments, prostatic hyperplasia, reflux esophagitis, xerostomia	Worsening of symptoms
Seretonin reuptake inhibitors	Anorexia	Worsensing symptoms Weight loss
Antipsychotics	Parkinsonism	Worsening of immobility
	Seizure disorder	Lower seizure threshold and may increase seizures
Psychotropics	Dementia	Further impairment of cognitive function

condition being treated. Orders for the numbers of times per day are generally sufficient. These types of orders allow the nursing staff flexibility and minimize the potential to disrupt the residents' routines (e.g., sleep, social and recreational activities). When a drug is ordered for an acute condition, the order should contain a stop date so that drugs are not continued for longer than necessary (e.g., cough/cold preparations for 7 to 10 days). All drug orders should be reviewed monthly and all unnecessary drugs discontinued. Appropriate drug-order formats can facilitate this process by listing the drug orders separately from other orders and by listing the original starting date of each order. Although monitoring is extremely important (see discussion under "Monitoring" below), unnecessary or excessive orders for monitoring should be avoided. For example, monitoring orders are frequently written for cardiovascular medications (e.g., "hold if systolic blood pressure less than 100 mmHg"). These types of orders may be necessary and appropriate for the first several days of drug therapy in order to monitor response and adjust dosages. But continuing them unnecessarily after the resident's condition is stable creates a substantial amount of time-consuming, unnecessary work for nursing staff.

One other consideration is important in prescribing drugs for NH residents: cost. The majority of NH residents are either on Medicaid or very close to qualifying for it. State Medicaid programs vary as to what drugs they will cover. Increasingly, NH residents are enrolled in Medicare health maintenance organizations (HMOs), which have limited formularies. Because most NH residents cannot afford to pay out of pocket for drugs, primary physicians should be familiar with the drugs that are covered by Medicaid or other programs and only prescribe other drugs (for which the residents or their families will have to pay) when absolutely necessary.

MONITORING

Careful monitoring of drug therapy is essential in order to minimize the number of unnecessary medications, improve the appropriateness of drug orders, and document efficacy of therapy. Monitoring consists of three basic activities:

1. Assessment of the clinical effectiveness of the drug and identification of side effects
2. Periodic measurement of various clinical parameters (e.g., pulse, blood pressure, postural blood pressure changes)
3. Periodic laboratory studies.

Progress notes of both primary physicians and licensed nurses should document the results of these monitoring activities. Primary physicians should write specific orders for monitoring clinical parameters and laboratory studies. The nature of these orders depends on the drug being monitored and the condition being treated. It is important to emphasize that these orders should be clinically reasonable and not result in excessive busy work for nursing staff or overuse of laboratory tests. There are no data from clinical trials that can provide guidelines for the monitoring of specific drug therapies in the NH setting. **Table 23-5** lists several examples of guidelines for monitoring drugs commonly prescribed in the NH. These examples are not based on data or on the guidelines of any state or health professional organization but represent the authors' best judgment of what is reasonable, given the current state of knowledge.

Table 23-5 Examples of drug monitoring for nursing home residents[a]

Analgesics
1. Document effectiveness regularly
   a. If p.r.n. doses are being used regularly for chronic pain syndromes, consider switching to routine orders
2. For nonsteroidal anti-inflammatory drugs (NSAIDs):
   a. Regularly (e.g., monthly) check stool for occult blood and/or measure blood hemoglobin level
   b. Renal function test should be monitored (e.g., every 2–3 months)

Antiarrhythmics
1. Blood levels should be monitored regularly (e.g., every 3 months when stable)
2. Pulse should be taken regularly (e.g., daily) if a supraventricular tachyarrhythmia is being treated
   a. Parameters can be set to monitor effectiveness (e.g., "Notify MD if pulse >100 or <60")
3. Periodic 24-hour electrocardiographic monitoring may be appropriate if malignant ventricular arrhythmias are being treated

Antibiotics
1. Temperature should be taken regularly (e.g., every shift)
2. Culture and sensitivity reports should be checked to ensure appropriateness of antibiotic

Anticoagulants
1. Prothrombin time should be checked regularly (e.g., monthly)

Anticonvulsants
1. Blood levels should be checked regularly (e.g., every 3 months when stable)
2. For carbamazepine, complete blood count should be checked regularly (e.g., every 2 weeks initially, then every 3 months); liver function tests should also be monitored periodically

Antidepressants
1. Blood levels may be helpful, especially if there is poor response or side effects (e.g., nortriptyline)
2. For tricyclics:
   a. Postural blood pressure and pulse should be checked for the first few days after initiating treatment or increasing dose
   b. Electrocardiogram should be done after initiation of therapy to detect new onset of heart block, especially if dose is adjusted upward
3. For lithium:
   a. Blood levels should be checked regularly (e.g., monthly when stable)
   b. Thyroid function should be measured periodically (e.g., every 6–12 months)
   c. Electrolytes should be monitored regularly (e.g., monthly) with concomitant diuretic therapy
4. Clinical response should be assessed and documented regularly

Antihypertensives
1. Blood pressure should be checked regularly (e.g., weekly when stable)
   a. Parameters can be set to monitor effectiveness (e.g., "Notify MD if systolic BP >180 or <100, or if diastolic BP >100")
2. Postural blood pressure and pulse should be checked after initiating treatment or dosage increases
3. For drugs that affect cardiac conduction (e.g., verapamil, diltiazem), an electrocardiogram should be done to detect new onset of heart block

Table 23-5 (*Continued*)

Antipsychotics

1. Clinical effectiveness should be assessed and documented regularly (e.g., weekly) by determining the frequency of target behaviors (see **Tables 23-6, 23-7, 23-8, and 23-9**)

Diuretics

1. Electrolytes and renal function tests should be checked regularly (e.g., every 1–3 months depending on dose and condition)
2. When an acute illness decreases fluid intake, diuretics should be held

Hematinics

1. Blood hemoglobin should be checked regularly (e.g., monthly)
   a. When hemoglobin becomes normal after acute blood loss, hematinics can be discontinued if nutritional intake adequate

Hypoglycemics

1. Fasting blood sugar and/or glycosylated hemoglobin should be monitored regularly (e.g., monthly) in stable diabetics
2. For unstable diabetics, finger stick glucose monitoring should be done more often until stable
3. Parameters should be set to monitor therapy (e.g., "Notify MD if glucose >250 or <60")

Respiratory Drugs

1. Blood levels of theophylline should be monitored periodically (e.g., every 3 months)
2. Periodic pulmonary function testing and/or pulse oximetry may be appropriate for residents with severe or unstable chronic lung disease

Sedative/hypnotics

1. Clinical effectiveness should be assessed and documented regularly (e.g., weekly) by reviewing frequency and severity of target symptoms and side effects (see **Tables 23-6**, **23-7** and **23-8**)

Thyroid replacement

1. When initiating therapy serum thyroid stimulating hormone (TSH) should be measured regularly (e.g., every 2–4 weeks) and dose adjusted until the TSH is normal
2. Serum TSH should be monitored regularly to detect over or under treatment (e.g., yearly when stable)
   a. Measurement of other thyroid function tests (e.g., T_3, T_4) is generally unnecessary

[a]These recommendations are those of the authors, and are not based on well designed clinical trials (which are lacking), or on any particular state or association guidelines.

PSYCHOTROPIC DRUGS

General Principles

Psychotropic drugs—including antidepressants, antipsychotics, and sedative-hypnotics—are probably the most inappropriately used drugs in the NH. Close to half of all NH residents are given at least one psychotropic drug and a substantial proportion receive more than one. The vast majority of these prescriptions are written without any input from a mental health professional. In a small but important subgroup of NH residents, psychotropic drugs and especially antidepressants may be underused. As mentioned earlier in this chapter, the federal government, via the 1987 OBRA legislation, has intervened to create specific rules regarding the use of antipsychotics. **Table 23-6** summarizes these rules.

Table 23-7 lists several general principles of prescribing psychotropic drugs for NH residents. Other chapters in this book discuss details of the diagnosis and management of dementia, depression, and related behavioral disorders (Chapters 11 and 12). When a psychotropic drug is prescribed, a specific diagnosis should be made whenever possible, and the nature and frequency of target symptoms and behaviors should be documented. Although an increasing number of physicians with training in geriatrics (including geropsychiatry) are becoming available, most primary care physicians who look after NH residents have not had such training. Thus, a consultation from an experienced psychiatrist or psychologist should be obtained whenever possible to provide input into diagnosis and management. In some settings, clinical nurse specialists and social workers can also provide valuable input. Because depression is common, often unrecognized, and treatable, it should be on the top of the differential diagnosis list. Depression commonly accompanies chronic medical illnesses among frail, cognitively intact NH residents and also commonly coexists with dementia. Like those of many medical conditions, the symptoms of depression may be nonspecific or atypical and a variety of medications may contribute to depression in this population (see Chapter 12). NH staff frequently describe a wide variety of behaviors ranging from wandering to yelling to physical aggression as agitation. It is critical to recognize that agitation, like delirium, may be the manifestation of a variety of underlying medical conditions. Any resident who becomes agitated or whose agitated behaviors suddenly worsen should be evaluated to rule out an underlying treatable medical condition before a psychotropic medication is prescribed.

Once a diagnosis is made and specific target symptoms and behaviors are identified, consideration should be given to nonpharmacologic approaches to treatment. A variety of nonpharmacologic approaches—such as socialization, activities, environmental manipulation, altering the way staff interacts with the resident, and behavior modification techniques—may be helpful for selected residents (see Chapter 12).

If a psychotropic drug is prescribed, it is important to choose the most appropriate drug for the specific target symptoms and behaviors in view of the condition of the resident. **Table 23-8** lists several common clinical indications for psychotropic drug therapy and appropriate types of drugs for each indication. The lowest possible dose should be prescribed initially and the dose gradually increased until target symptoms and behaviors respond or intolerable drug side effects occur.

Table 23-6 Summary of OBRA rules relevant to drug prescribing in nursing homes

Rules	Key aspects of interpretive guidelines
1. Each resident's drug regimen must be free from unnecessary drugs. An unnecessary drug is any drug when used: a. in excessive dose (including duplicate therapy); or b. for excessive duration; or c. without adequate monitoring; or d. without adequate indications for its use; or e. in the presence of adverse consequences which indicate the dose should be reduced or discontinued; or f. any combinations of the reasons above.	Long-acting benzodiazepines should not be used unless an attempt with a shorter-acting drug has failed Benzodiazepine or other anxiolytic/sedative drugs should only be used for specific indications (e.g., generalized anxiety, panic disorders, phobias, anxiety associated with depression) or organic mental syndromes (including dementia) with associated agitation as *defined by specific behaviors* which are quantitatively and objectively documented as representing a danger to the resident or others Drugs used for sleep induction should only be used if other treatable causes of sleep disorders (e.g., depression, pain) have been addressed, and the use of the drug maintains or improves the functional status of the resident Dosage guidelines for sedatives and hypnotics Selected drugs should not be used, such as barbiturates, glutethimide, ethchlovynol, meprobamate, and paraldehyde
2. *Antipsychotic drugs* Based on a comprehensive assessment of a resident, the facility must ensure that: a. Residents who have not used antipsychotic drugs are not given these drugs unless antipsychotic drug therapy is necessary to treat a specific condition as diagnosed and documented in the clinical record	Antipsychotic drugs should not be used unless the clinical record documents that the resident has one or more of the following "specific conditions": 1. Schizophrenia 2. Schizo-affective disorder 3. Delusional disorder 4. Psychotic mood disorders (including mania and depression with psychotic features) 5. Acute psychotic episodes 6. Brief reactive psychosis 7. Schizophreniform disorder 8. Atypical psychosis 9. Tourette's disorder 10. Huntington's disease 11. Organic mental syndromes (including dementia and delirium) *with associated psychotic and/or agitated behaviors*: – which have been quantitatively (number of episodes) and objectively (e.g., biting, kicking, scratching) documented

	– Which are not caused by preventable reasons; and
	– Which are causing the residents to:
	  – Present a danger to her/himself or to others
	  – *Continuously* cry, scream, yell, or pace if these specific behaviors cause an impairment in functional capacity (to evaluate functional capacity)
	  – Experience psychotic symptoms (hallucinations, paranoia, delusions) not exhibited as dangerous behaviors or as crying, screaming, yelling, or pacing but which cause the resident distress or impairment in functional capacity
	12. Short term (7 days) symptomatic treatment of hiccups, nausea, vomiting or pruritus
	
	Antipsychotics should not used if one or more of the following is/are the **only** indication:
	
	1. Wandering
	2. Poor self care
	3. Restlessness
	4. Impaired memory
	5. Anxiety
	6. Depression (without psychotic features)
	7. Insomnia
	8. Unsocialability
	9. Indifference to surroundings
	10. Fidgeting
	11. Nervousness
	12. Uncooperativeness, or
	13. Agitated behaviors which **do not** represent danger to the resident or others

b. Residents who use antipsychotic drugs receive gradual dose reductions, and behavioral interventions, unless clinically contraindicated, in an effort to discontinue these drugs	Residents must, unless clinically contraindicated, have gradual dose reductions of the antipsychotic drug. The gradual dose reduction should be under close supervision. If the gradual dose reduction is causing an adverse effect on the resident and the gradual dose reduction is discontinued, documentation of this decision and the reasons for it should be included in the clinical record. Gradual dose reductions consist of tapering the resident's daily dose to determine if the resident's symptoms can be controlled by a lower dose or to determine if the dose can be eliminated altogether. "Behavioral interventions" mean modification of the resident's behavior or the resident's environment, including staff approaches to care, to the largest degree possible to accommodate the resident's behavior

Table 23-7 Basic principles of prescribing psychotropic drugs for nursing home residents

1. Make a specific diagnosis and identify target symptoms and behaviors before prescribing a drug
   a. Consult an experienced psychiatrist or psychologist if necessary to provide input on diagnosis and treatment
   b. Depression is common and treatable
      (1) It frequently coexists with dementia
      (2) Clinical presentation may include a variety of symptoms or behaviors
   c. Residents who become "agitated" should be assessed to rule out delirium caused by treatable medical conditions, drugs or depression
2. Using non-pharmacologic approaches to manage target behaviors whenever possible
3. If a drug is prescribed, choose the drug that is most appropriate for the specific clinical indications and condition of the resident (see **Table 23-4**)
4. Start with low doses
5. Monitor and document response of target symptoms and behaviors, and side effects
6. Increase the dose gradually until:
   a. Target symptoms and behaviors are improved
   b. Intolerable drug side effects occur
7. Continue to monitor response of target symptoms and behaviors, and observe for side effects
8. If symptoms and behaviors are eliminated and remain stable over several weeks (e.g. 8–12 weeks), consider dose reduction and eventual discontinuation of the drug

One of the major problems with the use of psychotropic drugs in NHs is the lack of adequate monitoring after the drug is prescribed. **Table 23-9** lists several of the key elements of monitoring psychotropic drug use. Each of these issues should be addressed and documented on a regular basis in nursing and physician progress notes. During the initial phase of drug therapy, it may be necessary to summarize these data daily. After symptoms have stabilized, a weekly summary in the nursing notes would be an appropriate method of documentation. Routine physician progress notes should also summarize these data. Facilities with computers may want to incorporate the elements listed in **Table 23-9** into a database that can be used for quality assurance purposes.

If target symptoms and behaviors are improved and the resident's condition remains stable, consideration should be given to reducing the dose and discontinuing the drug. For some psychiatric conditions, such as depression and psychosis, it is appropriate to stabilize symptoms for a period of at least several weeks (e.g., 8 to 12) before beginning to withdraw the drug. For some residents, it may not be possible or clinically indicated to withdraw the drug at all (e.g., those who have failed previous attempts to withdraw drug therapy). If the drug is to be withdrawn, it is generally best to reduce the dose

Table 23-8 Clinical considerations in prescribing psychotropic drugs

Clinical indications	Most useful drugs	Comments
Depression with psychomotor retardation[a]	Less sedating antidepressant (e.g., desipramine, nortriptyline, serotonin reuptake inhibitor, nefazodone, venlafaxine, buproprion	Anticholinergic effects, potential cardiovascular effects, and potential interactions with antihypertensives are important considerations
Depression with psychomotor agitation[a]	More sedating antidepressant (e.g., doxepin, trazodone)	
Agitation without psychosis	Short-acting sedative (e.g., alprazolam, oxazepam, lorazepam, buspirone[a])	Should generally be used on prn basis Nonpharmacologic interventions may be more appropriate Buspirone is not effective acutely; chronic dosing rather than prn use necessary
Psychosis without prominent agitation (e.g., delusions and hallucinations in patients with depression or dementia)	Less sedating antipsychotic (e.g., haloperidol, thiothixene)	Extrapyramidal effects may be prominent Akathisia can make patient appear agitated
Severe agitation poorly controlled by a sedative	More sedating antipsychotic (e.g., thioridazine, molindone)	Stronger antipsychotics (haloperidol, thiothixene) sometimes needed Extrapyramidal effects may be prominent Akathisia can make patient appear more agitated
Insomnia	Chloral hydrate, temazepam, triazolam	Underlying cause(s) should be sought Nonpharmacologic interventions often helpful Benzodiazepines should be used on an intermittent rather than a nightly basis

[a]See Chapter 12.

gradually. Ongoing monitoring, as described above, is extremely important during these attempts to reduce or discontinue psychotropic drug use.

Specific information about the use of antidepressants can be found in Chapter 12. The sections that follow briefly discuss the use of antipsychotic and sedative/hypnotic drugs.

Table 23-9 Key elements of monitoring and documenting responses to psychotropic drugs

1. Specific target symptoms and/or behaviors for which drug was prescribed
2. Frequency of the target symptoms and/or behaviors
3. Number of p.r.n. doses given (if applicable)
4. Frequency and nature of any potential drug side effects
5. Plans for dosage adjustment, i.e.:
   a. Increase dose to improve symptoms or behaviors
   b. Keep dose stable (adequate response)
   c. Decrease dose
      (1) Due to side effects
      (2) After symptoms or behaviors have been improved for several weeks to try to minimize or eliminate drug use

Antipsychotics

Among the psychotropic drugs, antipsychotics are the most controversial with respect to NH residents. There is a general sense that antipsychotics are frequently used as "chemical restraints" in this population. This concern, as well as the possibility of permanent side effects such as tardive dyskinesia, is probably responsible for the specific attention given antipsychotics in the 1987 OBRA legislation. In addition to this concern, there is a lack of data from controlled trials on the efficacy of these drugs in the NH population.

Under the rules outlined in OBRA antipsychotics should no longer be used if the only indication is a nonspecific one, such as wandering, agitation, or uncooperativeness. They can be prescribed for specific psychotic conditions as well as in organic mental syndromes (including dementia) when the syndrome includes psychotic or agitated features, and when specific behaviors are objectively and quantitatively documented that cause resident to present a danger to themselves or others (see **Table 23-6**).

When dementia and/or depression is complicated by psychosis (e.g., paranoid delusions), an antipsychotic drug is generally indicated. The more common situation, however, is that a resident with dementia presents with agitated behaviors that are a danger to others or significantly interfere with care. In these situations (assuming the resident is not depressed or medically ill), the choice of drug therapy is between an antipsychotic and a short-acting sedative. There are advantages and disadvantages to each, and each class of drugs has its proponents. Data from well-controlled clinical trials comparing antipsychotics to short-acting sedatives for agitated behaviors among NH residents are not available at the present time. Whichever approach is taken, careful monitoring of the target symptoms and behaviors as well as careful observation for side effects are critical.

Table 23-10 lists examples of antipsychotic drugs. The major advantage of using the more potent antipsychotics (e.g., haloperidol, thiothixene) is that they

Table 23-10 Examples of antipsychotic drugs

Drug	Relative potency/ equivalent dose (mg)	Approximate dosages (mg)[a]	Relative sedation	Potential for side effects: Hypotension	Potential for side effects: Extrapyramidal effects[b]
Chlorpromazine (Thorazine, others)	50	10–300	Very high	High	Moderate
Thioridazine (Mellaril)	50	10–300	Moderate	Moderate	Low
Loxapine (Loxitane)	7.5	10–100	High	Moderate	Moderate
Molindone (Moban)	5	5–100	Moderate	Moderate	Moderate
Thiothixene (Navane)	2.5	1–5	Low	Low	Very high
Haloperidol (Haldol)	1	0.25–6	Low	Low	Very high
Rispiridone (Risperdal)	N/A[c]	0.5–3	Low	Moderate[d]	Low

[a]Per day in two to four divided doses.

[b]Rigidity, bradykinesia, tremor, akathisia.

[c]No dose equivalency published. Manufacturer recommends starting at 0.25 or 0.5 mg twice per day and titrating up weekly to a total daily dose of up to 3 mg.

[d]Usually occurs at beginning of dose titration; patients tend to accommodate to hypotensive effects.

are generally not sedating and do not have significant cardiovascular side effects. They are contraindicated in residents with parkinsonism. Even in very small doses (e.g., 0.5 mg of haloperidol), they can have significant extrapyramidal side effects, the most disabling of which are bradykinesia and rigidity. These side effects can result in immobility and can predispose already immobile residents to complications such as aspiration, pressure sores, and incontinence. Another important but commonly unrecognized side effect is akathisia. Manifested by motor restlessness, akathisia may be mistaken for a failure of response to the drug or even a worsening of symptoms. As a result, the dose may be increased until the resident is so bradykinetic and rigid that she or he appears less agitated. This is obviously the wrong approach to using these drugs, and primary physicians who prescribe potent antipsychotics should be very familiar with these potential side effects. Anticholinergics should not be routinely prescribed to prevent these extrapyramidal side effects. It is probably better to change the drug rather than add an anticholinergic agent because of the potential for anticholinergic side effects. Anticholinergic side effects may be especially bothersome in NH residents. They include dryness of the mouth, blurring of vision, constipation and fecal impaction, exacerbation of gastroesophageal reflux, and delirium. More sedating antipsychotics (e.g., thioridazine, loxapine, and molindone) may be appropriate for very agitated, psychotic residents. Low doses of thioridazine (e.g., 10 mg) may be effective, but anticholinergic and cardiovascular side effects (hypotension) may limit its usefulness. If mild sedation is the therapeutic goal, a short-acting sedative is probably a better choice.

Sedative/Hypnotics

Table **23-11** lists examples of sedative/hypnotic drugs. If the therapeutic goal is mild sedation for disabling anxiety or intermittent severe agitated behaviors, then it is appropriate to use a short-acting drug that has a relatively short onset of action (e.g., lorazepam, which can also be given intramuscularly). Antihistamines have been used for this purpose, but they probably should be avoided in NH residents with dementia because of their anticholinergic effects. Buspirone appears to have a low side-effect profile, but it may take several days of chronic therapy for its therapeutic effects to become apparent. Unlike short-acting benzodiazepines, buspirone is not useful as a hypnotic.

Before a hypnotic is prescribed, a careful assessment of complaints of insomnia is essential. First, self-reports of insomnia among NH residents are often unreliable, and this complaint should be verified by nighttime nursing staff. Second, insomnia may be caused by a lack of activity and naps during the day or by the “sundowning” associated with sensory deprivation. These factors are potentially amenable to nonpharmacologic approaches such as activity programming during the day and the use of night lights to diminish sensory deprivation. The nighttime NH environment has been shown to be noisy and disruptive to

Table 23-11 Examples of sedatives and hypnotic drugs

	Approximate dose equivalent (mg)	Relative rapidity of effect after oral administration	Half-life (h)	Active metabolites
	Benzodiazepines			
Longer-acting[a]				
Diazepam (Valium)	5	Very fast	20–100	Yes
Clorazepate (Tranxene)	7.5	Fast	30–100	Yes
Flurazepam[b] (Dalmane)	15	Fast	40–200	Yes
Clonazepam (Klonopin)	0.5	Intermediate	18–50	Yes
Shorter-acting				
Triazolam[b] (Halcion)	0.25	Fast	2–5	No
Lorazepam (Ativan)	1	Intermediate	10–20	No
Oxazepam (Serax)	15	Intermediate	5–15	No
Temazepam[a] (Restoril)	15	Intermediate	5–15	No
Alprazolam (Xanax)	0.25	Fast	6–20	No
	Antihistamines[c]			
Diphenhydramine[a] (Benadryl, others)	25	Fast	4–7	No
Hydroxyzine (Vistaril, Atarax)	10	Very fast	Unknown[d]	Unknown
	Other			
Chloral hydrate[a] (Noctec, others)	500	Fast	7–10	Yes
Busprione (BuSpar)[e]	10	Fast	2–3	Yes

[a]Use of long-acting benzodiazepines should be avoided.
[b]More commonly used as hypnotics.
[c]Anticholinergic side effects may be problematic.
[d]Duration of action: 4 to 6 hours.
[e]Must be used chronically to be an effective antianxiety agent.

sleep as well. Efforts should be made to keep noise to a minimum at night. Finally, insomnia may be caused by medical conditions such as nocturia, orthopnea, gastroesophageal reflux, and nocturnal myoclonus. A careful history may be necessary to detect these symptoms, and specific therapy should be initiated when appropriate.

Whenever sedative/hypnotic drugs are prescribed, it is best to use them intermittently rather than chronically (with the possible exception of buspirone). Intermittent use may lead to less tolerance to drug effects. In addition, withdrawal syndromes—with increased insomnia, anxiety, or agitation—can occur when chronic treatment is discontinued.

SUGGESTED READINGS

Avorn J, Gurwitz JH: Drug use in the nursing home. *Ann Intern Med* 123:195–204, 1995.

Beers M, Avorn J, Soumerai SB, et al: Psychoactive medication use in intermediate-care facility residents. *JAMA* 260:3016–3020, 1988.

Beers MH, Ouslander JG, Fingold SF, Morgenstern H, Reuben DB, Rogers W, et al: Inappropriate medication prescribing in skilled-nursing facilities. *Ann Intern Med* 117:684–689, 1992.

Beers MH, Ouslander JG, Rollingher I, Reuben DB, Brooks J, Beck JC: Explicit criteria for determining inappropriate medication use in nursing home residents. *Arch Intern Med* 151:1852–1832, 1991.

Carlson MA, Fleming KC, Smith GE, Evans JM: Management of dementia-related behavioral disturbances: Nonpharmacologic approach. *Mayo Clin Proc* 70:1108–1115, 1995.

Dement WC: Rational basis for the use of sleeping pills. *Pharmacology* 27(suppl 2):3–38, 1983.

Helms PM: Efficacy of antipsychotics in the treatment of the behavioral complications of dementia: A review of the literature. *J Am Geriatr Soc* 33:206–209, 1985.

Montamat SC, Cusack BJ, and Vestel RE: Management of drug therapy in the elderly. *N Engl J Med* 321:303–310, 1989.

Ouslander JG: Drug therapy in the elderly. *Ann Intern Med* 95:711–722, 1981.

Schneider LS, Pollock VE, Lyness SA: A meta-analysis of controlled trials of neuroleptic treatment in dementia. *J Am Geriatr Soc* 38:553–563, 1990.

Thapa PB, Meador KG, Gideon P, Fought RL, Ray WA: Effects of antipsychotic withdrawal in elderly nursing home residents. *J Am Geriatr Soc* 42:280–286, 1996.

Thompson TL, Moran MG, and Niles AS: Psychotropic drug use in the elderly (two parts). *N Engl J Med* 308:134–138, 194–199, 1983.

CHAPTER

TWENTY-FOUR

REHABILITATION IN THE NURSING HOME

Rehabilitation is the continuing and comprehensive team effort to restore an individual to his or her former functional status or to maintain or maximize remaining function. In the care of nursing home (NH) residents, rehabilitation should not necessarily be viewed as an episodic intervention for a definite period of time or as being appropriate only after the onset of a major disabling illness (e.g., stroke, hip fracture). Rather, rehabilitation involves a plan of care that may need to be continuous and an ongoing team effort. The concept of restoring functioning and/or maximizing remaining function is critical to providing a plan of care to any disabled or potentially disabled older person. Viewed in this way, rehabilitation becomes a process of delivering the minimal services which help maintain the highest possible level of function. On the other hand, it should be stressed that for short-stay residents, intensive rehabilitation services may be indicated to allow a rapid return to the home environment.

Table 24-1 describes the principles of rehabilitation in the NH setting. The potential benefits from rehabilitation include improvements in physical and psychological status and quality of life. Successful rehabilitation will lessen perceived dependency as well as reduce the burdens of existing disabilities. The process of rehabilitation follows the same principles outlined in **Table 24-1**. In order to carry out these principles and achieve the benefits of rehabilitation, a multidisciplinary team must evaluate the resident; establish a problem list with measurable goals; and work out a clear, realistic plan of rehabilitation to achieve these goals.

Table 24-1 Basic principles of rehabilitation in the nursing home

Treatment of the underlying disease(s)
Prevention of a secondary disability
Treatment of primary disabilities
Enhancement of residual function
Realistic goals
Emphasis on functional independence
Attention to motivation and other psychological factors
Provision of adaptive tools
Alteration of the environment to maximise function
Team approach

REHABILITATION TEAM

Central to the concept of rehabilitation is the rehabilitation team. This team must be multidisciplinary in membership and interdisciplinary in process. Members of the team traditionally represent the disciplines of physical therapy (PT), occupational therapy (OT), speech therapy (ST), medicine (physician trained in geriatrics or physiatry), social work, nursing, nutrition, and recreational therapy. **Table 24-2** describes the role of each member. Chapter 9 discusses the role of teams in NH care in greater detail.

THE PHYSICIAN'S ROLE

The physician's role is to review the assessment and impressions of all team members and to prescribe interventions. The clarity and accuracy of his or her orders is critical for proper compliance and appropriate reimbursement for rehabilitative interventions. The prescribing physician should adhere to the principle of defining a problem (which relates to an ICD-9 diagnosis) and have preferentially a measurable outcome in terms of time line and function. For example, for a resident with a poststroke contracture with measured limitation of range of motion, the physician must document the limitations and functional disability as well as set a goal to improve range of motion by set degrees, with the ability to perform a certain function (e.g., combing) to be attained within a given time (e.g., 7 days). The prescription should include the diagnosis, the treatment modality, and the treatment's frequency and duration. Keep in mind that in the NH setting the intensity of intervention for a given dysfunction should be realistic and geared toward achieving the measurable goals; otherwise payment may be denied because of an inappropriate intervention. For example, a resident with the new onset of hemiplegia should have at least three rehabilitation treatments per week, using several physical modalities, for 4 to 5

Table 24-2 Rehabilitation team members in the nursing home

Physical therapist	Focuses on improvement of range of motion, strength, endurance, balance, and mobility through exercise and training with assistive devices
Occupational therapist	Focuses on activities of daily living (ADL) such as eating, grooming, dressing, and bathing as well as improving upper extremity function; may also help to compensate for visual perceptual or sensory deficits
Speech therapist	Evaluates and treats disorders of communication, speech, and swallowing Limited cognitive evaluation
Nurse/restorative nurse's aide	Reinforces the techniques learned in physical and occupational therapy and helps to develop bowel and bladder training programs
Geriatrician/physiatrist	Provides comprehensive medical and functional evaluation and prescribes the program of therapy
Nutritionist	Provides nutritional assessment, makes recommendations for interventions, and implements interventions as prescribed
Social worker	Provides a psychosocial evaluation and assessment of mood and motivation, maintains liaison with family members; provides family support, and coordinates discharge planning
Recreation therapist	Provides evaluation for leisure-time activities; assists resident in adjusting to new situation and learning new recreational activities, utilizes music, exercise, arts and crafts
Clinical psychologist	Performs formal testing and provides staff education Short-term psychotherapy

weeks. One therapy session per week for a NH resident may be determined by a Medicare Part B intermediary as too little therapy for the level of function expected. In contrast, therapy daily may be disallowed because the resident is too impaired and should be a candidate for an acute care hospital rehabilitation center or a subacute rehabilitation unit where therapy is delivered five to six times per week. Issues surrounding reimbursement for rehabilitation are discussed at the end of this chapter.

TYPES OF REHABILITATION

Rehabilitation can involve either restorative or maintenance therapy. In restorative therapy, the goal is to reverse disability and improve function. *Restorative* therapy is exemplified by the NH resident disabled by a hip fracture or stroke with hemiplegia who needs rehabilitation in order to regain function and/or compensate for functional impairments. This therapy is usually quite

Table 24-3 Secondary complications preventable by rehabilitation in the nursing home

Anorexia
Confusion/delirium
Contractures
Deconditioning
Depression
Falls
Fecal impaction/incontinence
Pneumonia
Pressure sores
Psychological dependency
Urinary incontinence
Urinary tract infection
Venous thrombosis

intense, taking at least one to four hours per day for a determined period of time (e.g., 4 to 12 weeks). *Maintenance* therapy has the goal of preserving the present level of function and preventing secondary complications (see **Table 24-3**). It may be less intense and of longer duration than restorative therapy. For example, ongoing bi-weekly therapy may be given to a resident who had a stroke 4 months earlier and has already had a restorative therapy program but for whom continuing therapy can prevent contractures and a "frozen" shoulder. Similarly, maintenance therapy for the acutely ill bed-ridden resident might include bedside range-of-motion exercises, frequent changes of position to prevent pressure sores, and progressive active assistance and exercise to provide easy ambulation and prevent severe deconditioning. These tasks are frequently delegated to restorative nurse's aides (RNA) and certified nurse's aides (CNA). **Table 24-4** lists some examples of specific orders for common conditions requiring rehabilitation in the NH.

REHABILITATION POTENTIAL

While cure or complete restoration of function may sometimes be an unrealistic goal in the geriatric population, most NH residents may achieve benefits from the rehabilitation process. The resident and family may gain psychological benefit because they perceive that something can be done to improve function. This may also result in increased self-esteem for the resident. Quality of life may be enhanced as the resident regains control over bodily functions and interacts with therapists or other caregivers. The burden of disability may be diminished by small improvements in the ability to perform activities of daily living. For example, even an improvement in the ability to transfer from bed to chair can

Table 24-4 Examples of specific physician orders for conditions commonly requiring rehabilitation in the nursing home

Condition	Speech therapy disorders
Swallowing disorder due to Parkinson's disease (ICD9–787.2)	Dysphagia (swallowing) evaluation by speech therapy Dysphagia treatment by speech therapy five times weekly (twice per day) for 30 days to increase oral motor strength and control and safety of swallow
Aphasia due to stroke (ICD9–784.3)	Speech therapy evaluation Speech and language therapy five times weekly for 30 days to increase functional receptive and expressive language, cognition, and memory
Dysarthria (slurred speech) due to stroke (ICD9–784.5)	Speech evaluation and follow-up treatment as indicated Speech therapy five times weekly for 30 days to increase oral motor strength/control and functional speech intelligibility
Hearing loss (ICD9–388.01)	Speech and language evaluation Speech and language therapy three times weekly for 30 days to increase use of amplification device and improve lip-reading and functional communication skills
Condition/problem	**Physical therapy order**
Acute vertebral fracture (ICD9–805.0)	Physical therapy evaluation Hot packs, massage, ultrasound, electrical stimulation three times a week for 30 days for diagnosis of acute vertebral fracture
Proximal muscle weakness due to arthritis (ICD9–726.5)	Physical therapy for gait and transfer exercises three times a week for 30 days for diagnoses of right hip arthritis
Right femur fracture, status post ORIF (ICD9–820.0)	Transfer and gait training and exercise five times a week for 30 days for diagnosis of right hip fracture
CVA with right hemiplegia (ICD9–346.0)	Gait training and transfer exercises five times a week for 30 days
Lumbosacral spondylosis without radiculopathy (ICD9–721.3)	Hot packs, massage, ultrasound, exercise three times a week for 30 days
Gait disturbance due to weakness after acute hospitalization (ICD9–780.7)	Gait training and exercise three times a week for 30 days
Parkinson's disease (ICD9–332.0)	Gait training and exercise three times a week for 30 days
	Occupational therapy
Acute flareup of left shoulder arthritis with acute decreased ADLs (ICD9–716.91)	Compensatory ADL training Use of adaptive equipment as needed Upper extremity therapeutic activities three times a week for 30 days

Table 24-4 (*Continued*)

Condition/problem	Occupational therapy
Acute decreased ADLs and weakness due to acute hospitalization (ICD9–799.3)	Therapeutic activities to increase functional endurance Feeding program Compensatory ADL training three times a week for 30 days Use of adaptive equipment as needed
Left hip fracture (ICD9–820.8)	Compensatory ADL training Use of adaptive equipment as needed to assist with ADL performance
Acute decreased ADLs due to acute vertebral compression fractures	Compensatory ADL training with safety instruction three times a week for 30 days Instruction in use of adaptive equipment as needed

greatly affect quality of life and the burden of care. Subjective feelings of dependency may be alleviated by increased self-confidence and reduced perceived dependency. Some studies have alluded to the fact that individuals who undergo rehabilitation live longer than those who have not attempted rehabilitation. While data are limited, a rehabilitation program may also reduce the future costs of institutionalized care. Accordingly, the prospect of long-term institutionalization should not exclude NH residents from rehabilitation services.

Because of the possibility of benefiting from either restorative or maintenance rehabilitation therapy, all residents should be assessed for their rehabilitation potential. The most common impairments in older NH residents that may benefit from rehabilitation therapy are best quantified by a comprehensive functional assessment. Rehabilitation is most useful in trying to restore and/or maintain independence in basic activities of daily living (ADL), including: (1) mobility; (2) transferring; (3) feeding; and (4) grooming and dressing. These functions are critical in determining the resident's degree of independence and need for assistance. The rehabilitation potential for each resident should be assessed within 7 days of admission by the physician and a note to this effect should be placed in the medical record. The physician should estimate the resident's capability of cooperating with a rehabilitation program and making a measurable, functional gain. Consideration should also be given to whether or not the resident's quality of life can be improved. Physical, psychological and socioeconomic status all interact in determining rehabilitation potential.

Coexisting medical conditions such as peripheral vascular disease, arthritis, and neurologic disease (e.g., peripheral neuropathy) may adversely affect rehabilitation potential. Dementia may also have a significant adverse effect on the potential to benefit from rehabilitation, especially restorative forms of therapy. NH residents with dementia should not, however, automatically be excluded from restorative therapy (e.g., gait training after hip fracture), because many residents with moderately or even severely advanced dementia may benefit. Virtually all NH residents, regardless of how cognitively impaired, can benefit from an ongoing maintenance rehabilitation program, designed to maintain mobility and function and prevent deconditioning and the many other potential complications of immobility.

The following sections will briefly discuss principles of rehabilitation for common impairments of basic ADL function in the NH population.

CHAIR-BOUND RESIDENTS

The person most often forgotten in a rehabilitation program is the bedfast or chair-bound resident. The first goal of rehabilitation in these residents is to prevent contractures. These residents should have their upper and lower limbs moved through a complete range of motion on a twice-daily basis. To maintain functionality, the upper limbs should be actively or passively moved so that the hand touches the back of the head and the chest. For the lower limbs, it is important that the resident lie on his or her stomach and that the leg be lifted backward, at least 10°. This maintains adequate hip movements for walking. If pain occurs during range-of-motion exercises, an evaluation to determine the cause of the pain should be undertaken. This may require a consultation by a physiatrist or rheumatologist. If the resident already has contractures, passive stretching or the use of weights and/or splints may be helpful. In some of these residents, surgery may restore some function and prevent complications.

For chair-bound residents, a 15 to 20 min group exercise program should be provided four to five times a week. For some of these residents, supervised aerobic exercises in a swimming pool may be especially helpful. Recently it was reported that a strength-training program (lower extremity weight lifting) had a major impact on gait and balance in 90-year-old NH residents. In a program carried out by one of us, we found highly positive responses to a once-a-week walking program among residents who had been chair-bound for 3 months or longer. This program resulted in an improvement in gait and balance, an increase in morale, and a decrease in use of restraints. Integrating walking protocols with toileting may be a creative and, perhaps, efficient way of rehabilitation for chair-bound residents.

IMPAIRMENT OF GAIT AND MOBILITY

Normal gait is characterized by smooth, symmetrical movement of arms, trunk, and legs. A normal gait requires coordination of weight shifts and pelvic rotation to achieve elongation of the weight-bearing side and flexion of the non-weight-bearing side. Pelvic mobility, balance, and adequate base of support are important factors influencing gait. Normal gait is composed of two phases. The stance phase occurs when the foot contacts the floor and bears weight. It begins when the heel strikes the floor, the midfoot and forefoot bear weight, and the heel and midfoot leave the floor as hip and knee flexion begin and the foot pushes off. This phase comprises 60 percent of normal gait. The swing phase of gait is the time during which the foot swings through and is clearing the floor. This phase begins when the forefoot leaves the floor and ends when the heel strikes the floor. During this phase the pelvis remains level and the hip and knee sweep through flexion and extension (see **Fig. 16-1**).

An important problem in NH residents is backward leaning. This often develops when a resident spends a period of time in a chair, with resulting contractures in the back muscles. These contractures can, in turn, result in backward leaning and poor standing balance. Having the resident move objects around on a table in front of the chair for 15 to 20 min per day will help to prevent and treat back contractures. For ambulatory NH residents, muscle strengthening exercises have been shown to improve gait velocity with an objective increase in muscle mass and endurance.

Table 24-5 describes common conditions leading to functional impairments of gait in NH residents. Interventions to improve ambulation consist of physical and occupational therapy, both utilizing assistive devices. **Table 24-6** summarizes the most commonly used devices and their indications. **Figure 24-1** depicts examples of some devices. The assessment of gait and balance is discussed further in Chapter 16.

Table 24-5 Common conditions leading to functional impairment among nursing home residents

	Functional impairment
Right hemispheric stroke	Visual loss, sensory loss, distortion of spatial relations, lack of motivation, hemiplegia
Left hemispheric stroke	Disturbances of communication (e.g., asphagia) hemiplegia
Hip fracture	Gait instability
Spinal stenosis	Gait instability, proximal muscle weakness
Peripheral neuropathy	Loss of perception, hand-grip weakness
Arthritis (pain, contractures)	Gait instability, muscle weakness
Peripheral vascular disease	Limited mobility, muscle weakness
Parkinsonism	Rigidity, impaired coordination, gait instability, muscle weakness

Table 24-6 Examples of assistive devices for impaired mobility

Assistive devices	Characteristics	Indications	Advantages/disadvantages	Caveats
Single-pronged cane	Simplest device for ambulation Minimal support (25% of body weight is supported)	Unilateral deficits such as arthritis, fracture, or hemiplegia	Light, socially acceptable	Should be held on the unaffected side
Tripod/quad cane	Significantly more support	Same as single-pronged cane	Clumsy to maneuver; physically unattractive	Length of cane should allow 30° of elbow flexion
Pickup walker or hemiwalker	Provides substantial balance	More than localized impairment of function	Energy-consuming; requires upper extremity strength to coordinate a step forward with lifting the walker	Environmental hazards become obstacles; resident must be trained
Front-wheeled roller walker	Provides slightly less balance than pickup walker	For more impaired individuals	Requires less energy, strength, and standing balance	Environmental hazards become obstacles, resident must be trained
Walker with forearm troughs or handles; crutches	Good support	For individuals with painful and deformed hand, wrist, or elbow joint (e.g., rheumatoid arthritis)		Same as for other walkers

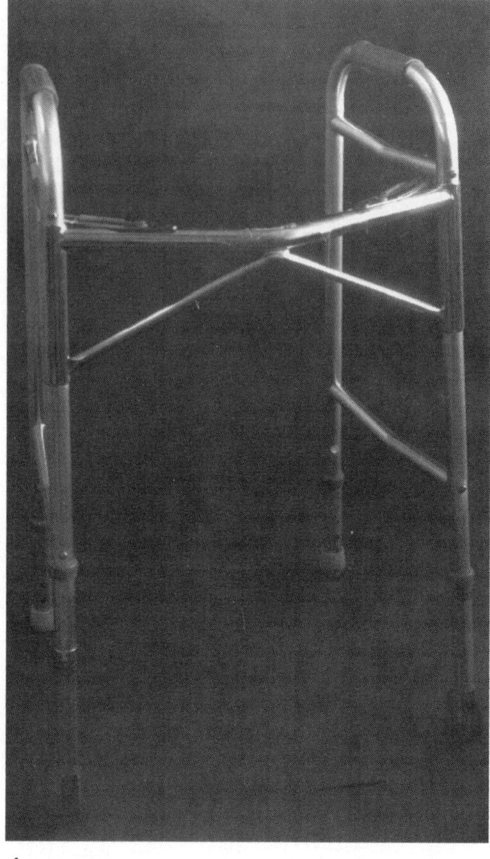

A

Figure 24-1 Examples of assistive devices for ambulation: A. Front-wheeled walker.

BALANCE TRAINING

Balance is important for stability in chair-bound residents during transfers, while standing, and while walking. Physical therapy techniques are now available to improve balance in all of these residents. Catching a beach ball while in a chair improves balance for the chair-bound. Stability devices that fit around the waist and allow residents to stand safely while they catch a ball or work on a pegboard in front of them can improve standing balance, as can exercises done with the assistance of parallel bars. Walking between parallel bars can lead to marked improvement of balance and confidence. Abnormalities of posture can also lead to balance problems. These abnormalities can be detected using a plumb line suspended from the ceiling. Specific exercise programs can help correct defects in posture. Muscle weakness can also contribute to instability, and this is

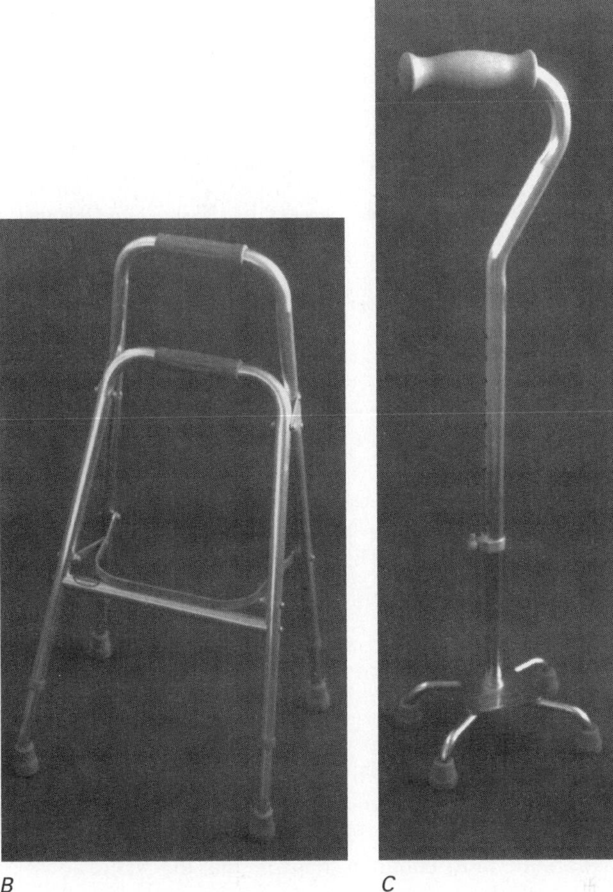

B C

Figure 24-1 (*Continued*) B. hemi-walker, C. quad cane.

responsive to strength-building exercises. Tai Chi has recently been shown to improve balance and possibly prevent falls in older individuals.

TRANSFERRING

As mentioned earlier, the ability to transfer may be critical to a NH resident's quality of life, his or her need for institutional care, and the burden of that care. A transfer is a movement by which the resident goes from one surface to another. Safe and efficient transfers require a combination of physical and perceptual capabilities, proper equipment, and training techniques that are suitable for the resident's abilities. Sitting balance is also an important prerequisite for safe

Table 24-7 Transfer techniques

	Process	Aids	Barriers
Bed to wheelchair (stand-pivot transfer)	Sitting position: Lock brakes Grasp side rails of bed Standing position: Grasp to wheelchair with unaffected side and sit down	Sliding board; person with belt	Dementia, obesity Neglect or affected side Upper- or lower-extremity disability Orthostatic hypotension
Wheelchair to toilet	Rise from wheelchair Stand Pivot onto toilet Must be able to manage clothing and undergarments	Toilet seat 20 in. from floor or raised toilet seat Hand rails on unaffected side	Dementia, depression, obesity Neglect of affected side Upper- or lower-extremity disability Orthostatic hypotension
Tub transfer (rarely required in NH because supervision is mandated)	Transfer from wheelchair to bench Move lower extremity with normal hand into tub	Tub transfer bench	Dementia, obesity Neglect of affected side Upper- or lower-extremity disability Orthostatic hypotension

transfers. To transfer safely, the resident must be free of or have only minimal orthostatic hypotension and be capable of maintaining the hip and knee in a position of extension. Strong shoulder adduction and abduction, elbow flexion and extension, and hand or wrist function on one side are also required. **Table 24-7** summarizes the most common transfers that the NH resident may need to learn and techniques for training for such transfers.

FEEDING, BATHING, AND DRESSING

The evaluation of a resident for feeding, grooming, and dressing rehabilitation should determine whether weakness, limited range of motion, incoordination, spasticity, or perceptual loss is the primary or sole impairment. This evaluation is usually conducted by the physician and the occupational therapist. Interventions generally consist of exploiting the preserved functions and enhancing the affected functions as much as possible.

Awareness of subtle deficits such as visual and perceptual spatial distortions or lack of motivation associated with right hemispheric stroke may guide the rehabilitation program by exploiting the unaffected side and providing assistance for those with impaired judgment and safety awareness. Left hemispheric stroke victims usually have preserved perceptual functions but may suffer from aphasia and communication problems that can affect their rehabilitation. In these cases, use of communication boards, picture books, and gestures may be necessary.

Impaired feeding, grooming, and dressing can also result from rigidity and lack of coordination, as seen in Parkinson's disease. Therapy consists of gradual resistive exercise to increase the strength of muscles governing gross motor activity as well as mobility. Energy-saving techniques are also an important component of rehabilitation in these areas, since fatigue aggravates incoordination. Foods that eliminate the need for cutting, chopping, or mixing may be a useful consideration. Weighted utensils and items with double handles that can easily be gripped will also partially counteract the effects of incoordination. Stabilization can be achieved by using a spike board, rubber mat, or sponges. Oversized bowls can be used to avoid spillage by extension movements or tremor. **Figure 24-2** depicts examples of eating utensils that may be beneficial in helping functionally impaired individuals regain independence in feeding.

For cognitively impaired residents who have difficulty with eating, feeding programs may be very valuable. Initiation of a feeding program should be preceded by a thorough swallowing and nutritional history as well as feeding trials to ascertain the resident's food preferences and the optimal food textures. This type of approach may prevent irreversible malnutrition in NH residents. Speech therapists are often well trained to assess and participate in the management of NH residents with feeding problems. Impairment in grooming and dressing (i.e., ADL impairment) often results from limited range of motion related to a frozen shoulder, arthritis or spasticity, or contracture

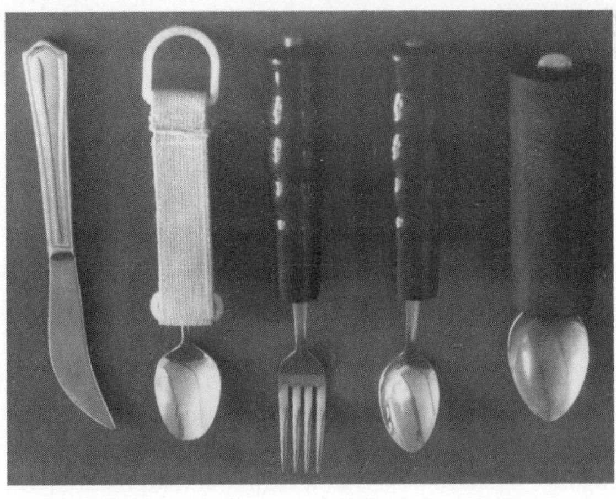

A

Figure 24-2 Examples of utensils for handicapped individuals. A. Utensils including a rocking knife for use by a single hand and spoons and forks for individuals with difficulty grasping.

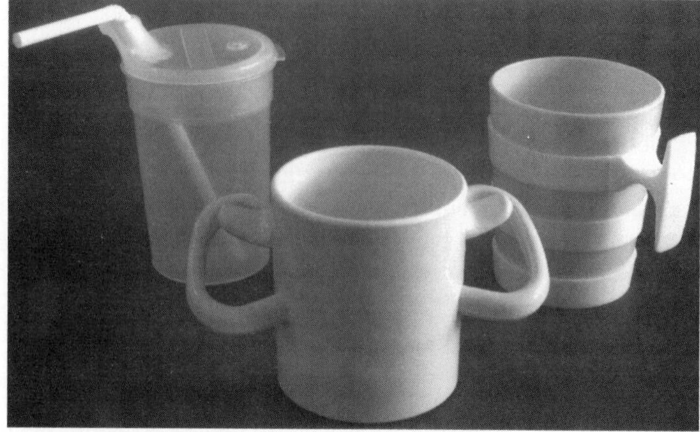

B

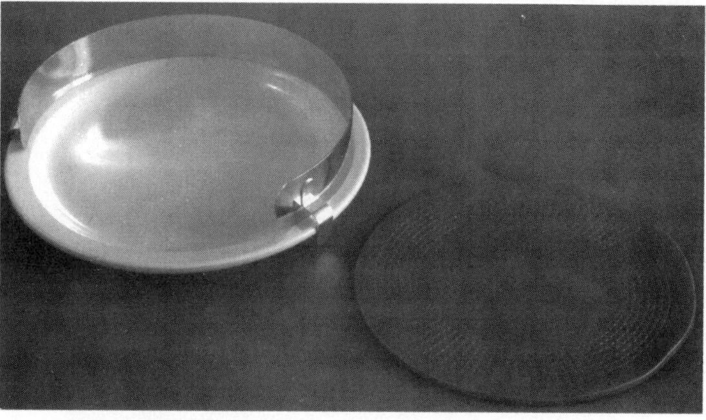

C

Figure 24-2 (*Continued*) B. Drinking cups for individuals with difficulty holding a cup. C. Plate with guard to facilitate cutting and skidless mat to prevent plate from moving, used mainly for individuals with hemiparesis.

from a previous stroke. The act of reaching as well as manual dexterity may be impaired, so that functions such as buttoning clothes are a problem. The goal of rehabilitation in these situations is to enhance the ability to reach and to enhance manual dexterity. Environmental alteration and devices may be helpful. Velcro closures in lieu of buttons, slip-on dressing aids (especially for socks), and long-reach zipper pulls are examples of devices that may help some residents regain independence in these functions.

HEAT AND COLD MODALITIES

Heat and cold modalities can play an important role in alleviating pain while undergoing physical therapy. Ultrasound can be particularly useful for pain associated with movement of the hip or shoulders. Local heat is used to allow immediate movement and to decrease pain following movement, while cold is applied for some time (10 to 15 min) before movement to anesthetize the area to be moved.

ORTHOTICS

An orthotic is an externally applied device used to modify structural and functional characteristics of the musculoskeletal system. The goals of orthotics are to:

- Relieve pain
- Immobilize and protect weak, painful, or healing musculoskeletal structures
- Reduce axial load
- Prevent and correct deformity
- Improve function.

A nomenclature has been devised for orthotics consisting of a series of letters that are the first letters of the English anatomic name of the joints that are crossed by the device, ending with the letter "o." **Tables 24-8** and **24-9** describe various types of orthotics that may be useful in the NH.

PROSTHETICS

The most common cause of amputation in the geriatric population is peripheral vascular disease. Thus, the majority of prostheses are prescribed for the lower extremities. The site of anatomic amputation is an important consideration. Preserving the knee joint decreases the energy required for walking and preserves proprioception.

The decision to perform a lower extremity amputation in an older individual is a major issue that requires careful weighing of risks and benefits. It involves a thorough preoperative assessment and interventions to stabilize any active medical problems. Postoperative care should be discussed before the operation, and potential problems such as pain and phantom-limb sensation should be mentioned.

Fitting protheses in the elderly in general, and in NH residents in particular, calls for some special considerations. In below-knee amputations, a

Table 24-8 Lower limb orthotics

Orthotics	Indication	Purpose/comments
Ankle/foot orthosis (AFO)	Limited weight bearing Alignment	Limb weakness due to stroke
Knee/ankle/foot orthosis (KAFO)	Essentially an AFO with additional joint surrounding the knee Provides more stability	Severe weakness of lower extremity (e.g., hemiplegia); resident needs to be able to lock/unlock a simple hinge
Cervico-thoracic lumbosacral orthosis (CTLSO; Milwaukee Brace)	Worn 23 h a day to correct vertebral compression fracture, cervical disk disease	Pain relief Maintain adequate posture
Simple corset	Vertebral compression fracture	Pain relief Should be fitted Sold over the counter
Rigid brace	Multiple vertebral fractures	Stability Pain relief Reduce deconditioning by early mobilization Not well suited for older patients
Cervical collar (may include occipital and mandibular projections	Cervical disk disease	Limit range of motion Should be fitted to prevent ischemia

Table 24-9 Upper extremity orthotics

Orthosis	Indication	Purpose
Wrist/hand orthosis	Stroke, carpal tunnel syndrome	Immobilize Improve alignment Assist in restoring function
Splint	Stroke Lower motor lesions Rheumatoid arthritis	Maintain position of flaccid or paretic extremity
Cockup splint	Carpal tunnel syndrome	Reduce nerve entrapment at night
Heat-moldable plastic orthosis	Interphalangeal joint immobilizer	Reduce tendency to subluxation and prevent ulnar deviation
Static interphalangeal joint orthosis	Proximal interphalangeal joint movement	Prevent "swan neck" deformities

Table 24-10 Basic principles of postoperative rehabilitation for amputees

1. Prevent contractures by range-of-motion exercises
2. Use compression bandages to prevent hemorrhage and decrease edema (be cautious not to obliterate arterial flow)
3. Meticulous local care to suture site to keep stump clear of infection
4. Provide adequate nutrition
5. Control concomitant medical conditions (e.g., diabetes, heart failure)
6. Mobilize stump as soon as possible
7. Socket of prosthesis should evenly contact the entire skin surface and fit snugly
8. Observe stump carefully for breakdown when ambulation with prosthesis begins

prosthesis decreases energy requirements but still requires one-third more energy than before the amputation. Proprioception is more likely to be preserved with below-knee amputation, which helps to maintain balance. Above-knee amputations should be avoided, because thereafter ambulation requires two-thirds more energy than before the amputation. **Table 24-10** outlines some general principles of postoperative care of amputees. Adequate nutrition, controlling blood sugar in diabetics, and meticulous local care to the suture site are important for fitting a prothesis successfully. Intensive physical therapy should begin even before the prosthesis is fitted, because it may take weeks for the edema to subside to the point where the prosthesis can be fitted. Some NH residents with moderate to severe dementia may not be candidates for a prosthesis if the eventual goal of ambulation is unrealistic due to impaired cognitive function.

Table 24-11 The Barthel Index

	Points for performance[a]	
Activities rated by examiner	**Independently**	**With help**
Feeding (if food needs to be cut = help	10	5
Moving from wheelchair to bed (includes sitting up in bed)	15	10–5
Personal toilet (wash face, comb hair, shave, clean teeth)	5	0
Getting on and off toilet (handling clothes, wipe, flush)	10	5
Bathing self	5	0
Walking on level surface	15	10
Propel wheelchair (score only if unable to walk)	5	0
Ascend and descend stairs	10	5
Dressing (includes tying shoes, fastening fasteners)	10	5
Controlling bowels	10	5
Controlling bladder	10	5

[a]Total possible points = 100.

MEASURING REHABILITATION OUTCOMES

Measuring progress toward the goal or goals of a restorative rehabilitation program is critical to planning subsequent therapy as well as to reimbursement. While progress can be measured in a semistructured manner, some of the standardized instruments used to assess function are suitable for measuring

Table 24-12 Katz Index of independence in activities of daily living

The index of independence in activities of daily living is based on an evaluation of the functional independence or dependence of patients in bathing, dressing, going to the toilet, transferring, continence, and feeding. Specific definitions of functional independence and dependence appear below the index.

A. Independent in feeding, continence, transferring, dressing, and bathing.
B. Independent in all but one of these functions.
C. Independent in all but bathing and one additional function.
D. Independent in all but bathing, dressing, and one additional function.
E. Independent in all but bathing, dressing, toileting, and one additional function.
F. Independent in all but bathing, dressing, toileting, transferring, and one additional function.
G. Dependent in all six functions.
Other Dependent in at least two functions but not classifiable as C, D, E, or F. Independence means without supervision, direction, or active personal assistance except as specifically noted below. This is based on actual status and not on ability. Patients who refuse to perform a function are considered as not performing the function, even though they are deemed able.

Bathing (sponge, shower, or tub)
Independent: needs assistance only in bathing a single part (as back or disabled extremity) or bathes self completely
Dependent: needs assistance in bathing more than one part of the body and in getting in or out of tub or does not bathe self

Dressing
Independent: gets clothes from closets and drawers; puts on clothes, outer garments, braces; manages fasteners; act of tying shoes is excluded
Dependent: does not dress self or remains partly dressed

Toileting
Independent: gets to toilet; gets on and off toilet; arranges clothes, cleans organs of excretion (may manage own bedpan used at night only and may not be using mechanical supports)
Dependent: uses bedpan or commode or receives assistance in getting to and using toilet

Transfer
Independent: moves in and out of bed independently and moves in and out of chair independently (may or may not be using mechanical supports)
Dependent: assistance in moving in or out of bed and/or chair; does not perform one or more transfers

Continence
Independent: urination and defecation entirely self-controlled
Dependent: partial or total incontinence in urination or defecation, partial or total control by enemas, catheters, or regulated used of urinals and/or bedpans

Feeding
Independent: gets food from plate or its equivalent into mouth (precutting of meat and preparation of food, as buttering bread, are excluded from evaluation)
Dependent: assistance in act of feeding (see above); does not eat at all or receives parental feeding

baseline function and change with time during the rehabilitation process. Some of these instruments are discussed throughout this text and will be mentioned only briefly here in the context of rehabilitation.

The Barthel Index (**Table 24-11**) assesses self-care and ambulation in slightly broader ranges than Katz ADL scale (**Table 24-12**). It includes stair climbing and wheelchair use, is administered by an interviewer on the basis of judgment or observation, and is particularly useful in the rehabilitation setting. It is not as useful as scales such as the Katz for detecting and following progress of minor impairments. The Minimum Data Set (MDS), also contains items that may be useful for following the functional status of a resident undergoing rehabilitation (**Table 24-13**). Other comprehensive instruments are complex and time-consuming, and some have limited use in cognitively impaired individuals.

The Functional Independence Measure (FIM) is the most widely used outcome measurement method in acute rehabilitation centers, and is being used increasingly in hospital-based subacute units and skilled nursing facilities. Its main limitation is the need for extensive training of examiners in its use in order to obtain reliable assessments. **Table 24-14** describes the elements and scoring of the FIM. The FIM is comprised of 18 items covering motor functioning (13) and cognitive function (5), and uses a seven-point scale for each function. The ratings are used in team conferences to discuss progress, identify needs and to decide when a plateau in the patient's progress has been reached. The FIM is also being used increasingly by payors to measure performance.

Because dementia can influence the outcomes of rehabilitation and cognitive function can change during rehabilitation, some type of cognitive assessment should be performed. Cognitive function can be assessed by the Folstein Mini-Mental State Examination (MMSE), which has a fairly broad range of sensitivity and will detect moderate—but not mild or subtle—impairment (see Chapter 11). This test is fairly quick to administer and is helpful for detecting changes over time. Other tests are either insensitive to change over time or able to detect only gross cognitive dysfunction (e.g., Short Portable Mental Status Questionnaire) or are too long to administer repeatedly to NH residents (e.g., Wechsler Memory Scale). The MDS also contains a Cognitive Performance Scale, which correlates well with the MMSE (see Chapter 11). Its sensitivity to change in a rehabilitiation setting is, however, not known. For a geriatric rehabilitation center or skilled nursing facility, the MMSE is a reasonable choice. More in-depth mental function assessments should be reserved for selected residents with mild cognitive impairment who score well on the MMSE.

Assessment of mood or emotional state may be important because of the prevalence of depression after major medical illnesses (e.g., stroke) and the importance of motivation to the rehabilitation process. The geriatric depression scale (GDS) can be either self-administered or administered by an interviewer, is quick and reliable, and avoids somatic questions. It is good for establishing a baseline description and for monitoring progress in frail NH residents (see Chapter 12).

Table 24-13 Selected items from the Minimum Data Set relating to functional status and rehabilitation

Customary routines

1. Cycle of daily events
   - ______ Stays up late at night (e.g., after 9 p.m.)
   - ______ Goes out 1 or more days a week
   - ______ Stays busy with hobbies, reading, or fixed daily routine
   - ______ Spends most time alone or watching TV
   - ______ Moves independently indoors (with appliances, if used)
   - ______ None of above
2. Eating patterns
   - ______ Distinct food preferences
   - ______ Eats between meals all or most days
   - ______ Use of alcoholic beverage(s) at least weekly
   - ______ None of above
3. ADL patterns
   - ______ In bedclothes much of day
   - ______ Wakens to toilet all or most nights
   - ______ Has irregular movement pattern
   - ______ Prefers showers for bathing
   - ______ None of above
4. Involvement patterns
   - ______ Daily contact with relatives/close friends
   - ______ Usually attends church, temple, synagogue (etc.)
   - ______ Finds strength in faith
   - ______ Daily animal companion/presence
   - ______ Involved in group activities
   - ______ None of above
   - ______ Unknown—resident/family unable to provide information

Cognitive patterns

1. Comatose (no discernible consciousness/persistent vegetative state)
   0. No   1. Yes
2. Memory (recall of what was learned or known)
   a. Short-term (seems/appears to recall after 5 min.)
      0. Memory OK   1. Memory problem
   b. Long-term (seems/appears to recall long past)
      0. Memory OK   1. Memory problem
3. Memory/recall ability (check all that resident normally able to recall during last 7 days)
   - ______ Current season
   - ______ That he/she is in a nursing home
   - ______ Location of own room/facility
   - ______ Staff names/faces
   - ______ None of above are recalled
4. Cognitive skills for daily decision making (decisions regarding tasks of daily life)
   0. Independent—decisions consistent/reasonable
   1. Modified independence—some difficulty in new situations only
   2. moderately impaired—decisions poor; cues/supervision required
   3. Severely impaired—never/rarely makes decisions

Table 24-13 (*Continued*)

Cognitive patterns (*Continued*)

5. Indicators of delirium (periodic disordered thinking/awareness)
   ______ Less alert, easily distracted
   ______ Changing awareness of environment
   ______ Episodes of incoherent speech
   ______ Judgment less reliable
   ______ None of above
6. Change in cognitive status
   0. No change 1. Improved 2. Deteriorated

Communication/hearing patterns

1. Hearing (with hearing appliance, if used)
   0. Hears adequately—normal talk, TV, phone
   1. Minimal difficulty when not in quiet listening conditions
   2. Hears in special situation only—speaker has to adjust tonal quality and speak distinctly
   3. Highly impaired/absence or useful hearing
2. Communication devices/techniques
   ______ Hearing aid, present and used
   ______ Hearing aid, present and not used
   ______ Other receptive communication technique used (e.g., lip reading)
   ______ None of above
3. Modes of expression
   ______ Speech
   ______ Writing message to express or clarify needs
   ______ Signs/gestures/sounds
   ______ Communication board
   ______ Other
   ______ None of above
4. Making self understood (express information content—however able)
   0. Understood
   1. Usually understood
   2. Sometimes understood
   3. Rare/never understood
5. Ability to understand others (understanding verbal information content, however able)
   0. Understand
   1. Usually understood
   2. Sometimes understood
   3. Rare/never understood
6. Change in communication
   0. No change 1. Improved 2. Deteriorated

Vision patterns

1. Vision (ability to see in adequate light and with glasses if used)
   0. Adequate—sees fine detail, including regular print in newspapers/books
   1. Impaired—sees large print but not regular print in newspapers/books
   2. Highly impaired—limited vision, not able to see newspaper headlines, appears to follow objects with eyes
   3. Severely impaired—no vision—e.g., may/appear to see light, color, or shapes
2. Visual limitations/difficulties
   ______ Side vision problems—decreased peripheral vision; e.g., leaves food on one side of tray, difficulty traveling, bumps into people and objects, misjudges placement of chair when seating self
   ______ Experience any of following: see halos or rings around lights, sees flashes of light, sees "curtains" over eyes
   ______ None of above
3. Visual appliances (glasses, contact lenses, lens implant)
   0. No 1. Yes

Table 24-13 (*Continued*)

ADL

1. Basic ADL (code for most support provided)
    0. No setup or physical help from staff
    1. Setup help only
    2. One-person physical assist
    3. Physical assist from two or more persons
    a. Bed mobility: How resident moves to and from lying position, turns from side to side, and positions body while in bed
    b. Transfer: How resident moves between surfaces—to/from bed, chair, wheelchair, standing position (*exclude* to/from bath/toilet)
    c. Locomotion: How resident moves between locations in his/her room and adjacent corridor on same floor. If in wheelchair, self-sufficiency once in chair
    d. Dressing: How resident puts on, fastens, and takes off all items of street clothing, including donning/removing prosthesis
    e. Eating: How resident eats and drinks (regardless of skill)
    f. Toilet use: How resident uses the toilet room (or commode, bedpan, urinal); transfers on/off toilet, cleanses, changes pad, manages ostomy or catheter, adjusts clothes
    g. Personal hygiene: How resident maintains personal hygiene, including combing hair, brushing teeth, shaving, applying makeup, washing/drying face, hands, and perineum (exclude baths and showers)
2. Bathing (how resident takes full-body bath, sponge bath, and transfers in/out of tub/shower)
    0. Independent—no help provided
    1. Supervision—oversight help only
    2. Physical help limited to transfers only
    3. Physical help in part of bathing activity
    4. Total dependence
3. Body-control problems
    ______ Balance—partial or total loss of ability to balance self while standing
    ______ Bedfast all or most of the time
    ______ Contracture to arms, legs, shoulders, or hands
    ______ Hemiplegia/hemiparesis
    ______ Quadriplegia
    ______ Arm—partial or total loss of voluntary movement
    ______ Hand—lack of dexterity (e.g., problem using toothbrush or adjusting hearing aid)
    ______ Leg—partial or total loss of voluntary movement
    ______ Leg—unsteady gait
    ______ Trunk—partial or total loss of ability to position, balance, or turn body
    ______ None of above
4. Mobility appliances/devices
    ______ Cane/walker
    ______ Brace/prosthesis
    ______ Wheels self
    ______ Other person wheeled
    ______ Lifted (manually/mechanically)
    ______ None of above
5. ADL functional potential (check all that apply during last 7 days)
    ______ Resident believes he/she capable of increased independence in at least some ADLs
    ______ Direct-care staff believe resident capable of increased independence in at least some ADLs
    ______ Resident able to perform tasks/activity but is very slow
    ______ Major difference in ADL self-performance or ADL support in mornings and evenings (at least a one-category change in self-performance or support in any ADL)
    ______ None of above
6. Change in ADL function
    0. No change   1. Improved   2. Deteriorated

Table 24-13 (*Continued*)

Continence in last 14 days (code as follows):

0. Continent—complete control
1. Usually continent—bladder, incontinent episodes once a week or less; bowel, less than weekly
2. Occasionally incontinent—bladder, two or more times a week but not daily; bowel, once a week
3. Frequently incontinent—bladder, tended to be continent daily, but some control present (e.g., on day shift); bowel, two to three times a week
4. Incontinent—Had inadequate control. For bladder, multiple daily episodes; for bowel, all (or almost) of the time

1. Bowel incontinence (control of bowel movement, with appliance or bowel continence program if employed)
2. Bladder continence (control of urinary function (if dribbles, volume insufficient to soak through underpants), with appliances (e.g., Foley) or continence programs if employed)
3. If incontinence of bladder (skip if resident's bladder continence code equals 0 or 1 and no catheter is employed)
   ______ Resident has been tested for a urinary tract infection
   ______ Resident has been checked for presence of a fecal impaction, or there is adequate bowel elimination
   ______ None of above
4. Appliances and programs
   ______ Any scheduled toileting plan
   ______ External (condom) catheter
   ______ Indwelling catheter
   ______ Intermittent catheter
   ______ Did not use toilet room/commode/urinal
   ______ Pads/briefs used
   ______ Enemas/irrigation
   ______ Ostomy
   ______ None of above
5. Change in urinary continence
   0. No change 1. Improved 2. Deteriorated

Oral/nutritional status

1. Oral status
   ______ Chewing problem
   ______ Swallowing problem
   ______ Mouth pain
   ______ None of above
2. Height and weight ____________
3. Nutritional problems
   ______ Complains about the taste of many foods
   ______ Insufficient fluid; dehydrated
   ______ Has not consumed all liquids provided at/between meals during last 3 days
   ______ Regular complaint of hunger
   ______ Leaves 25% or more of food uneaten at most meals
   ______ None of above
4. Nutritional approaches
   ______ Parenteral/IV
   ______ Feeding tubes
   ______ Mechanically altered diet
   ______ Therapeutic diet
   ______ Supplement between meals
   ______ None of above

Table 24-13 (*Continued*)

Activity pursuit patterns	
1. Average time involved in activities	
0. Most	2. Little
1. Some	4. None of above
2. Preferred activity settings	
______ Own room	______ Outside facility
______ Day/activity room	______ Inside NH/off unit
______ None of above	
3. General activities preference	
______ Cards/other games	______ Crafts/arts
______ Spiritual/religious	______ Trips/shopping
______ Exercise	______ Music
______ Read/write	______ Walking/wheeling outdoors
______ Watch TV	______ None of above

REIMBURSEMENT FOR REHABILITATION

Rehabilitation services are reimbursed predominantly by Medicare and to a lesser degree by other programs. Familiarity with the basic principles that govern these programs is essential for the primary physician and the medical director. Knowledge of Medicare guidelines will facilitate appropriate and realistic care planning.

Rehabilitative services after an acute hospitalization for conditions such as stroke, hip fracture, major abdominal surgery, or infection requiring ongoing parenteral antibiotics (e.g., osteomyelitis) are usually covered by Part A of the Medicare program. **Table 24-15** describes the criteria currently used by Medicare to determine eligibility for reimbursement for skilled nursing care. **Table 24-16** describes requirements for rehabilitation services under Medicare. Rehabilitation for residents who do not qualify for Part A coverage can be provided under Medicare Part B. Most diagnoses can, however, be treated for only a limited time (e.g., 12 to 30 sessions) under Part B.

Appropriate documentation by all team members is critical for a successful rehabilitation program as well as for reimbursement. Physicians must write appropriate orders for rehabilitation (see **Table 24-4**). Ongoing communication by all team members about the progress of therapy and function of the resident are essential. This communication can be carried on by way of legible notes as well as by regular team conferences. Medicare as well as other third-party payers require frequent reevaluations, at least monthly. These reevaluations are generally accomplished by the NH's utilization review committee. This committee usually includes the director of nursing, the medical director and two other physicians, the administrator, and a medical records staff person. In

Table 24-14 The Functional Independence Measure (FIM)

Items

Self care
- grooming
- bathing
- dressing upper body
- dressing lower body
- toileting

Sphincter control
- bladder
- bowel

Mobility
- transfer to/from
- bed/chair
- toilet
- tub
- shower

Locomotion
- walk
- wheelchair
- stairs

Communication
- comprehension
- expression

Social cognition
- social integration
- problem solving
- memory

Scoring

Independence	7	Completely independent
	6	Modified independence (with device)
Modified	5	Supervised
Dependence	4	Minimal assistance (subject performs >75 percent of tasks)
	3	Moderate assistance (subject performs 50–74 percent of tasks)
Complete	2	Maximal assistance (subject performs 25–49 percent of dependence tasks)
	1	Total dependence (Subject performs <25 percent of tasks)

hospital-based skilled nursing facilities—usually referred to as transitional care units (TCU) or facilities with a "distinct part"—the review meeting takes place weekly. These meetings determine the resident's progress and therefore eligibility for ongoing program benefits. The success of any rehabilitation program in a NH depends on the Utilization Review Committee's familiarity

Table 24-15 Criteria for Medicare reimbursement for skilled nursing care[a]

- Patients admitted for rehabilitation should be alert enough to participate and benefit from a program or require skilled nursing procedures/observation at least on a daily basis.
- Intravenous feedings, fluids, or medication
- Enteral tube feedings
- Fractures of femur, pelvis, pubic ramus, vertebrae, or multiple fractures
- Injectables (e.g., intramuscular antibiotics)
- Wound care
- Ostomy care and teaching
- Skilled ostomy care
- Acute diabetic observation (e.g., unstable blood sugars, sliding-scale insulin coverage)
- Dialysis in unstable patient
- Radiation therapy
- Pain management with parenteral medications
- Blood transfusions
- Respiratory services
- Frequent laboratory studies
- Frequent diagnostic testing
- Physical, occupational, and/or speech therapy (less than 3 h/day)
- Chest tubes (no wall suction)
- Postoperative supervision
- Traction
- Skilled nursing observation for an unresolved medical condition
- Procedures than cannot be done on an outpatient basis or at a lower level of care
- Bowel and bladder training

[a]Based on criteria for admission to a hospital-based skilled nursing unit.

Table 24-16 Basic criteria for Medicare coverage of rehabilitation services[a]

- Services that require registered therapists
- Services must be required daily
- The resident must require an in-patient treatment program
- The treatment modalities, frequency, and duration must be specifically ordered by the physician
- The resident must have a reasonable potential and make significant improvement in a reasonable, generally predictable time period

[a]Physical therapist, occupational therapist, speech therapist.

with Medicare guidelines. Lack of this knowledge may deprive many NH residents of their legitimate right to a trial of rehabilitation.

In the next decade, the NH may become the center for rehabilitation of most geriatric patients, replacing other in-patient rehabilitation programs. The NH is conducive for geriatric rehabilitation by providing the option of graded interventions, as opposed to the rigid 3-hour-per-day therapy required in acute rehabilitation units. The cost-effectiveness of rehabilitation in the NH should be measured in terms of the reduction in the burden of care achieved by improved self-care and improved quality of life for residents and families. The cost-effectiveness of standard physicial therapy for long-stay NH residents has been questioned. Some authors suggest utilizing a ratio, dividing the cost of physical therapy by an observed improvement in physical functioning as a way of assessing the financial viability of the intervention.

SUGGESTED READINGS

Cook L, Smith DS, Truman G: Using functional independence measures profiles as an index of outcome in the rehabilitation of brain-injured patients. *Arch Phys Med Rehabil* 75:390–393, 1994.

Department of Health and Human Services, Health Care Financing Administration: *Outpatient Physical Therapy and Comprehensive Outpatient Rehabilitation Facility Manual*. Revised Material, Chapter 5, Sec. 501, Transmittal No. 79, Washington, DC, August 1988.

Erickson RV: Principles of rehabilitation, in *Geriatrics Review Syllabus*. New York, American Geriatrics Society, 1988.

Fiatarone, MA, O'Neill, EF, Ryan, ND, et al: Exercise training and nutritional supplementation for physical frailty in very elderly people. *New Engl J Med* 330:169–1775, 1994.

Granger, CV, Hamilton BB, Linacre, JM, Heinemann, AW, Wright BD: Performance profiles of functional independence measure. *Am J Phys Med & Rehab* 72:84–88, 1993.

Hoenig, H, Mayer-Oaks, SA, Siebens, H: Geriatric rehabilitation: What do physicians know about it and how should they use it? *J Am Geriatr Soc* 42:341–347, 1994.

Kalra, L, Crome, P: The role of prognostic scores in targeting stroke rehabilitation in elderly patients. *J Am Geriatr Soc* 41:396–400, 1993.

Mosqueda, LA: Assessment of rehabilitation potential. *Clinics in Geriatric Med* 9:689–703, 1993.

Mulrow, CD, Gerety, MB, Kanten, D, et al: A randomized trial of physical rehabilitation for very frail nursing home residents. *JAMA* 271:519–524, 1994.

Osterweil D: Geriatric rehabilitation in the long term care institutional setting, in Kemp B, Brummel-Smith K, Ramsdell JW (eds): *Geriatric Rehabilitation*. Boston, Massachusetts, Little, Brown & Co, 1990.

Rentz, DM: The assessment of rehabilitation potential: cognitive factors in Hartke RJ (ed). *Psychological Aspects of Geriatric Rehabilitation*, Gaithersburg, Maryland, Aspen 1991.

Wolf SL, Barnhart HX, Kutner NG, McNeely E, Coogler C, Xu T, Atlanta FICSIT Group: Reducing frailty and falls in older persons: An investigation of Tai Chi and computerized balance training. *J Am Geriatr Soc* 44:489–497, 1996.

Yew E, Kropsky B, Neufeld R, Libow L: The clinical utility of a comprehensive periodic assessment form for the geriatric rehabilitation patient. *Gerontologist* 29:263–267, 1989.

CHAPTER
TWENTY-FIVE

HOSPICE CARE AND PAIN MANAGEMENT

Francis Bacon said "it is as natural to die as to be born" the appropriate care of the dying is one of the most difficult tasks for the staff in a nursing home (NH). Societal concerns, regulations, and the problems of the staff in dealing with their own mortality can all interfere with allowing the NH resident a "good death." There is evidence that transfer of dying persons to a NH may lead to a shortfall in meeting the needs of the dying person and their relatives. The purpose of this chapter is to delineate management techniques that can improve the quality of the dying process. Many persons with dementia may benefit from hospice care during the last stages of the disease. In addition, this chapter discusses the vexing problem of pain management in NH residents.

HOSPICE CARE

Treatment decisions concerning a dying NH resident require the consensus of the staff as well as that of the resident and his or her family. This often necessitates people of different spiritual and philosophical backgrounds to find a common meeting place. Thus, the first rule of caring for the terminally ill should be that anyone who finds the consensus management plan unacceptable should be allowed to withdraw from the care of that resident. Unfortunately, in most NHs many staff do not accept such an approach in reality. In these situations the staff member should be required to carry out comfort and palliative care but not to actively administer therapies that seem objectionable. Careful education of the interdisciplinary team in the philosophies and principles of hospice care can obviate the development of some of these unpleasant situations. The hospice social worker can be particularly important in the education of the NH staff and also in negotiating and advocating for appropriate therapy for the resident.

Hospice care is a concept of helping the dying person and his or her family cope with the dying process in the least painful way possible. The central concept of hospice care is to relieve physical and psychological suffering and to alleviate unwanted symptoms. The objectives of hospice care are outlined in **Table 25-1**.

Identification of NH residents who should receive hospice care can be extremely difficult. The resident with end-stage untreatable cancer is easily identifiable as a candidate for hospice care. In other cases, however, the need for hospice care is often less apparent. Residents with end-stage dementia, severe weight loss, and recurrent infections are possible candidates for hospice care, as

Table 25-1 Objectives of hospice care

Objective	Providers
For the resident	
Provide high-quality care	Physician, nurse[a]
Provide adequate pain relief	Physician, nurse
Provide maximum comfort[b]	Nurse, family, physical therapist
Provide psychological support[b]	Physician, nurse, family, psychologist, pastoral case worker, social worker, clergy
Provide appropriate individualized understanding of the dying process	Physician, nurse, social worker
Provide appropriate spiritual support[b]	Clergy, pastoral case worker
Provide assistance with social and financial problems	Social worker
Respect wishes regarding terminal care	Physician, nurse
For the family	
Provide psychological support[b]	Physician, nurse, family, social worker, psychologist, pastoral case worker, clergy
Provide understanding of dying process	Physician, nurse, social worker
Help with interpersonal problems (i.e., resident-family; family-family)	Physician, nurse, social worker
Provide assistance with social and financial problems[b]	Social worker
Provide appropriate spiritual support[b]	Clergy, pastoral care worker
Provide support in the period immediately following death[b]	Physician, nurse, family, psychologist, pastoral care worker, social worker, clergy

[a] Includes nurse assistants.

[b] Volunteers may also play a role in these areas.

are those with amyotrophic lateral sclerosis, Huntington's disease, or end-stage heart, lung, kidney, or liver failure. A specific group of patients with a subset of unique problems comprises those suffering from acquired immune deficiency syndrome (AIDS). When an individual with AIDS is admitted to a NH, he or she is generally much younger than the other residents and thus may have greater problems accepting the situation.

Table 25-2 lists the major physical symptoms that may require management in order to maintain comfort among the dying. Treatment of weakness requires appropriate attention to passive and active physical therapy and nutritional status. Among those with a relatively long-term prognosis, testosterone enanthate, 200 mg intramuscularly every 2 weeks, may be useful. Short-term use of prednisone (15 mg daily) may produce euphoric effects.

Treatment of anorexia is difficult. The use of supplements, milk shakes, and favored foods may be helpful. Small meals and snacks should be offered on multiple occasions throughout the day. Antidepressants (except fluoxetine), in particular monoamine oxidase inhibitors, may enhance food intake. Medroxyprogesterone acetate may also increase food intake. Dry mouth can be alleviated

Table 25-2 Physical symptoms requiring management in order to maintain comfort among the dying

Pain

Constitutional symptoms
- Weakness
- Anorexia
- Thirst/dehydration/dry mouth
- Hypercalcemia
- Bleeding
- Fever

Gastrointestinal symptoms
- Xerostomia
- Nausea and vomiting
- Dysgeusia
- Dysphagia
- Diarrhea/constipation
- Ascites
- Abdominal pain
- Fecal incontinence

Cardiopulmonary symptoms
- Halitosis
- Cough
- Shortness of breath
- Moist, noisy respirations
- Hiccups
- Thrombosis
- Edema

Central nervous system symptoms
- Depression
- Anxiety/panic
- Insomnia
- Delirium
- Dementia
- Paralysis
- Seizures

Urinary tract symptoms
- Incontinence
- Urinary retention
- Bladder spasms
- Urinary tract infection

Skin and cosmetic problems
- Pressure sores
- Pruritis
- Alopecia
- Draining fistulas
- Fungating growths
- Colostomy

by sucking dry ice or candies. Glycerine and citric acid mouthwashes as well as artificial saliva (e.g., Salivart) may also help. Fever should be treated with aspirin or acetaminophen. If these agents are ineffective, indomethacin may be useful. A recent study has suggested that palliative management of fever among male NH residents with end-stage Alzheimer's disease yields the same mortality as when such individuals also receive antibiotics.

If hypercalcemia occurs late in the course of a disease, it may allow a relatively painless death. However, when hypercalcemia occurs early, it may be debilitating. Fluids, corticosteroids, and phosphates will generally control hypercalcemia. Mithramycin in low dosages (1–2 mg intravenously twice per week) may produce the best effects in those with terminal cancer.

For the treatment of nausea and vomiting, prochlorperazine syrup (5 mg every 4 h or 25 mg suppositories three times per day) or the serotonin antagonist, ondansetron, (8 mg orally or intravenously every 8 h) are the treatments of choice. Dopamine antagonists such as metoclopramide or cisapride can also be helpful. Dronabinol, the cannabinoid extract, often causes delirium in older persons, but can be useful for young cancer and AIDS patients. This drug may improve nausea but can have central nervous system side effects. Pain on swallowing due to radiation-induced esophagitis is best treated with oral viscous lidocaine. While nystatin (suspension or troches) remains the treatment of choice for oral candidiasis, clotrimazole troches or ketoconazole may be necessary to obtain symptomatic relief.

Cough can be treated with guaifenesin, hydrocodeine syrup, or benzonatate (tessalon). Use of a vaporizer in order to provide humidification of the air may be useful. Hiccups can be treated by inducing a Valsalva maneuver (this can be done by getting the resident to drink water from the opposite side of a glass). If this fails, chlorpromazine (25 mg three times per day) is the appropriate treatment. Residents with moist, noisy respirations ("death rattle") may respond to transdermal scopolamine or atropine to dry secretions. Severe air hunger during the last few hours of life is best treated with morphine. Sedation is an acceptable method of decreasing awareness of terminal suffocation.

Depression is best treated with low doses of desipramine (25–50 mg a day) or trazadone (50–100 mg at night) if the resident is agitated. Methylphenidate (Ritalin) can be utilized when short-term arousal from a depressive episode may be beneficial, as when a relative the person has not seen for a while comes to visit.

Hydroxyzine or short-acting benzodiazepines are used for anxiety. Haloperidol (0.5–1 mg once or twice per day) is useful for the treatment of hallucinations, delusions, or agitated behaviors that are interfering with care or comfort. An indwelling bladder catheter may be appropriate for the management of incontinence among the terminally ill. Painful bladder spasms due to irritation from the catheter may respond to oxybutynin (2.5 mg three times per day). Pruritus may respond to diphenhydramine, hydroxyzine, or topical triamcinolone cream. A wig should be used for the treatment of hair loss if the resident is upset about his or her appearance. Hydrogen peroxide may decrease the smell associated with fungating lesions, and topical application of epinephrine (1:1000 dilution) may decrease capillary bleeding associated with such lesions. Radiation therapy may produce symptomatic relief either by relieving pain or obstruction or shrinking cosmetically the unacceptable tumor.

Terminal dehydration appears to produce little additional suffering aside from a dry mouth which can be treated with ice chips and sips of water. Dehydration decreases secretions and urine output and thus decreases resident suffering. Approximately 16 to 50 percent of terminally ill residents may need sedation for intolerable symptoms. Barbiturates, benzodiazepines and morphine have all been used for this purpose. Paul Rousseau has pointed out that the ethical validity of this approach is derived from the ethical principle of double effect, an axiom which recognizes that the primary therapeutic intent of a therapy may unintentionally accelerate death.

Table 25-3 lists the most useful orders for NH residents receiving terminal care. For all concerned, adequate hospice care demands that the resident's appearance be maintained throughout the dying process. At all times staff should put comfort measures ahead of medical treatment. Care should be taken not to talk about the resident in a derogatory manner. Finally, the role of the care team does not end with the resident's death. Allowing the family to view the body for a sufficient period of time helps with the "letting go" process. Attendance at the funeral by members of the health care team can also be helpful for both family and caregivers if the dying process is prolonged. The health care team needs to help the family through the bereavement process. This is particularly important when the spouse has no close relatives.

Table 25-3 Example of orders for terminal care

Do not transfer to hospital
Do not resuscitate
No routine blood work or radiographs
Foley catheter for relief of urinary retention or incontinence
Turn every 2 h
Do not record intake/output or weights
Activity as tolerated
Ice cubes p.r.n.
Analgesics: ______
Analgesics must be given on schedule and p.r.n.s as requested.
(Do *not* make judgments that the resident does not need analgesic or is overreacting)
Antidepressant ______
Anxiolytic ______
Oxygen ______ liters/minute
Antiemetic ______
Allow family visits at all times
Do not restrain unless necessary for comfort

PAIN MANAGEMENT

Little is known about pain among elderly NH residents, although anecdotally it would seem fair to assume that pain is undertreated in NHs. The reasons for this include fear of addiction, fear of side effects of narcotics, problems associated with multiple medications and drug–drug interactions, and a failure to take complaints of pain seriously. Pain has been reported to occur in 71 percent to 83 percent of NH residents, while the National Nursing Home Survey of 1977 found that only 37 percent were given analgesic medications. In one study of long-term care residents with an average age of 88.4 years, pain was considered constant in approximately one-third. Fifty-two percent described their pain as severe, horrible, or excruciating. The most common causes of pain in older individuals in the NH are listed in **Table 25-4**. Pain has been shown to: impair involvement in recreational activities and to limit walking; impair posture; cause insomnia; produce anxiety, depression, and constipation; cause anorexia; and interfere with the ability to carry out basic activities of daily living.

Assessment of pain starts with the physician believing the complaint of pain. Older individuals are less likely to complain than younger individuals, yet their complaints are less likely to be taken seriously. Any NH resident with a complaint of pain is entitled to a careful history and examination and appropriate diagnostic tests. In addition, residents with pain should be carefully assessed for depression as well as for their level of anxiety. Although most pain complaints in older individuals are due to organic pathology rather than to psychological causes, identification and treatment of these psychological conditions may be important in the overall management of the pain.

In the geriatric population, several specific pain syndromes need to be considered (**Table 25-5**). Temporal headaches, with or without pain over the temporal arteries, should prompt consideration of the diagnosis of temporal (cranial) arteritis. Temporal artery biopsy is indicated, as this condition can lead

Table 25-4 Common types and causes of pain in the nursing home

Low back pain	Arthritis
Osteoporosis	knee
Vertebral fractures	hip
Disk disease	shoulder
Lumbar stenosis	Pain from fractures
Myeloma	Neuropathies
Metastatic bone tumors	Leg cramps
Epidural abscess	Claudication
Referred visceral pain	Foot pain
	Neck pain

Table 25-5 Specific pain syndromes common among nursing home residents

Syndrome	Management options
Temporal arteritis	Prednisone 60 mg daily
Herpes zoster	Analgesics Carbamazepine Desipramine Topical capsaicin TENS
Postamputation phantom limb pain	Local anesthetic blocks Narcotics TENS
Degnerative back pain	Analgesics Limited period of bed rest Topical ice or heat Local anesthetic injection Chymopapain injection TENS Surgery
Leg cramps	Potassium and magnesium supplementation (if indicated) Quinine Baclofen Short-acting benzodiazepines
Claudication	Exercise (graded) Lower blood sugar Pentoxifylline Consider evaluation for surgery
Osteoporosis	Flexion exercises Short-term back bracing (1 week maximum) Nonsteroidal anti-inflammatory agents Analgesics Calcitonin

to blindness. Treatment is with high-dose steroids (e.g., 60 mg of prednisone per day). Herpes zoster can be associated with severe pain. Shooting pains may respond to carbamazepine, while deep burning or aching pains respond better to desipramine. Topical capsaicin, a substance-P depleting agent, or transcutaneous electrical nerve stimulation (TENS) may be useful in some cases of post-herpetic neuralgia. Postamputation phantom limb pain is often very difficult to treat. TENS and local anesthetic blocks can be tried, but often narcotics are necessary. Degenerative changes in the spine (osteophyte formation, bulging intervertebral disks, and ligamentum flavum hypertrophy) can cause back pain and pain radiating down the buttocks. Diagnosis is made by computed tomography or magnetic resonance scanning. Treatment involves short periods of bed rest (no more than 4 days at a time), topical ice or heat, and injection of local anesthetics into "trigger points." Chymopapain injections into the disk space may be used. Surgery should be reserved for those with intractable pain or objective weakness due to nerve compression.

Management of leg cramps involves checking that the resident has adequate potassium and magnesium levels. Quinine's effectiveness has been questioned, and it may cause side effects, such as deafness and dizziness. Some residents with severe cramps respond well to muscle relaxants, such as short-acting benzodiazepines or baclofen. Claudication can be treated by normalizing glucose levels in diabetics and by the use of pertoxifylline. If there is no response, revascularization surgery may be useful in appropriately selected candidates. Osteoporosis associated with vertebral fractures can cause severe pain. Treatment consists of flexion exercises, short-term bracing of the back, and use of nonsteroidal anti-inflammatory agents. Fear of addiction should not lead to the withholding of narcotics for the short-term relief of pain associated with an acute vertebral fracture. Calcitonin may be effective in some instances for relief of pain related to osteoporosis. A nasal spray is now available. However, calcitonin therapy may cause hypocalcemia and/or anorexia among NH residents.

A useful strategy for the general management of pain is to have residents who are able to do so record the degree of pain using the present pain intensity scale of the McGill Pain Questionnaire (**Table 25-6**). The scale can be repeated just before each dose of pain medication. Where possible, pain should be treated by physical therapy methods such as splinting, exercise (active or passive), application of heat or cold, TENS, or ultrasound. Relaxation therapy and distracting techniques may also be helpful. When pain causes insomnia, the temporary use of short-acting benzodiazepines is appropriate.

Mild to moderate pain that is not inflammatory in nature is best treated first by acetaminophen. We have found that the use of Tylenol Extended Relief (ER), one or two tablets given regularly every 6 to 8 h have dramatically improved pain relief in many of our residents. If pain is associated with inflammation, it is best

Table 25-6 Present pain intensity scale of the McGill Pain Questionnaire[a]

1	=	Mild
2	=	Discomfort
3	=	Severe
4	=	Horrible
5	=	Excruciating

[a]This scale may be helpful in evaluating the need for or response to analgesics.

treated by enteric-coated aspirin. Nonsteroidal anti-inflammatory agents (ibuprofen, naproxen, etc.) are excellent for arthritic pain. Residents on nonsteroidal anti-inflammatory agents should be checked regularly (e.g., every 1 to 2 months) to exclude gastrointestinal tract bleeding by examining the stool for occult blood and/or by measuring the blood hemoglobin value. Among those who have had a bleed on these agents, the addition of misoprostol should be considered, but diarrhea often develops at doses that provide adequate cytoprotection.

Codeine is an excellent second-tier analgesic. It is best used in combination with aspirin or acetaminophen. The major side effect of codeine is constipation, which responds well to lactulose therapy. Propoxyphene hydrochloride is no more effective than acetominophen and has a high addiction potential. It provides only weak pain relief and should rarely if ever be used in NH residents. Tramadol is a centrally active analgesic with both opioid activity and inhibition of re-uptake of serotonin and norepinephrine. Side effects occur in 5 percent of resident and include nausea, dizziness, constipation and delirium. Tramadol dosing is 50–100 mg every 4 to 6 h with the total daily dose not exceeding 300 mg in residents over 75 years and 400 mg in younger residents. In renal failure the dose should be reduced to 100 mg every 12 h and those with liver dysfunction to 50 mg every 12 h.

For severe pain, morphine is the drug of choice. Morphine can be given orally at six times the intramuscular dose. Methadone, which can be given once a day because of its long half-life, is a useful drug for relief of chronic pain. The addition of a nonsteroidal anti-inflammatory drug to morphine or methadone therapy may increase the potency of these drugs. Medication for severe pain should be given regularly rather than on an as-needed basis. In residents undergoing hospice care,

Table 25-7 Examples of analgesic drugs for mild to moderate pain

	Equianalgesic dose (mg)	Duration of action (h)
Aspirin	650	4–6
Acetaminophen	650	4–6
Propoxyphene	65[a]	4–6[b]
Meperidine	50	4–6
Pentazocene	30	4–6
Codeine[c]	32	3
Tramadol[d]	25	4–6

[a]Potentially transformed to toxic metabolite norpropoxyphene and has high addiction potential—should be avoided in older persons.

[b]Plasma half-life is 12 h compared to 4 or less for all other drugs. This increases chances of toxic accumulation in older persons.

[c]Codeine is biotransformed to morphine and 130 mg intramuscularly is equivalent to 10 mg of morphine.

[d]Accumulates in renal failure and liver disease.

Table 25-8 Narcotic analgesics available for treatment of severe pain

Drug	Route of administration	Equianalgesic dose (mg)	Duration of action (h)	Sedation	Addiction	Respiratory depression
Morphine	i.m.	10	4–6	++	++	++
	p.o.	60	4–7			
	Rectally	5	2–4			
Controlled-release Morphine	p.o.	30	8–12	++	++	++
Meperidine[a]	i.m.	75	3–4	+	++	++
	p.o.	300	3–4			
Methoadone[b]	i.m.	10	4–6	+	+	++
	p.o.	20	4–24 ++			
Oxycodone[c]	i.m.	15	3–5	++	++	++
	p.o.	30				
Hydro-morphone (Dilaudid)[d]	i.m.	1.5	2–3	+	++	++
	p.o.	7.5	2–3			
Butorphanol[e] (Stadol)	i.m.	2	4–6	+	0	0
Fentanyl	Transdermal	5	72	+	+	+

[a]Not for use in renal disease; metabolite normeperidine produces agitation.
[b]Duration increases with repeated administration due to long half-life of 15 to 30 h.
[c]May be used in combination with aspirin or Tylenol.
[d]Also available in rectal suppository.
[e]May precipitate withdrawal in physically dependent patients; no oral form available.

the use of diluted intravenous morphine every 2 h until pain relief is obtained is a reasonable approach and can result in reduced narcotic dosages. In the NH this can be accomplished by placing a heplock rather than administering a continuous intravenous infusion. Sometimes switching from one narcotic to another improves pain relief, as one-to-one cross-tolerance does not occur with narcotics. **Tables 25-7** and **25–8** summarize drugs that are available to treat pain.

Finally, it should not be forgotten that radiation therapy can produce dramatic pain relief in some individuals with pain syndrome related to cancer. Corticosteroids may also produce pain relief when the tumor is compressing a nerve in a confined space.

SUGGESTED READINGS

Hospice

Amar DF: The role of the hospice social worker in the nursing home setting. *Am J Hospice & Palliative Care* 11:18–23,1994.

Cobbs E, Lynn J: The care of the dying patient, in Hazzard WR, Andres R, Burman EL, Blass JP (eds), *Principles of Geriatric Medicine and Gerontology*. New York, McGraw-Hill, 1990, pp 354–361.

Fabiszewski KJ, Volicer B, Volicer L: Effect of antibiotic treatment on outcome of fevers in institutionalized Alzheimer patients. *JAMA* 263:3168–3172, 1990.

Levy MM, Catalano RB: Control of common physical symptoms other than pain in patients with terminal disease. *Semin Oncol* 12:411, 1985.

Maccabee J: The effect of transfer from a palliative care unit to nursing homes—are patients' and relatives' needs met? *Palliative Med* 8:211–214, 1994.

Meares CJ: Terminal dehydration: A review. *Am J Hospice & Palliative Care* 11:10–14, 1994.

Pfeiffer E: Institutional placement for patients with Alzheimer's disease: How to help families with a difficult decision. *Postgrad Med* 97:125–132, 1995.

Rousseau P: Hospice and palliative care. *Disease-a-Month* 41:769–842, 1995.

Zimmerman JM: Hospice: *Complete Care for the Terminally Ill*. Baltimore, Urban & Schwarzenberg, 1986.

Pain Management

Dalgin PH: Use of tramadol in chronic pain. *Clin Geriatr* 3(6):17–30, 1995.

Ferrell BA, Ferrell BR, Osterweil D: Pain in the nursing home. *J Am Geriatr Soc* 38:409–414, 1990.

Ferrell BA, Ferrell BR, and Rivera L: Pain in cognitively impaired nursing home patients. *J Pain Symptom Manag* 10:591–598, 1995.

Foley KM: Pain management in the elderly, in Hazzard WR, Andres R, Bierman EL, Blass JP (eds), *Principles of Geriatric Medicine and Gerontology*. New York, McGraw-Hill, 1990, pp 281–295.

Hadzinski DM: An algorithmic approach to cancer pain/management. *Nurs Clin North Am* 30:711–723, 1995.

Morley GK, Erickson DL, Morley JE: The neurology of pain, in Jognt RJ (ed), *Clinical Neurology* (Vol 2). New York, Hoeber-Harper, Chapter 18, pp. 1–95.

Payne R, Pasternak GV: Pain and pain management, in Cassel CK, Riesenberg D, Sorensen LB, Walsh JR (eds), *Geriatric Medicine*. New York, Springer-Verlag, 1990, pp 583–601.

Sunshine A: New clinical experience with tramadol. *Drugs* 47(Suppl)1:8–18, 1994.

CHAPTER
TWENTY-SIX

COMPUTERS AND OTHER TECHNOLOGIES

THE NEED FOR AND ROLE OF COMPUTERS IN THE NURSING HOME ENVIRONMENT

In the last two decades, the nursing home (NH) industry has been characterized by increasing complexity of its operation and increasing regulatory requirements for documentation. As a result, the need for proper documentation, recording of changes, cost tracking, and cost reporting has grown considerably. The purpose of introducing computers into the NH environment is to meet the challenge raised by these requirements and at the same time improve the information flow in the long-term care setting. Since the introduction of the prospective payment system, there has been a shift toward care outside of hospitals; it is predicted that in the next decade, transitional care units and community-based skilled nursing facilities will play a major role in the health delivery system. Accurate and expeditious flow of information from acute care hospitals to these settings and vice versa will add significantly to the quality of care delivered. The implementation of the Minimum Data Set (MDS) across the nation has added to the challenges of organizing, communicating, and documenting a large amount of information.

The physician in the NH setting receives, reviews, and provides information via the NH medical record. The NH medical record is a combination of an acute care and ambulatory record. The NH environment has elements of both settings, and the requirements for information management bridge the gap between the two. Current NH records are significantly handicapped by factors which are "people dependent," such as handwritten, illegible, inaccurate, and unreliable notes. Much information is recorded, but the retrieval process is difficult and the information is frequently not usable. Clinical decisions may therefore be based on inaccurate and incomplete information. An inefficient information system also handicaps efforts to carry out quality assurance in a timely and cost-effective manner. In addition, lack of access to good data from the NH record interferes with the ability to perform clinical research.

In this chapter, we will describe basic principles of the flow of information in the NH setting, briefly review the design of an integrated computerized information system applicable to a NH, and address ways of selecting and implementing a computer system in a NH. Other uses of technology will be reviewed briefly. The "Suggested Readings" contain more detailed information regarding the use of computers in the NH.

INFORMATION AND THE FLOW OF INFORMATION IN THE NURSING HOME SETTING

The information used in a NH is basically similar to the information used in the acute hospital. It includes demographic information, clinical data, and information related to the resident's resources and financial status. In contrast to the acute care hospital, much of the information in the NH relates to functional status and daily care routines, and there is more of a multidisciplinary focus. **Table 26-1** describes the basic flow of information in a NH setting. Computers can provide an information center that can efficiently integrate the diverse inputs and help make data flow in an organized and efficient manner. **Figure 26-1** describes the desired flow of information in a NH with a computerized information system. In a typical NH, there are three major functions: (1) clinical, (2) administrative, and (3) business or accounting. An optimal information system integrates and creates an effective flow of information among all three functions.

Table 26-2 lists some basic terminology and definitions related to information and its flow in the NH. All information pertaining to the resident is considered the database. Different people use the database for different purposes and in different ways. Traditionally, health care institutions have relied primarily on a financial database. A financially oriented database, however, may not provide and integrate clinical information in an efficient and effective manner.

Table 26-1 The basic flow of information in a nursing home

Third-party payers to institution and vice versa
Regulatory agency to institution and vice versa
Regulatory agency to physician and vice versa
Physician to resident and vice versa
Physician to nurses and other health professionals and vice versa

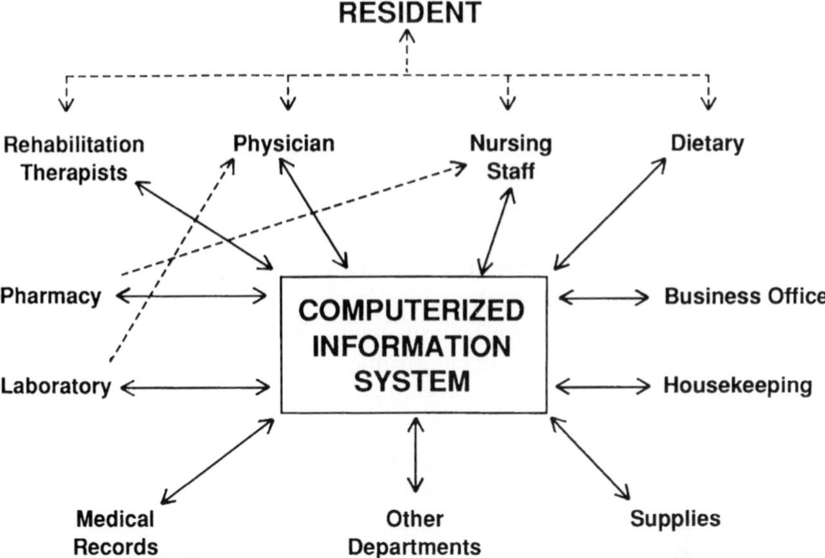

Figure 26-1 Basic flow of information in a NH with a computerized information system. Dotted lines indicate verbal/written communications which are not directly incorporated into the computer database.

Table 26-2 Terminology and definitions related to information systems and computers in the nursing home

Terminology	Definition
Database	Contains specific elements of information—demographic, financial, clinical, functional status, resources utilized
Clinical information system	A coordinated approach to the systematic collection, storage, and use of information concerning residents—their health and associated needs and problems
Medical record	A sequential chart that records the timing of events and all relevant clinical and administrative data related to a resident's care
Computerized information system	The use of computers to collect, store, organize, analyze, and generate reports for clinical, administrative, or financial purposes
Report	A computer-generated document that organizes and presents information in a predetermined format based on the user's objectives; it can become a part of the medical record

Thus, clinical information should be the centerpiece of a system that determines utilization of personnel and other types of financial information essential to the operations of a facility, rather than vice versa. Clinical information can be used to generate financial data relatively easily, but the opposite does not hold true. A clinical information system that collects and organizes clinical data in a usable fashion is therefore needed.

Computer databases can help in standardizing data collection and in avoiding multiple entries of the same data. In a NH, for example, much of the clinical and functional status information is collected by more than one discipline. The computerized information system can make this process more efficient by allowing the clinical information to be input only once; at the same time, it can integrate that clinical information into multiple reports. Reports can be used for clinical purposes (by incorporating them into the medical record) as well as for administrative and financial purposes. **Table 26-3** lists examples of clinical data categories that could be included into a computerized information system. Such data categories can allow for the generation of standardized reports (e.g., a medical face sheet (see "Appendix"), a structured progress note, an administrative face sheet—the storage of data to monitor progress and changes over time, and the organization of information in a manner that is helpful for quality assurance purposes. Standard coding systems, e.g., ICD-9 (International Classification of Disease, 9th Revision), DRG (Disease Related Group), are not as applicable in NH settings as they are in acute care hospitals. Thus, a list of diagnoses for use specifically in the NH must be developed. Where applicable, these diagnoses can then be linked to a standard code, such as ICD-9.

A computerized information system in a NH setting must also be a dynamic system. After the information is collected the first time, it must be continuously revised and updated by health professionals as new information related to the resident's progress is collected and entered into the database for ongoing review. Because much of the information is redundant, the computer can make this process much more efficient. In addition, the computer may help identify when significant changes occur that should, in turn, trigger revision of the care plan and new goals and approaches.

Table 26-3 Examples of clinical data categories

- Demographic information
- Age, sex, socioeconomic data, insurance status
- Functional status
- Diagnoses
- Progress notes
- Diagnostic studies and results
- Therapeutic interventions and results
- Medical problem list or face sheet

GENERAL PHILOSOPHY OF DESIGNING A COMPUTERIZED INFORMATION SYSTEM

A computerized information system should satisfy administrators, nursing staff, medical staff, and other health professionals. The system should integrate clinical, functional status, demographic, and financial data. It should be capable of generating reports that can be either incorporated into the medical record or used for administrative and financial purposes. A variety of quality assurance activities, discussed below, can be enhanced by properly managed computer-generated data.

Although sophisticated in its internal mechanism, the computer system must be user-friendly. It should be designed to allow the nurse, physician, physical therapist, occupational therapist, pharmacist, and social worker to enter and obtain data about the resident in a simple manner. The computer should encourage entry of data according to the true meaning (i.e., "raw data"), rather than storing it in an interpreted form. The data can then be structured and interpreted by one of several output programs to meet the focused needs of the user. Such an approach increases the variety of users who can be supported by the database and, to a degree, insulates the database from biases about the ways in which residents are classified.

Interactive terminals need to be available throughout a NH in order to facilitate data entry and retrieval. The system response time should be rapid and, to prevent loss, data must be simultaneously recorded on more than one device. Nursing home staff must come to view the system as providing enough payback to justify the time to learn the system.

It must be recognized that, realistically, all potential users will not be willing to interact directly with the terminal. Therefore, a system must be designed to work equally well in interactive and noninteractive modes. Thus, different forms of input that feed into the computer database are needed. Work sheets to be used by personnel who do not work at the terminal may be necessary. These work sheets must be user-friendly and at the same time easily coded into the computer. For personnel who do use the terminal, data entry screens must be complemented by systems that simplify the process of data entry.

Many standard software packages are available for a variety of uses in the NH. Although NHs may find many of these standard packages useful, they need to be able to tailor the software to meet different and changing needs in information content and practice over time. The more sophisticated systems can be user-defined to incorporate the rules under which a given institution must operate. Inflexible programs that focus on financial data will not be useful for clinical and quality assurance purposes.

EXAMPLES OF COMPUTER APPLICATIONS IN THE NURSING HOME

The potential applications of computers in NHs range from the generation of reports and progress notes to quality assurance. In this section we briefly review some applications that have particular relevance to primary care physicians and medical directors.

Resident Care Plan

The resident care plan is theoretically the pillar of the NH medical record. It is intended to guide the care that the individual resident receives. It consists of a synthesis of entries made by all members of the interdisciplinary team. Computer-based resident care planning can be a time saver by allowing almost instantaneous updating as the resident's condition changes and/or when goals of care are achieved and problems are resolved. Many commercially available software programs can generate triggers for the resident assessment protocols (RAPs) and contain libraries of goals and approaches from which resident care plans can be easily generated. These libraries also facilitate the association of a problem with a diagnosis and can suggest language for the goals and approaches—enforcing, when possible, the requirement of measurability. The resident care plan thus generated can be designed in accordance with regulations and, by its simple structure and legibility, facilitate its use by the multi-disciplinary team. For each problem and nursing diagnosis, there may be multiple goals (objectives); for each goal, one or more approaches. For each approach, one or more disciplines are identified and a reassessment date is determined. (A sample format of a standard care plan, which could be computer-generated, is illustrated in Chapter 10, Table 10-2.)

Higher-quality software programs have the ability to review and update the resident care plan in an interactive mode. When a resident is selected, his or her problem list is displayed in a brief form. The operator selects an existing problem category for review or adds a new one. The most recent history is automatically displayed. The operator may scroll through the complete history of the problem or any part of it. In addition to facilitating immediate updating of the care plan, many programs provided well-developed dictionaries of problems, goals, and approaches that can serve as a valuable training tool for the staff.

Utilization Review

Computers are easily used to retrieve information on various utilization patterns. One of the most important examples is the utilization of drugs. The computer can list drugs by type, frequency, potential interactions, and appropriateness in relation to diagnosis. This information may be utilized for quality assurance purposes, as discussed in the next section. Utilization of special diets and dietary supplements is another example. Utilization of resources and self-monitoring of case mix are important in states where case-mix reimbursement of NH care [e.g., resource utilization groups (RUGS)] has already been implemented. The national Minimum Data Set (MDS) for NHs lends itself to computerization, and assessments incorporated in this data set may serve many purposes, including care planning, monitoring trends in case mix, and clinical research. Currently, NHs are being required to computerize the MDS so that the data can be used to generate the RUGS (see Chapter 2) and quality indicators (see following section).

Quality Assurance

Computers can be an invaluable resource in a quality assurance program. The computer can help to monitor trends in critical clinical areas, such as pharmacy services and medication use, accidents, infections, and adherence to various clinical protocols. In order for the computer to be helpful in these areas, it is critical that key data elements for quality assurance purposes be incorporated into the database. Thus, when one is designing a database, it is helpful to think of the types of quality assurance reports that will be desirable (e.g., monthly trends in falls, medication use, infections, cultures, antibiotic use), so that required data can be output. One of the potential advantages of the computer for quality assurance is the ability to link various trends to resident outcomes. Although using a computer for these quality assurance purposes requires some up-front time to input relevant data, the capability to generate various reports will be worth this time if the database and report format are carefully planned. Examples of computer compatible data collection forms for incidents and infections are provided in the "Appendix." MDS data entered into a computer can be used to generate quality assurance data at a national, regional, state, local or individual facility level. Examples of quality indicators derived from the MDS which were developed by Zimmerman and colleagues under contract with the Health Care Financing Administration (HCFA) are illustrated in Chapter 8.

SELECTING A COMPUTER SYSTEM

Selecting hardware and software for a NH computer system may be an intimidating experience, especially for physicians, nurses, and administrators who are not versed in computer terminology and use. A computer for a NH needs to be a flexible system that serves multiple users. Clinical staff should have input into the decision-making process as it relates to the resident care components of the system. The choice of size, configuration, and sophistication of a system depends on the size of the facility and financial considerations as well as the stability and sophistication of the staff. The market offers a spectrum of systems for a broad range of needs—from personal-computer-based single-station systems that have single-module software (as for resident care planning and accounting) to microcomputer, integrated, multiple-module, and multiple-user systems. It is beyond the scope of this chapter to go into details about the various systems that are available. Systems that allow the most flexibility and are vertically integrated are the most suitable for facilities of 150 beds or larger, while the less complicated systems are better suited for smaller institutions with very specific needs (e.g., accounting, care planning).

FUTURE USES OF COMPUTERS IN THE NURSING HOME

As computers begin the transition to a "paperless" record, staff behavior will become a critical issue in successfully incorporating computers into NH care. As it stands now, nurses' aides provide most of the care and a significant portion of charting in a NH setting. Charting consists of reporting on several critical aspects of resident care, including food intake, toileting, and exercise. Staff observe and report verbally on residents' behavior, which is later recorded by either the aide or licensed staff. Computer technology can be used to enhance supervision and accountability for such resident care procedures and their documentation. Nurses' aides can carry hand-held computers, scan a resident's bar-coded band, and log in their observations and treatments in real time, very much as supermarket cashiers or package handlers do today. The resident-related information could then be entered electronically into the computer system. This type of approach could improve performance efficiency and reliability without compromising resource utilization.

Another potential use for computer technology may be direct monitoring of residents with behavioral problems such as wandering. Monitoring systems have been developed that report resident wandering patterns to a computer. This information can be utilized in care planning via adjustments in the environment, staffing, or medications. A similar approach may be used for monitoring recurrent fallers, whose beds or wheelchairs can be monitored with a fall-management mobility monitoring device (see Chapter 16).

In summary, computerized information systems will be increasingly important to the future of NH care. Many benefits can be derived, including improved documentation, increased accountability, better utilization of resources, quality assurance, education, research, and potential cost savings. With limited resources, NHs may be reluctant to get involved in any activity that cannot have a favorable effect on their bottom line and on resident care. Studies and demonstration projects that focus on human resource management, quality assurance, and the fiscal aspects of NH care are needed in order to introduce computer technology into the NH on a scale similar to that of the introduction of computerization to business and industry in the last two decades.

OTHER TECHNOLOGIES

The NH is a low-technology, high-touch industry. This has made it difficult for many NH staff to accept the possibility that technological innovations may improve the humanistic care of the resident. One example of technology that has great potential to improve the quality of that care is a voice-activated robotic arm, which can pick up objects and move them into an appropriate position in response to the resident's voice. Robots may also be particularly useful for helping dependent residents do passive exercises or for assisting nurses' aides in critical repetitive tasks, such as positioning residents or offering them water.

The introduction of high-tech environmental control systems may lead to significant improvements in NH residents' quality of life. A series of simple environmental control systems for persons with quadriplegia and poliomyelitis were first developed in Britain in 1960. A sophisticated environmental control system developed in a Canadian NH has given residents a heightened sense of independence, reduced frustration levels among both residents and nursing staff, and produced a saving of 1 h of nursing time per resident per day. These systems allow the resident to control the room lights, radio, and television set from a bed or chair and can be adapted to allow the resident to have control of any simple on/off system. Many hospital beds are now fitted with these systems, but their

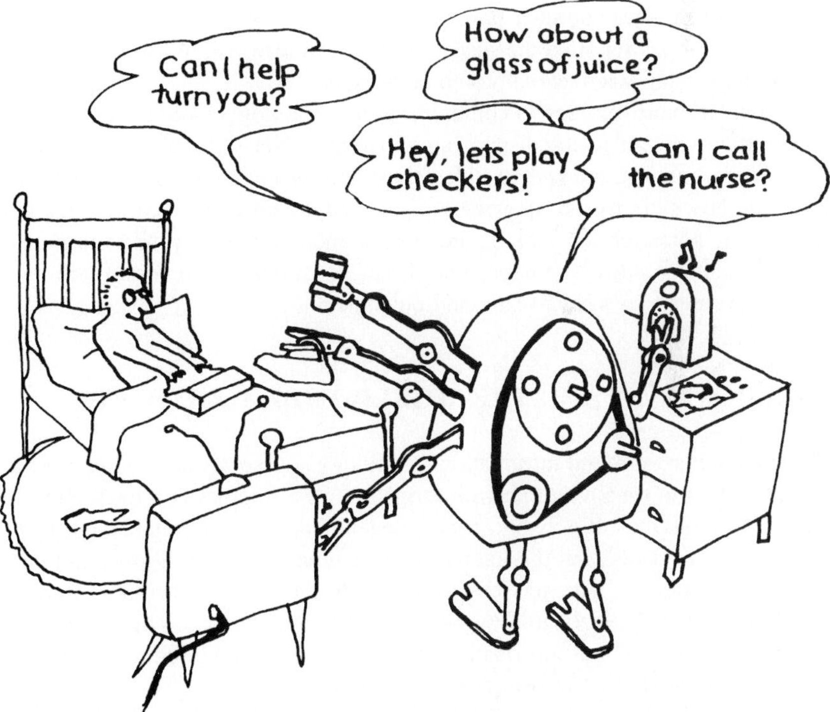

Figure 26-2 The future of NHs. Robotics could help improve the environment and quality of life for NH residents. They could reduce the nursing time needed for selected repetitive tasks—thereby freeing their time to interact with residents on a more social basis—and help restore a locus of control to dependent NH residents. (After Morley JE: New concepts of medical management of nursing home patients. *Ann Intern Med* 108:728, 1988.)

introduction into NHs has not been generalized. These innovative approaches can permit the resident to reestablish a level of control while allowing nursing staff more time to engage in meaningful dialog with the resident. The science-fiction potential of such environmental control systems and robotics is suggested in **Fig. 26-2.**

Improvements in communication technology are also beginning to have an impact on the NH environment. Fax machines may produce a major advance in the way in which information is communicated between NHs, hospitals, and laboratories as well as between physicians and nurses. Predetermined "panic" values for laboratory tests can be established; when such results are obtained, they can be faxed immediately back to the NH or directly to the physician. Fax transmissions may become viable substitutes for many telephone calls between physicians and nurses. These calls are time-consuming and a major source of frustration for all concerned. Nurses can use fax transmissions to inform physicians of subacute changes that do not require immediate notification, to report abnormal lab results, and to request changes in orders. Physicians could fax responses back to the NH. Administrative and legal issues surrounding the use of fax machines for such purposes will have to be worked out. The Mayo Clinic has already reported the successful and cost-effective use of fax machines in its relationship with several community NHs.

Finally, improvements in communication technology could lead to exciting opportunities for educational programs involving NH staff. Computer-assisted learning techniques, interactive videotapes, and teleconferences with opportunities for NH staff to ask questions of experts at different locations all hold significant potential for making the NH a more interesting and stimulating environment for staff. One hopes that these educational technologies will result in improvements in resident care and outcomes.

THE INTERNET AND THE WORLD-WIDE WEB (WWW)

Telecommunications and information technology are rapidly advancing, opening up new ways to obtain and share information. The Internet is a interconnected system of thousands of networks which began in the United States in the 1960s. It has been suggested that the Internet will eventually be "the ultimate library of public information". The services available on the Internet include: electronic mail (e-mail), bulletin boards, newsgroups, file-transfer protocol servers (free computer software), text information (gopher servers), and multimedia information servers for sharing information on the WWW.

There is a large volume of information relating to aging available on the WWW and the Internet. It is important to recognize that this information is unedited and uncensored. Misinformation abounds. Many NH chains and academic organizations are in the process of developing their own home pages and networks. These should be useful sources of information on NHs. The academic and government sites that are available tend to have more accurate information, but even information obtained from these cannot always be relied upon.

TELEMEDICINE

For those of us who work in NHs, telemedicine represents one of the most exciting aspects of the information superhighway. The technology now exists to allow the physician to visualize and directly talk to the resident from the office or home when a problem occurs. In addition, the physician will be able to obtain hard copies of any components of the chart necessary to make a diagnosis. This technology will not only improve the quality of care, but also has the potential to improve human interactions between the resident and the physician. When the resident has a problem they will be able to "see" their physician. In addition, it will become much easier to obtain consults through the medium of telemedicine.

SUGGESTED READINGS

Bluin BI (ed): *Information Systems for Patient Care*. New York, Springer-Verlag, 1984.

Haber PAL: Technology in aging. *Gerontologist* 36:350, 1986.

Ellis RD, Jankowski TB, Jasper JE, Abdul A: Gero-informatics and the internet: Locating gerontology information on the world-wide web (WWW). *Gerontologist* 36:100–105, 1996.

Levenson SA: *Medical Directions in Long-Term Care*. Owings Mills, Maryland, National Health Publishing, 1988, 235–276.

Morley JE: New concepts of medical management of nursing home patients. *Ann Intern Med* 108:727, 1988.

Post JA: Internet resources on aging. *Gerontologist* 36:11–12, 1996.

Schnelle JF, McNees P, Crooks V, Ouslander JG: The use of a computer-based model to implement an incontinence management program. *Gerontologist* 35:656–665, 1995.

Symington DC, Lywood DW, Lawson JS, MacLean J: Environmental control systems in chronic care hospitals and nursing homes. *Arch Phys Med Rehabil* 67:321, 1986.

Weiler GP, Thorpe L, Walters R, Chiziboga D: An automated medical record system for a skilled nursing facility. *J Med Systems* 11:367, 1987.

Williams ME: Geriatric medicine on the information superhighway: Opportunity or road kill. *J Am Geriatr Soc* 43:184–185, 1995.

Williams ME, Ricketts RC, Thompsson BG: Telemedicine and geriatrics: Back to the future. *J Am Geriatr Soc* 43:1047–1051, 1995.

CHAPTER

TWENTY-SEVEN

ETHICAL AND LEGAL ISSUES

A myriad of ethical issues are confronted on a daily basis in the nursing home (NH), ranging from the allocation of resources and access to care, to the individual rights of NH residents, to decisions involving the withholding or withdrawal of life-sustaining treatment. Ethical dilemmas in the NH setting commonly remain unresolved by residents, their loved ones, and their health care providers. Concerns about the process of making difficult ethical decisions are frequently couched in terms of fear of litigation. Medical–ethical issues and the law therefore frequently become muddled.

In this chapter we focus on important ethical issues faced by physicians and other health professionals who care for NH residents, and suggest strategies to deal with them. A brief section at the end of the chapter discusses some of the basic legal issues that are relevant to health care professionals in the NH. But it is our contention, as well as that of most physicians and lawyers, that ethical decisions about the care of NH residents should remain at the bedside and not be made in court. By resorting to the courts to make such decisions, we usurp the right of residents and their loved ones to decide for themselves, and compromise the ability of health care professionals to serve the best interests of their patients. We hope the principles and strategies outlined in this chapter will be helpful in this regard.

OVERVIEW OF MEDICAL–ETHICAL ISSUES

Table 27-1 lists the major principles of medical ethics. These form the basic foundation of medical practice and should be considered when ethical dilemmas

Table 27-1 Major principles of medical ethics

Autonomy
Respect for a person's right to self-determination regarding his/her life, body, mind, and medical care

Beneficence
The obligation to do good and act in the best interests of others

Justice
Duty to treat individuals fairly and without discrimination, and to distribute resources in a non-arbitrary and fair manner

Nonmaleficence
The obligation to avoid harm

Fidelity
Duty to keep promises

in the care of NH residents are being faced. The most discussed and debated medical–ethical issues in the care of NH residents involve decisions about the intensity of treatment provided to frail, dependent, usually cognitively impaired elderly NH residents in the end stages of life. To be sure, these are critical issues that must be addressed in a careful, ethical manner in light of growing concerns over the costs of health care. Before discussing these "life and death" ethical dilemmas further, it is important to take a step back and emphasize that there are

Table 27-2 Common ethical issues in the nursing home

Ethical issues	Examples
Preservation of autonomy	Choices in many areas are limited in most nursing homes (see Table 27-3) Families, physicians, and nursing home staff tend to become paternalistic
Quality of life	This concept is often mentioned in relation to decision making, but it is difficult to measure, especially among those with dementia Ageist biases can influence perceptions of nursing home residents' quality of life
Decision making capacity	Many nursing home residents are incapable or questionably capable of participating in decisions about their care There are no standard methods of assessing decision-making capacity in this population
Surrogate decision making	Many nursing home residents have not clearly stated their preferences or appointed a surrogate before becoming unable to decide for themselves Family members may be in conflict, have hidden agendas, or be incapable of or unwilling to make decisions
Intensity of treatment	A range of options must be considered, including cardiopulmonary resuscitation and mechanical ventilation, hospitalization, treatment of specific conditions (e.g., infection) in the nursing home without hospitalization, enteral feeding, comfort and support care only

many other, more fundamental ethical issues that must be addressed in the care of NH residents. **Table 27-2** lists common ethical issues confronted in the NH. Because the vast majority of NH residents are admitted with diminished functional capacities and/or cognitive impairment, they are especially vulnerable and susceptible to having their decisions made by others (paternalism). This includes the right not to be in a NH. To the extent possible, people should be given the choice about entering a NH and information about noninstitutional resources which might be available should they prefer not to enter the NH. The limits imposed by generally inflexible care routines in NHs reinforces this tendency toward paternalism. Clearly when an individual moves into a communal living environment there will be tension between the autonomy of the individual and the larger "community"—in this instance—of NH residents. Thus, one of the most difficult challenges in caring for NH residents is to attempt to preserve their autonomy and maintain their personhood and rights as individuals. Many of the recommendations made in the Institute of Medicine's

Table 27-3 Basic ethical issues in daily care: the rights of NH residents

1. Access to and choice of medical and other health related care
2. Opportunity to participate in resident and family groups (e.g., a Resident Council)
3. The right to non-disruptive care routines that account for individual preferences, e.g.:
    a. Bed and awakening times
    b. Avoidance of routines that disrupt sleep
    c. Choice of when to get dressed and what to wear
    d. Freedom from unnecessary medications and physical restraints
4. Choices about eating
    a. Freedom from unnecessarily restrictive diets
    b. Opportunity to eat non-institutionalized foods of preference when available
    c. Right to eat at other than mealtimes, e.g., bedtime snacks
5. Opportunity and freedom to participate in activities, including activities outside the facility
6. The right to have visitors
7. The right to manage finances when capable
8. The right to security of personal property
9. The right to voice complaints and grievances
10. The right to privacy
    a. Mail
    b. Use of telephone
    c. Bathroom and bathing
    d. Non-intrusive roommate(s)
    e. Confidentiality of medical and other records
    f. Access to private area for appropriate sexual expression

Based on Kane, RA, Kaplan, A (eds): *Everyday Ethics: Resolving Dilemmas in Nursing Home Life*. New York, Springer, 1990.

1986 report on improving the quality of care in NHs focus on this issue, and residents' rights are a fundamental component of the new rules for NH care defined in OBRA 1987. A book edited by Rosalie Kane and Arthur Kaplan (*Everyday Ethics: Resolving Dilemmas in Nursing Home Life*. New York, Springer, 1990) uses case examples to highlight the importance of these more fundamental and mundane ethical issues to the lives of NH residents. **Table 27-3** lists examples of these basic ethical issues. A specific section of the Minimum Data Set (MDS) is dedicated to documenting residents' daily preferences related to these issues (Section AC, Customary Routine). Although most of these issues are more dependent upon institutional policies and care routines than on medical care, it is important for primary physicians to consider them when writing orders, and to work with the NH to maximize the individual rights of the residents under their care. The primary physician may, in fact, be in the best position to serve as an advocate for residents in maximizing their individual rights and should take advantage of the opportunity to do so whenever possible.

DECISION-MAKING CAPACITY AND INFORMED CONSENT

A fundamental premise of the practice of medicine is that each individual who is capable of making decisions for himself or herself regarding his or her medical care has the right to do so. This right is no different for NH residents than for any other population, but; for a variety of reasons, it is more difficult to uphold in the NH setting.

Table 27-4 outlines several key principles relevant to decision-making capacity and informed consent among NH residents. The right to make decisions regarding medical care is implemented by the process of informed consent. (The requirements for informed consent are outlined in **Table 27-4**.) It is often difficult to fulfill these requirements among NH residents because:

1. Impaired vision, hearing, and cognitive function often make it difficult to communicate the information the resident needs in order to make an informed decision.
2. Dependent NH residents may be afraid that their decisions will result in unfair treatment in the NH.
3. Impaired cognitive functioning and other factors (such as depression, pain, medical illness) may interfere with the resident's ability to make an informed decision based on his or her preferences and best interests.

Thus, an absolutely critical determination that must be made is whether or not residents are capable of playing a meaningful role in making decisions about their care. This turns out to be very tricky business. Much of the literature refers to competence, a legal term that may only confuse the issue. Decision-making capacity is a better way of describing what needs to be determined. Some of the

Table 27-4 Key principles about decision making among nursing home residents

1. Informed consent requires:
   a. The communication of relevant, understandable and unbiased information about the potential risks and benefits of a given intervention
   b. Freedom from coercion and other factors that might unduly influence a decision
   b. The ability to:
      (1) Understand the information
      (2) Weigh the risks and benefits
      (3) Make a reasoned decision based on information and on individual values and preferences

2. Decision making should be done *prospectively*
   a. Written documentation, via an advance directive or other format, is critical (see Table 27-7)
   b. Because many NH residents are incapable of decision making at the time of NH admission, prospective decision making should be discussed *before* NH admission whenever feasible
   c. Specificity regarding all possible medical interventions in an advance directive is often impractical
      (1) More general statements about various levels of intensity of care and common treatment decisions may be more appropriate

3. Decision making capacity relates to the ability to make specific decisions
   a. Dementia and other causes of cognitive impairment do *not* necessarily render NH residents incapable of making decisions regarding their care
   b. Legal competence (or incompetence) is *not* the equivalent of being incapable of participating in care decisions

4. There is no standardized test to determine if NH residents are capable of making specific decisions about their care
   a. Scores on standard mental function tests do *not* predict a resident's ability to participate in care decisions

5. A variety of factors, some of which fluctuate over time and are reversible, can have an important influence on the ability to make decisions, e.g.:
   a. Delirium and other reversible acute confusional states
   b. Depression
   c. Pain
   d. Medication side effects
   e. Perceived quality of life
   f. Perceived wishes of family and other loved ones
   g. Economic considerations

6. The primary physician and interdisciplinary team should regularly review, and document, whether the resident is:
   a. Capable of making their own health care decisions
   b. Capable of participating in health care decisions with involvement of a proxy
   c. Incapable of participating and health care decisions should be make by proxy

7. When a resident is determined to be incapable of making a particular decision:
   a. His/her prior expressed wishes relevant to the decision should be taken into account whenever known
   b. A surrogate or proxy decision maker, preferably assigned by the resident, who is known to be acting in the best interests of the resident, should be consulted

key principles relevant to determining decision-making capacity are outlined in **Table 27-4**. Several of these principles are worthy of special emphasis.

First, unlike legal competence (or incompetence), the ability to make a decision about one's health care should be considered specific to the situation at hand. For example, a NH resident may be legally declared to lack testamentary competence (the ability to execute a will). This, however, has nothing to do with determining whether that same resident is capable of deciding if she or he should have a surgical procedure. Decision-making capacity must be determined in relation to the resident's ability to meet the criteria for informed consent about a specific diagnostic or therapeutic procedure. Second, there is no standardized test that determines the capacity of a NH resident to make a specific decision. Scores on standardized mental status tests are not predictive of decision-making capacity and should not be used in this manner. Third, the fact that a NH resident is known to have a dementia syndrome does not automatically imply that he or she is incapable of participating meaningfully in decisions about his or her care. Even NH residents with moderate or severe dementia are capable of expressing preferences, and an attempt should be made to elicit these preferences whenever feasible. Fourth, a variety of factors, many of which fluctuate over time and are reversible, may influence a NH resident's decision-making capacity. These factors include delirium due to acute medical conditions, depression, pain, and medication side effects. These factors must be identified and managed in order to optimize the resident's ability to express preferences and participate in making decisions.

In the final analysis, the determination of a NH resident's decision-making capacity must rest on a careful clinical judgment that takes into account all the factors discussed above. Psychiatrists and neuropsychologists may be helpful in making this determination. In most situations, however, a primary care physician can make this determination in conjunction with others who know the resident well, including family and other loved ones, nursing staff, and the resident's social worker and representative of the clergy. The MDS contains an item on general decision making capacity (Cognitive Skills for Daily Decision-Making). As a practical strategy related to health care decisions, we recommend that the primary care physician regularly review the residents' decision making capacity and document whether the resident is either:

1. Capable of making their own health care decisions without involvement of a proxy
2. Capable of participating in health care decisions with involvement of a proxy
3. Incapable of participating and decisions should be made by a proxy.

This determination should be reviewed regularly by the interdisciplinary team (e.g., at the quarterly care plan meeting) and any disagreements discussed with the primary physician.

If the resident is found to lack the capacity to make a specific decision, then a proxy or surrogate decision maker must be identified. As discussed below, the surrogate is preferably chosen in advance by the resident. Generally the surrogate is a relative; even if the relative has not been legally identified as the attorney-in-fact or conservator, his or her input is generally sought. Whether or not the surrogate is a relative or is legally identified, it is important to ensure that he or she is accounting for the resident's preferences if known and acting in the best interests of the resident. In situations where a legally identified surrogate is not available, there is disagreement among potential surrogates, or the physician suspects that the surrogate is not acting in the best interests of the resident consideration should be given to consulting to an ethics committee. Involvement of the legal system should be avoided in dealing with these issues.

One other critical aspect of decision making among NH residents is timing. Under optimal circumstances important treatment decisions should not be made at a time of crisis. The decision to place a resident on a respirator should not be made on the spur of the moment, as when a physician is called in the middle of the night about acute respiratory distress, nor should the decision about surgery for a gangrenous extremity be delayed until the resident is septic and delirious. Prospective decision making is discussed further in subsequent sections of this chapter.

DECISIONS ON INTENSITY OF TREATMENT

When one is helping NH residents and their surrogate decision makers to arrive at decisions on medical care, it is generally helpful to categorize various treatment options systematically. **Table 27-5** lists examples of levels of intensity of medical care. Decisions about desired intensity of care should preferably be made prospectively, when residents are still capable of expressing their preferences and before a crisis occurs. The mechanisms to accomplish this, advance directives, are discussed further in the following section of this chapter.

Table 27-5 Examples of levels of intensity of medical care that might be included in advance directives of NH residents

1. Cardiopulmonary resuscitation (CPR)
2. Mechanical ventilation (respirator care)
3. Care in intensive care unit (ICU)
4. Care in an acute hospital, but without CPR, respirator, or ICU care
5. Care in the nursing home only, including specific treatments when indicated (e.g., antibiotics, blood transfusions)
6. Comfort and supportive care only, with enteral ("tube") feeding if necessary for nutrition and/or hydration
7. Comfort and supportive care only, without enteral feeding

Categorizing treatment options, as illustrated in **Table 27-5**, is helpful in giving relatively specific guidance to health care providers and may be helpful in meeting legal requirements for clearly documenting an individual's preferences. However, it is not absolutely necessary, and it may be problematic in certain situations. Many individuals may find it difficult to understand all the potential risks and benefits of the specific treatments, especially when they are being asked to decide about them under hypothetical future conditions. Precluding specific types of care may not always be in the best interests of a resident, even if he or she is severely impaired or terminally ill. For example, acute care hospitalization may be necessary under certain circumstances to provide maximum comfort (e.g., pain control, management of respiratory distress). Similarly, antibiotics may be necessary to provide maximum comfort when a resident has a painful urinary tract infection, cellulitis, or other infection.

In making decisions about the intensity of medical treatments, several basic principles in addition to those outlined in **Table 27-4**, should be considered:

1. In addition to any decisions about specific interventions, a more general statement should be included that (a) alludes to the resident's condition (e.g., irreversible illness, coma) and (b) allows for treatment when the potential benefits outweigh the risks, especially with regard to comfort (e.g., hospitalization, antibiotics).
2. When decisions about specific treatments are made, they must be consistent (e.g., deciding for cardiopulmonary resuscitation (CPR) but against respirator or intensive care unit (ICU) care is not reasonable because in many instances these latter interventions are necessary after a cardiac arrest).
3. Decisions to forego the specific treatments do not imply that other forms of care should be withheld (e.g., a "No CPR" order does not preclude hospitalization for pneumonia). Ventilation needs to be separated from CPR as some studies suggest good outcomes in older persons with respiratory arrest who are ventilated for short periods.
4. In many situations, a time-limited therapeutic trial may be helpful in determining the benefits and risks of a specific treatment (this is especially true for enteral feeding; see below).

A great deal of attention has been focused on decisions about CPR in the NH setting. Although CPR provides a good model for decision making, it has become clear that decisions about CPR for NH residents are less important than decisions about the other categories of treatment listed in **Table 27-5**. This is because CPR has been shown to be an ineffective procedure in the vast majority of NH residents. Its ineffectiveness relates to the overall medical condition of the residents, the survivability of CPR in this population (which is between 0 percent and 5 percent), and the ability, generally limited, of NH staff to provide effective CPR. Some have discussed reversing the standing order in NHs (i.e., a NH resident should be on "No CPR" status unless there is an order to perform CPR).

It should be emphasized, however, that a "No CPR" order may be inappropriate for some NH residents, such as those who are generally healthy and are in the NH for rehabilitation after an acute illness. With the increased development of subacute care units, which should be staffed with nurses trained in advanced resuscitation, outcomes of frail older patients in these settings should be better than in a typical NH.

Decisions to forego acute hospitalization and specific treatments such as antibiotics and blood transfusions may be appropriate for some NH residents. Noted medical ethicist Daniel Callahan has addressed the difficult issues surrounding limiting life-sustaining treatment of demented individuals (See "Suggested Readings" for citation). He discusses the importance of trying to understand the "selfhood" of demented people as their illness progresses, and how this concept might influence decision making. He defines full selfhood as the capacity to have feelings and be aware of them, to reason and be able to make decisions, and to enter into relationships with other persons. He proposes three standards for making decisions to withhold or terminate life-sustaining treatment:

1. No one should have to live longer in the advanced stages of dementia than he would have in a pre-technological era.
2. The likely deterioration in late-stage dementia should lead to a shift in the usual standard of treatment, that of stopping (or withholding) rather than continuing treatment.
3. There is as great an obligation to prevent a lingering, painful, or degrading death as there is to promote health and life.

The American Geriatrics Society has published a position statement which embodies many of the key principles of caring for dying patients, such as those with advanced dementia in a nursing home. This position statement is outlined in **Table 27-6**.

Decisions to limit care imply that the NH staff is able and willing to provide the care that is necessary to ensure the comfort of such residents if they become subacutely ill. Residents for whom these decisions have been made often require substantial nursing time to monitor their comfort and to provide care such as suctioning, hydration, nutrition, and prevention of skin breakdown. In addition, such decisions should not compromise appropriate medical care. If, for example, a NH resident develops pneumonia that is complicated by dehydration, congestive heart failure, or other conditions, optimal medical treatment generally requires care in a "subacute" unit or in an acute care hospital. Treating such complicated conditions in the NH without intravenous fluids and medications and close nursing monitoring is rarely effective and serves no real purpose. Thus, if a specific medical condition such as pneumonia is to be treated, treatment should be provided in an optimal manner, not compromised by limitations that preclude appropriate care.

Table 27-6 Key points in the American Geriatric Society's position statement on the care of dying patients

1. The care of the dying patient, like all medical care, should be guided by the values and preferences of the individual patient.
2. Palliative care of dying patients is an interdisciplinary undertaking that attends to the needs of both patient and family.
3. Care for dying patients should focus on the relief of symptoms, not limited to pain, and should be addressed by both pharmacologic and nonpharmacologic means.
4. Dying patients should be guaranteed access to comprehensive, interdisciplinary palliative care across the spectrum of care settings as part of any federal or state health care reform plan, without care being conditioned on the financial status of the patient.
5. Reimbursement policies should be modified to enhance the availability of palliative care.
6. Administrative and regulatory burdens that may serve as barriers to palliative care should be reduced.
7. Physicians, as well as other health care professionals, at all levels of training should receive concrete, insightful, and culturally sensitive instruction in the optimal care of dying patients.
8. The public, including our patients and our colleagues, needs to be educated regarding the availability of palliative care as an important and desirable option for dying patients.
9. Adequate funding for research on the optimal care of dying patients should be provided.

The most difficult and controversial decisions about intensity of care center around nutrition and hydration. It is beyond the scope of this book to discuss this very complex issue in great detail. Readers are encouraged to review the suggested readings at the end of this chapter, which provide detailed analyses of the complex issues involved. A book edited by Joanne Lynn (*By No Extraordinary Means: The Choice to Forego Life-Sustaining Food and Water*, Indianapolis, Indiana University Press, 1986) is probably the most comprehensive work on this topic.

Several general principles related to decisions about withholding or withdrawing nutrition and hydration are outlined in **Table 27-7**. It should be emphasized that these decisions must be made at an appropriate time, before the resident becomes so malnourished that artificial feeding will not be of any benefit. Because several cases have been ruled on in the courts, physicians must be aware of federal and state rules that bear on these decisions. We believe that it is appropriate to withhold artificial feeding and hydration only for a carefully selected group of NH residents (see **Table 27-7**). When such a decision is made, the NH staff must be comfortable in providing the necessary supportive measures without instituting artificial feeding or hydration. When there is any ambivalence on the part of the resident or their proxy, we recommend that artificial feeding and hydration be implemented. It may be appropriate to do so on a time-limited basis as a therapeutic trial, so that the benefits and risks can be assessed objectively. This might involve providing fluids, nutrition, and medications through a small-caliber nasogastric tube for 1 to 2 weeks in order to determine whether the resident can benefit from and tolerate enteral feeding. Many

Table 27-7 Important considerations about artificial nutrition and hydration

1. Sound decision making practices are critical when considering withholding or withdrawing artificial nutrition and hydration (see Table 27-4)
2. Although generally considered a medical intervention, a myriad of emotional, religious and legal issues are involved
   a. Physicians should become familiar with relevant federal and state rules
3. Decisions about artificial nutrition should be made before a resident becomes so malnourished that artificial feeding will be of no benefit
4. If artificial nutrition and hydration is begun, proper techniques should be employed (see Chapter 13)
5. It may be appropriate to withhold or withdraw artificial feeding and hydration from carefully selected residents who:
   a. Are severely or terminally ill with a limited life expectancy
   b. Have clearly expressed a preference not to have this type of intervention given their condition
   c. Have no reversible causes of inability to obtain adequate oral hydration and nutrition (e.g., depression, pain)
   d. Are unlikely to derive meaningful benefit compared to the risks
6. NH staff who provide day-to-day care must be comfortable in providing supportive care without artificial hydration and nutrition when such decisions are made
7. When there is any ambivalence about the decision:
   a. A time-limited therapeutic trial may be appropriate
   b. It may be more appropriate to provide the artificial hydration and nutrition and withhold other types of treatment (e.g., antibiotics for pneumonia or sepsis)
8. Some residents who are severely malnourished (but not demented) can have dramatic improvements after short-term artificial nutrition (3 weeks to 4 months) while other conditions are being treated.
9. Malnutrition is commonly associated with depression. Short-term artificial nutrition may be appropriate while waiting the results of the treatment for depression.

residents tolerate enteral feeding through a gastrostomy better than an NG tube and the option should be offered even if it is believed that the feeding may only be short term. Of course, proper techniques for providing artificial feeding and hydration should be employed (see Chapter 13). In many situations involving severely impaired residents, it may be most appropriate to use artificial feeding and hydration (because of the complex medical, emotional, religious, and legal issues involved) and to forego other life-sustaining treatments when acute conditions develop (e.g., withhold antibiotics if sepsis occurs and use supportive and comfort measures only). Most ethicists believe that there is no difference between decisions not to initiate feeding or to withdraw it. Dehydration is usually a more comfortable and quicker way to die than malnutrition. When artificial nutrition is withdrawn this should be coupled with withdrawal of artificial hydration.

POLICY AND PROCEDURAL CONSIDERATIONS

Policies and Guidelines

Nursing homes should develop policies and/or guidelines about common ethical dilemmas. This may be accomplished by a joint effort among administrative staff, the medical director, the director of nursing, other disciplines (e.g., social work, clergy), and residents or by a biomedical ethics committee (see below). Such policies and guidelines should, at a minimum, address resident rights and autonomy, informed consent and decision-making capacity, the use of advance directives and surrogate decision makers, procedures for resolving conflicts, and appropriate documentation practices. An example of a policy on artificial nutrition and hydration is included in the Appendix.

Advance Directives

The importance of attempting to make health care decisions in advance, when an individual still has the capacity to express preferences and before a medical crisis occurs, cannot be overemphasized. Linda Emanuel and her colleagues have written extensively on the structure and importance of advanced directives (see "Suggested Readings"). They identify five key steps of advance care planning:

1. Introducing the topic and giving information
2. Facilitating the discussion
3. Completing directives and recording the statements
4. Reviewing and updating the directives
5. Applying directives to actual circumstances.

There is now available, in most states, a useful instrument for prospective decision making: an advance directive for decision making. Advance directives include living wills, which are generally limited to situations involving terminal illness, and the durable power of attorney for health care (DPA), which is a more general document. The Patient Self Determination Act requires that NHs inform residents about advance directives.

The DPA is a legal document executed when an individual is still capable of making decisions. It allows the individual to document two important items: (1) an attorney-in-fact whom the resident trusts as his or her surrogate decision maker in the event that the resident becomes unable to make his or her own health care decisions and (2) the types of decisions the resident would want to have made on his or her behalf. Although the DPA is a potentially powerful tool for ascertaining an individual's treatment preferences before he or she becomes incapable of expressing them, it is by no means a panacea. There are some practical problems with the use of a DPA. First, as already mentioned, it may be very difficult for an individual to think about, no less specifically identify, various treatment options under a given set of abstract circumstances and to choose among them. Some people do not want to deal with these issues and may not be able to understand all the implications of opting for or against specific treatments that are generally not relevant to their present state of health. On the other hand, several surveys suggest that elderly people are willing to take part and interested in such discussions, and they do not find them emotionally upsetting.

The biggest practical problem with the DPA or any other written advance directive is that most NH residents have not executed such a directive before entering a NH and becoming incapable of doing so. The basic ethical principles outlined earlier in this chapter as well as several legal precedents (which require clear and convincing evidence of an individual's preferences in order to withhold or withdraw life-sustaining treatment) demand that primary care physicians take a proactive stance in this area. Discussions about advance directives must become a routine component of the practice of geriatric medicine and should occur, when possible, before or shortly after an individual enters a NH.

The "Appendix" contains examples of advance directives. Physicians should become familiar with laws about advance directives in their state and encourage their geriatric patients to execute one if available. Even if the patient does not sign a legal advance directive, the physician should carefully document in the patient's medical records any discussions regarding future treatment decisions and the patient's preferences. This documentation may later be of critical importance in helping to preserve the autonomy of that patient, whether or not he or she enters a NH. In Missouri one of us (JEM) has found it useful to develop a three tie "code" status for all patients to allow rapid communication of the patient's (or proxy's) wishes in emergencies. This is signed by the patient (or proxy) and a witness. Code 1 is full resuscitation. Code 2 is do not resuscitate, but hospitalize and give all other necessary treatment. Code 3 is do not hospitalize or resuscitate.

Documentation

Many of the dilemmas and conflicts about decisions to withhold or withdraw life-sustaining treatment arise from inadequate documentation procedures. Although it is impossible to eliminate the fear of litigation and to prevent lawsuits, adequate documentation is critical in order to convince whoever needs to be convinced that thorough and appropriate procedures were followed in making these decisions. The existence of proxy decision makers and advance directives must be recorded in the MDS. **Table 27-8** lists some of the key aspects of documenting decisions to withhold or withdraw life-sustaining treatment. It is essential that such documentation be clear, kept in a specific location in the medical record, and transferred with the resident when he or she leaves the NH to enter another health care institution (i.e., an acute care hospital or another NH). Various procedures can be developed to accomplish these goals. We have developed a "treatment status sheet" that is used for all such documentation; it is

Table 27-8 Medical record documentation of decisions to withhold or withdraw life-sustaining treatment

1. All official documents (e.g., durable power of attorney for healthcare) and other written documentation relevant to treatment decisions should:
   a. Be kept in a defined area of the chart
   b. *Not* be thinned from the chart, if for example the resident is hospitalized and readmitted to the nursing home
   c. Be copied and sent with the resident if she or he is transferred to another health care institution
2. When a decision has been made to withhold a specific form of treatment (e.g., "No CPR"), this information should be clearly identified by:
   a. An order in the physician's orders
   b. Appropriate labelling of the medical record
   c. Maintaining a list readily accessible to nursing staff, so that paramedics or ambulances are not called for residents who have decided against CPR or hospitalization
3. A physician's note, placed in a specified location in the medical record (and not thinned), should clearly and concisely address several issues:
   a. Clinical data relevant to the treatment decision including diagnosis and prognosis
   b. The treatment decision(s) made
   c. Who was involved with the treatment decision
      (1) If the resident, the note should include a statement about the resident's ability to make the decision
      (2) If a surrogate decision maker, the note should state:
         (a) Who the surrogate is
         (b) Their legal status if applicable (e.g., attorney-in-fact, conservator)
         (c) That the surrogate is acting in the best interests of the resident
   d. The basis for the decision
      (1) Any written or verbal expression of the resident's prior know wishes should be mentioned (e.g., statements made in Durable Power of Attorney for Healthcare)
   e. The treatment plan to be implemented
   f. Discussion of the decisions and treatment plan with NH staff and other family members

kept next to the medical face sheet and not thinned from the medical record. The "Appendix" contains the medical face sheet and an example of a specific form developed for documentation purposes by the California Medical Association. In addition to the documentation, it is critical to develop strategies to communicate these decisions to the interdisciplinary team that cares for the resident.

Biomedical Ethics Committees

Many NHs have developed biomedical ethics committees, although most facilities are still without them. Many NHs do not have the resources or expertise to form such a committee. Options for these NHs might be to join with other local NHs to form a committee, utilize the committee of a nearby larger institution, develop a city or countrywide committee, encourage a corporate owner of several facilities to form a committee, or adopt the guidelines of local medical and legal societies.

A biomedical ethics committee should include representatives from the NH's administration as well as its medical, nursing, and social service departments. It should also include a member of the clergy, a lawyer, and someone representing the community the NH serves. The NH biomedical ethics committee should devote itself to:

1. Self-education about medical ethical principles and common ethical dilemmas
2. Education of NH staff, residents, and families
3. Development of policies, guidelines, and procedures to handle ethical dilemmas
4. Quality assurance activities to ensure that policies, guidelines, and procedures are implemented and are being followed.

A question frequently arises as to whether such a committee should be involved in reviewing individual cases. While the committee may often be helpful in clarifying difficult issues, there are several potential problems with expecting NH ethics committees to help resolve conflicts and make specific recommendations about an individual case. First, many committees do not have enough expertise to do this. Second, even if the committee does have members with sufficient expertise, they may not be available to meet at the time a conflict must be resolved. Third and most important, a committee, like a court, should not be used in a manner that removes the decision-making process from its proper place: with the resident, his or her loved ones, and the health professionals responsible for his or her care. For these reasons, it is more appropriate and practical for NH biomedical ethics committees to confine their activities to those listed above and not become involved in individual cases. Only in the rare circumstance when conflicts arise that cannot be resolved any other way should a committee be involved in an individual case. In such situations, it is better for a committee to become involved than to resort to the court system. One of us (JEM) consistently involves an ethicist or ethics committee to help mediate as a neutral person where resident, family and/or physician disagree. In most cases such mediation can lead to mutual agreement on the appropriate action. The medical director can also play this role if a NH does not have an ethics committee.

LEGAL CONSIDERATIONS

It is beyond the scope of this book to discuss the many varied legal issues that are relevant to NH care. Readers who are interested in this area should review the "Suggested Readings" for further sources of information. The most comprehensive reference on legal issues in geriatrics is a text edited by Marshall Kapp and Arthur Bigot (*Geriatrics and the Law*, New York, Springer, 1985). A few brief comments about legal considerations are worthy of special emphasis.

The need to adhere to federal and state laws and the risk of lawsuits are facts of life. But they should not usurp the medical profession's ability to provide optimal, humane, and compassionate care or an individual's right to make decisions about his or her own health care. Medical care in the NH should not be practiced on the basis of fear of litigation. We believe that the strategies outlined in this chapter are ethically sound and in compliance with the law. Development of clear, specific, and appropriate policies and procedures, adequate documentation, and quality assurance activities to ensure that policies and procedures are being adhered to are the best protection against litigation.

There will always be test cases that reach the courts and are highly publicized. But test cases and federal and state laws should not be over-interpreted. Much of the fear of litigation stems from ignorance of what, in fact, is the relevant law. Physicians who practice in NHs should become familiar with federal and state laws, especially as they relate to decisions to forego life-sustaining treatment. Many medical journals regularly publish articles relevant to health care law, including briefs presented to the courts by professional societies and interest groups on specific cases. Federal and state laws should be reviewed when necessary, as should interpretive guidelines. It should be emphasized, however, that the latter are not the law but only an interpretation of it, which may or may not be appropriate in an individual case.

The role of the legal system should optimally be to set up and oversee an environment in which appropriate procedures can be followed that uphold the rights of individuals and their loved ones to make decisions about their care, and to enable health professionals to act in their patients' best interests given the patients' preferences. If health professionals who work in NHs work diligently to develop, implement and monitor appropriate policies and procedures, we should avoid the unnecessary intrusion of the legal system in decisions that belong in the clinical arena, not the courts. Unfortunately the unreasonable expectations and sometimes frank greed of relatives and the cost of lawsuits (both monetary and emotional) has resulted in many cases being settled out of court, and has made the legal system presently governing care in NHs very difficult for providers.

SUGGESTED READINGS

General

American Geriatrics Committee: The care of dying patients: A position statement from the American Geriatrics Society. *J Am Geriatr Soc* 43:577–578, 1995.

Besdine RW: Decisions to withhold treatment from nursing home residents. *J Am Geriatr Soc* 31:602–606, 1983.

Callahan D: Terminating life-sustaining treatment of the demented. *Hastings Center Report* 25–31, November–December, 1995.

Eddy DM: A conversation with my mother. *JAMA* 272:179–181, 1994.

Hilfiker D: Allowing the debilitated to die. *N Engl J Med* 309:716–719, 1983.

Kane RA, Caplan AL (eds): *Everyday Ethics: Resolving Dilemmas in Nursing Home Life*. New York, Springer, 1990.

Libow LS, Olson E, Neufeld RR, et al: Ethics rounds at the nursing home: An alternative to an ethics committee. *J Am Geriatr Soc* 40:95–97, 1992.

Kapp MB, Bigot A: *Geriatrics and the Law*. New York, Springer, 1985.

Lynn J: Dying and dementia. *JAMA* 256:2244–2245, 1986.

Rango H: The nursing home resident with dementia: Clinical care, ethics and policy implications. *Ann Intern Med* 102:835–841, 1985.

Sachs GA, Ahronheim JC, Rhymes JA, et al: Good care of dying patients: The alternative to physician-assisted suicide and euthanasia. *J Am Geriatr Soc* 43:553–562, 1995.

Uhlman RF, Clark H, Pearlman RA, et al: Medical management decisions in nursing home patients: Principles and policy recommendations. *Ann Intern Med* 106:879–885, 1987.

Advance Directives and Decision Making

Danis M, Southerland LI, Garrett JM, Smith JL, et al: A prospective study of advance directives for life-sustaining care. *N Engl J Med* 324:882–888, 1991.

Emanuel LL, Danis M, Pearlman RA, Singer PA: Advance care planning as a process: Structuring the discussions in practice. *J Am Geriatr Soc* 43:440–446, 1995.

Freedman M, Stuss DT, Gordon M: Assessment of competency: The role of neurobehavioral deficits. *Ann Intern Med* 115:203–208, 1991.

Gillick MR: A broader role for advance medical planning. *Ann Intern Med* 123:621–624, 1995.

Holtzman J, Pheley AM, Lurie N: Changes in orders limiting care and the use of less aggressive care in a nursing home population. *J Am Geriatr Soc* 42:275–279, 1994.

Mott PD, Barker WH: Hospital and medical care use by nursing home patients: The effect of patient care plans. *J Am Geriatr Soc* 36:47–53, 1988.

Murphy DJ: Do-not-resuscitate order: Time for reappraisal in long-term-care institutions. *JAMA* 260:2089–2101, 1988.

Volicer L, Rheaume Y, Brown J, et al: Hospice approach to the treatment of patients with advanced dementia of the Alzheimer type. *JAMA* 256:2210–2213, 1986.

Intensity of Treatment and Outcomes

Applebaum GE, King JE, Finucane TE: The outcome of CPR initiated in nursing homes. *J Am Geriatr Soc* 38:197–200, 1990.

Fabiszewski KJ, Volicer B, Volicer L: Effect of antibiotic treatment on outcome of fevers in institutionalized Alzheimer patients. *JAMA* 263:3168–3172, 1990.

Ghusn HF, Teasdale TA, Pepe PE, Ginger VF: Older nursing home residents have a cardiac arrest survival rate similar to that of older persons living in the community. *J Am Geriatr Soc* 43:520–527, 1995.

Murphy DJ, Murray AM, Robinson BE, Campion EW: Outcomes of cardiopulmonary resuscitation in the elderly. *Ann Intern Med* 111:199–205, 1989.

Artificial Feeding

Finucane TE: Malnutrition, tube feeding and pressure sores: Data are incomplete. *J Am Geriatr Soc* 43:447–451, 1995.

Lo B, Dornbrand L: Guiding the hand that feeds: Caring for the demented elderly. *N Engl J Med* 311:402–404, 1984.

Lo B, Dornbrand L: The case of Claire Conroy: Will administration review safeguard incompetent patients? *Ann Intern Med* 104:869–873, 1986.

Lynn, J (ed): *By No Extraordinary Means: The Choice to Forego Life-Sustaining Food and Water.* Indianapolis, Indiana University Press, 1986.

McCann RM, Hall WJ, Groth-Juncker A: Comfort care for terminally ill patients. *JAMA* 272:1263–1266, 1994.

McNabney M, Beers MH, Siebens H: Surrogate decision-makers' satisfaction with the placement of feeding tubes in elderly patients. *J Am Geriatr Soc* 42:161–168, 1994.

Steinbrook R, Lo B: Artificial feeding; Solid ground, not a slippery slope. *N Engl J Med* 318:286–290, 1988.

Economics at the End of Life

Emanuel EJ, Emanuel LL: The economics of dying: The illusion of cost savings at the end of life. *N Engl J Med* 330:540–544, 1994.

Lubitz J, Beebe J, Baker C: Longevity and medicare expenditures. *N Engl J Med* 332:999–1003, 1995.

CHAPTER

TWENTY-EIGHT

EDUCATION AND RESEARCH

The continued growth of multidisciplinary educational programs in nursing homes (NHs) and of research studies that target the management of conditions common in the NH are of vital importance to improving NH care. The purpose of this chapter is to provide primary care physicians and medical directors with a brief overview of key issues involved in educational and research programs in the NH setting. Although most primary care physicians and medical directors are only indirectly involved in them, it is critical that they understand the importance and objectives of such programs so that the programs will be accepted by NHs and have a chance to be successful in meeting their goals.

EDUCATION

In this chapter we focus on medical education in the NH. We want to emphasize, however, the importance of undergraduate and postgraduate educational programs for all health professionals who work in or relate to NHs. NHs with qualified staff should be encouraged to participate in the training of nurse's aides, licensed nurses, social workers, rehabilitation therapists, pharmacists, and administrators. Multidisciplinary rounds and conferences highlighting common clinical conditions and management issues are an effective method of involving such trainees. Participation in undergraduate and graduate education offers the NH an excellent opportunity to improve its image in the community, enhance the education of its own staff, and make the NH a more vital and stimulating environment. NHs may also benefit by attracting interested and well-trained students to jobs in the facility.

The need to educate medical students and postgraduate physician trainees in long-term care has been increasingly recognized over the last several years. The vast majority of medical schools now have at least some opportunity for medical students, internal medicine residents, and family practice residents to have an educational experience in NHs. To date, most of these programs are elective, quite limited in scope, and infrequently subscribed compared to other elective activities. Relatively few programs require rotations for medical students or house staff in a NH. Training opportunities at the fellowship level have increased dramatically over the last several years. There are now at least 84 geriatric medicine fellowship training programs and 55 in geropsychiatry. The Veteran's Administration has played a leadership role in developing and supporting these fellowships. Medical schools and teaching hospitals have also provided substantial support, boosted by special provisions in Medicare to support training in geriatric medicine. The National Institutes of Health, other governmental agencies, some private foundations, and a small number of pharmaceutical companies also provide support for geriatric fellowship programs, especially those with a research focus. Most fellowship programs have well-established relationships with one or more NHs, and some larger NHs have supported fellowship positions. Although these fellowship programs now graduate over 100 trainees per year, they are still far behind projected needs for academic geriatricians. As is the case with most other subspecialty fellowships, at least half the trainees have pursued clinical careers outside academic institutions. Two developments should serve to enhance training in geriatrics: the formal accreditation of geriatric medicine fellowship programs and the development of a joint examination by the American Board of Internal Medicine and the American Board of Family Practice for a Certificate of Added Qualification in Geriatrics.

In view of the rapid changes in the American health care delivery system, geriatrics is included in the renewed interest in primary care specialties. Managed care, Medicare risk programs seek physicians and NPs well versed in caring for the frail and subacutely ill. Older patients who previously were cared for in acute hospitals are now treated in subacute units of the nursing homes, requiring staff to provide hands-on care. Hospitals in aging communities have recognized the need for practitioners skilled in efficient and appropriate utilization of the whole continuum of care. Thus, they are seeking practitioners with geriatric training to manage the system as well as to provide direct care. Demonstration projects funded by private foundations have attempted to increase geriatric content (including NH care) in the curriculum of general internal medicine and family practice residency. The program's Bureau of Health Professions has funded 14 Geriatric Educational Centers, some of which have initiatives to train mid-career physicians, nurses and social workers in skills required to practice in institutional and community-based long-term care. Curriculum recommendations for resident

Table 28-1 General educational objectives of a nursing home rotation for trainees in geriatric medicine

1. Enhance the ability to care for elderly, chronically ill, and dependent residents of NHs
2. Improve understanding of appropriate evaluation and management of common problems in the NH setting
3. Further develop perspectives on and understanding of the rehabilitative, psychological and socioeconomic aspects of caring for NH residents
4. Enhance effectiveness of the multidisciplinary team in providing institutional long-term care
5. Understand the administrative issues involved in nursing home and the role of the medical director

training in NHs have been developed by a joint task force of national organizations involved in geriatric education and emphasize content areas such as rehabilitation, organization and financing of services, and coordination of care between acute and chronic settings.

Table 28-1 lists several general educational objectives for trainees in a NH. These objectives focus on the care of chronically ill and functionally dependent NH residents, the limitations and advantages of the NH setting, the importance of psychological and socioeconomic factors, and their role in relation to a multidisciplinary team. Most educational programs for medical students and house staff fight an uphill battle against negative attitudes toward the geriatric population that are often engendered by experiences in medical school—such as caring for frail, dependent elderly when they are acutely ill, delirious, difficult to manage, uninteresting, and a "placement problem." Educational experiences in a NH must expose trainees to attitudes and situations that are more conducive to providing humane, compassionate, and effective care to the NH population. **Table 28-2** lists several attitudinal objectives for a NH experience. Trainees must come to understand that common geriatric syndromes—such as dementia, immobility, and incontinence—are not inevitable consequences of growing old. Even in long-term care settings, active and appropriate medical care of specific disease processes and chronic illnesses can optimize health, function, and overall well-being. They should recognize the importance of functional assessment and

Table 28-2 Attitudinal objectives of a nursing home rotation for trainees in geriatric medicine

1. Illness and disability are not an inevitable consequence of growing old
2. The goals of NH care are often different than those in other settings
3. Caring rather than curing is most often the appropriate overall goal
4. Small changes in function can make major differences in well-being
5. A multidisciplinary approach is essential for effective care
6. Ethical and legal issues are common in the NH

Table 28-3 Specific knowledge and skills objectives of a nursing home rotation for trainees in geriatric medicine

Knowledge

Long-term care
- Definition and demographic considerations
- Community services
- Federal and state policies
- Economics
- Nursing home administration
- Organization and financing of services
- Coordination of long term care services
- Administrative role of medical director
- Utility of continuous quality improvement principles in enhancing nursing home care

Aging
- Physiological changes that affect clinical evaluation and management of NH residents
- Altered presentation of disease in the NH

Assessment and treatment of common disorders
- Cancer
- Dementia and related behavioral disturbances
- Depression
- Diabetes
- Falls/gait disorders/postural hypotension/syncope
- Hypertension
- Incontinence
- Infection (especially pneumonia and urinary tract infection)
- Nutrition/malnutrition
- Osteoporosis
- Parkinson's disease
- Pressure sores
- Rehabilitation—stroke, hip fracture, amputations, other
- Sensory impairment
- Surgical interventions—preoperative evaluation, altered risk/benefit considerations
- Terminal illness

Pharmacology
- Geropharmacology of drugs commonly used in the NH
- Psychotropic drugs

Role of members of the multidisciplinary care team
- Nursing—aides, LVNs, RNs
- Social work
- Physical therapy
- Occupational therapy
- Nurse practitioner
- Geriatricians
- Others

Ethical and legal issues
- Decisions to limit care
- Decision-making capacity
- Advance directives
- Role of family caregivers
- Examples of case law relevant to NH care
- Functions of an institutional ethics committee

Table 28-3 (*Continued*)

Skills
Comprehensive history and physical examination of frail elderly, including chronically ill and dependent NH residents, with emphasis on in-depth assessments of mental and functional status
Ability to perform telephone consultation for subacute problems in the nursing home
For medical direction, ability to formulate policies and procedures, and design and implement quality assurance studies based on principles of continuous quality improvement

rehabilitation and that even small changes in function (e.g., the ability to transfer) may have a major impact on the health and quality of life of a frail NH resident and the caregiver and can sometimes even affect the need for institutional care. At the same time, they must also understand that, unlike the goals of the acute care hospital and ambulatory clinic, those of NH care are generally not to cure but to manage conditions in a way that maximizes functional capabilities, prevents complications, and enhances quality of life. These goals vary depending upon characteristics of individual residents and whether rehabilitation, terminal care, or maintenance and preventive care are emphasized. A multidisciplinary approach that encompasses the psychological and socioeconomic aspects of residents' illnesses and disabilities—as well as the medical aspects—is essential for effective care of the NH population. In working with a multidisciplinary team, trainees should also come to understand the critical importance of the nonmedical aspects of NH care, such as many ethical and legal dilemmas that are confronted on a daily basis in the NH setting.

Table 28-3 lists more specific educational objectives for trainees in a NH, including both knowledge and skills. While it is impossible to meet all these objectives in a single student or house staff rotation, fellowship trainees are generally expected to develop substantial expertise in these knowledge and skill areas.

One issue that frequently arises in the design of educational experiences in a NH is the complicated logistics of attempting to meet the educational objectives involved in caring for chronically ill residents over a long period of time. It is difficult to meet these objectives if the exposure of the trainee occurs over a short time span. Most medical student and house staff rotations are scheduled for blocks of 4 to 6 weeks. An alternative which many fellowship and some residency programs have developed is a longitudinal experience. **Table 28-4** outlines some of the advantages and disadvantages of block versus longitudinal NH rotations. We believe that in most NHs, longitudinal rotations are preferable, especially for residents and fellows, because they afford the trainee an opportunity to meet more of the objectives, to observe the time course of various subacute and chronic conditions common in a NH, and to assume a primary-care role for a cohort of NH residents. To make a longitudinal rotation effective, several important details must be attended to:

Table 28-4 Advantages and disadvantages of block versus longitudinal rotations in the nursing home

Block Rotations
- Advantages
  - Concentrated exposure
  - More opportunity to observe
    - Interdisciplinary process
    - Management of acute problems
    - Administrative issues
- Disadvantages
  - Difficult to obtain exposure to all objectives
  - May miss some of the course of acute/subacute problems
  - Difficult to integrate into primary care
  - Frequent reorientation of new trainees necessary

Longitudinal Rotations
- Advantages
  - Primary care role possible
  - Chance to meet more objectives
  - Opportunity to observe time course of various conditions
- Disadvantages
  - May miss interdisciplinary and administrative aspects
  - Set time for rounds may be difficult to integrate with other responsibilities
  - Availability for management of interim problems may be difficult

1. A regular time must be scheduled for primary care activities and for attending rounds with a faculty member who is experienced in long-term care. The best way to accomplish this is to substitute monthly NH rounds for another regularly scheduled activity, such as a longitudinal ambulatory clinic.
2. There should be planned exposure to the major objectives of the NH rotation over the course of the longitudinal experience.
3. Trainees should have the opportunity to meet with the administrator, medical director, and the multidisciplinary team on one or more occasion.
4. If trainees assume a primary care role, they should have close supervision by a faculty attending and should have backup coverage for acute problems when they are busy on other rotations. The latter can be provided by the faculty, a fellow, a nurse practitioner or physician's assistant, the medical director, or an interested member of the NH medical staff.
5. Exacerbation of chronic conditions which do not require immediate attention can be communicated to medical residents utilizing e-mail or facsimile, allowing the resident to call or fax his or her response within one working day.

Block rotations may offer some advantages in an academic NH with enough faculty to provide continuous on-site supervision. An intensive in-depth exposure will allow the trainee to interact with multidisciplinary staff more frequently, get an idea of the day-to-day routines in a NH, and become a functioning member of the multidisciplinary team—albeit for a short period of time. If the block rotation is chosen, faculty should make sure that the trainee receives a broad exposure to the various aspects of NH care. He or she should also be helped to gain a perspective on the overall time course of conditions and situations that commonly occur in the NH setting (of which the trainee may observe only a small portion).

The main challenge facing geriatric education in the next decade is to train generalists. The main thrust is skill acquisition and management style that will address interdisciplinary team functioning and time-efficient management of complex, very old patients with increased acuity of illness and functional disabilities.

RESEARCH

Research is absolutely vital if NH care is to be improved. There remains a paucity of data from well-designed studies that scientifically demonstrate the most effective methods of managing common conditions in the NH. But it is not easy to implement research in the NH successfully. **Table 28-5** lists several of the major challenges faced by researchers who embark on studies in the NH setting. Many researchers, including ourselves, have encountered the pitfalls outlined in **Table 28-5.** Although many NHs now participate in a wide variety of research studies, most do not, and there remains a great deal of apprehension about research among NH administrators, staff, residents, and residents' families. Of particular concern to administrators, owners, and governing bodies is the potential cost of participating in research. There are, in fact, many potential costs, some of which may not be obvious either to the researchers or the NH. **Table 28-6** lists these potential costs. It is incumbent upon researchers to address these costs thoroughly when planning a study and preparing a budget. NHs should be made aware of these costs and be assured that adequate resources are available to support a study before it is implemented.

Table 28-5 Major challenges faced by researchers in the nursing home setting

1. General apprehension among administrators, staff, residents, and families about research
2. Potential costs to facilitate (see Table 28-6)
3. Assessment of NH residents is time-consuming compared to research in other settings
4. Logistical difficulties in performing various tests that require specialized equipment (e.g., radiographic studies, complex urodynamics, electrophysiologic studies)
5. Informed consent may be problematic in the cognitively impaired
6. Nursing home medical records often contain scant and inaccurate data for research purposes
7. Sample size may be limited by informed consent, failure to meet screening criteria, and dropouts due to illness, death, or discharge

Table 28-6 Potential costs of research for nursing homes

1. Disruption of usual care routines
2. Preparing and transporting residents to research activities
3. Identifying surrogates and witnessing informed consent
4. Providing information on functional status
5. Answering questions of residents and families
6. Minor supplies, space, and telephones used by research staff
7. Assisting in administering treatment protocols
8. Assisting in assessing outcomes

More NHs must become involved in research for at least two reasons. First, the results of research that is carried out in "teaching" NHs, which often have more resources and staff than nonteaching facilities, may not be translatable to the typical American NH. Thus, research studies should include typical as well as teaching NHs, so that research findings will be generalizable to the former as well as the latter. Second, the nature of the NH population, especially its heterogeneity and high turnover rate, and the types of outcomes being sought require relatively large sample sizes in order to obtain scientifically valid data. Many studies, therefore, will require the involvement of several different NHs. As a result, an increasing number of primary care physicians and medical directors will be asked to assist in facilitating research in the their own NHs. Thus, it is important for practicing physicians to become familiar with some of the key issues that must be addressed if NH research is to be successful.

Because NH residents are an especially vulnerable population, it is essential that research in the NH setting conforms to the highest possible scientific and ethical standards. Just because NH residents are vulnerable, however, does not mean that they should be precluded from participation in research that may benefit them as individuals while also leading to improvements in NH care in general. **Table 28-7** lists several guidelines that we believe, on the basis of our experience as well as that of others, are critical if NH research is to succeed. Research in the NH, as all other settings, should be scientifically sound. It should undergo peer review and be approved by a federally sanctioned institutional review board or human subjects protection committee. Pilot studies are extremely important in developing efficient, nonintrusive methods of screening potential subjects, refining the research protocol, and determining sample sizes. In general, research that involves minimal risk to subjects (i.e., no more risk than they normally incur in the NH), is of potential benefit to individual subjects, and is generalizable to typical NHs is more likely to be accepted than research that does not meet these criteria. Educational and discussion sessions should be held with NH staff, residents, and families to convey the importance, objectives, and anticipated benefits of the proposed research. The potential costs of the research to the facility (see **Table 28-6**) should be addressed in detail with the administrator. A written list

Table 28-7 Keys to success of research in the nursing home

1. Plan research that is
    - Scientifically sound
    - Poses minimal risk
    - Is of potential benefit to individual subjects
    - Is clinically relevant
    - Is generalizable to typical NHs (as opposed to teaching facilities affiliated with universities)
2. Educate and enlist the support of facility administration and staff, governing body, residents, and families
3. Address the potential costs of the research to the facility before starting the study (see Table 28-6)
4. Develop explicit and detailed procedures for informed consent
    - Enlisting and reimbursing a staff member (nurse or social worker) for assistance in determining decision-making capacity, identifying surrogates, and witnessing the consent process is very helpful
5. Develop efficient, nonintrusive screening procedures
6. Perform pilot studies
    - Data-collection instruments
    - Assessment procedures
    - Treatment protocols
    - Determination of sample size
7. Provide feedback to facility staff
    - Present progress reports and results to staff meetings

of mutual expectations is helpful in this regard. Because many NH residents are not capable of providing informed consent, procedures for obtaining informed consent must be developed. Meetings with families may be especially important, because most often one or more family members provide the informed consent required for the resident's participation. We have found that enlisting and reimbursing a NH staff member to assist in determining a resident's capacity to consent, identifying an appropriate surrogate, and witnessing the consent process is extremely helpful and may go a long way toward assuaging fears of exploitation. Finally, it is very important that the research team provide feedback about the results of the research to NH staff. A conference that describes the results and their implications for care in the NH, along with written materials, will be an effective means of accomplishing this objective.

SELECTED READINGS

Education

Aiken LH, Mezey MD, Lynaugh JE, et al: Teaching nursing homes: Prospects for improving long-term care. *J Am Geriatr Soc* 33:196–201, 1985.

Breitenbacher RB, Schultz AL: Extended care in nursing homes: A program for a country teaching medical center. *Ann Intern Med* 1:96–100, 1983.

Counsell, SR, Sullivan GM: Curriculum recommendations for resident training in nursing home care: A collaborative effort of the Society of General Internal Medicine Task Force on Geriatric Medicine, the Society of Teachers of Family Medicine Geriatrics Task Force, the American Medical Directors Association, and the American Geriatrics Society Education Committee. *J Am Geriatr Soc* 42:1200–1201, 1994.

Counsell SR, Katz PR, Karuza J, et al: Resident training in nursing home care: Survey of successful educational strategies. *J Am Geriatr Soc* 42:1193–1199, 1994.

Grady MJ, Earll JM: Teaching physical diagnosis in the nursing home. *Am J Med* 88:519–521, 1990.

Kane R, Solomon D, Beck J, Keeler E: The future need for geriatric manpower in the United States. *N Engl J Med* 302:1327–1332, 1980.

Kapp MB: Nursing homes as teaching institutions: Legal issues. *Gerontologist* 24:55–60, 1984.

Libow LS: Geriatric medicine and the nursing home: A mechanism for mutual excellence. *Gerontologist* 22:134–141, 1982.

McVey LJ, Davis DE, Cohen HJ: The 'aging game': An approach to education in geriatrics. *JAMA* 262:1507–1509, 1989.

Pawlson LG: Education in the nursing home: Practical considerations. *J Am Geriatr Soc* 30:600–602, 1982.

Rosenthal MS, Marshall CE, Martin SE, et al: Nursing home rounds as a format for teaching residents and medical students. *J Med Educ* 62:975–980, 1987.

Rowe JW, Grossman E, Bond E, et al: Academic geriatrics for the year 2000: An Institute of Medicine report. *N Engl J Med* 316:1425–1428, 1987.

Schneider EL, Ory M, Aung ML: Teaching nursing homes revisited: Survey of affiliations between American medical schools and long-term-care facilities. *JAMA* 257:2771–2775, 1987.

Woolliscroft JO, Calhoun JG, Maxim BR, et al: Medical education in facilities for the elderly: Impact on medical students, facility staff, and residents. *JAMA* 252:3382–3385, 1984.

Research

Cohen-Mansfield J, Kerin P, Pawlson G, et al: Informed consent for research in a nursing home: Processes and issues. *Gerontologist* 28:355–359, 1988.

Lipsitz LA, Pluchino FC, Wright SM: Biomedical research in the nursing home: Methodological issues and subject recruitment results. *J Am Geriatr Soc* 35:629–634, 1987.

Melnick VL, Dubler NN (eds): *Alzheimer's Dementia: Dilemmas in Clinical Research.* Clifton, New Jersey, Humana Press, 1985.

Ouslander JG, Schnelle JF: Research in the Nursing Homes: Practical Aspects. *J Am Geriatr Soc* 41:182–187, 1993.

Palumbo FB, Magaziner JS, Tenney JH, et al: Recruitment of long-term care facilities for research. *J Am Geriatr Soc* 35:154–158, 1987.

Warren JW, Sobal J, Tenney JH, et al: Informed consent by proxy: An issue in research with elderly patients. *N Engl J Med* 315:1124–1128, 1986.

Zimmer AW, Calkins E, Hadley E, et al: Conducting clinical research in geriatric populations. *Ann Intern Med* 103:276–283, 1985.

APPENDIX

1 EXAMPLES OF POLICIES AND PROCEDURES

1.1 Jewish Home for the Aging—Policy and Procedures Regarding Advance Directives and Treatment Decisions (Effective September 1, 1995)

Policy

I. The Jewish Home (the Home) supports a resident's right to participate in health care decision-making. Through education and inquiry about advance directives, the Home will encourage residents to communicate their health care preferences and values to others. Such communication will guide others in health care decisionmaking for the resident if the resident is incapacitated. For purposes of this policy, an advance directive refers to a written instruction that relates to the provision of health care when the resident is incapacitated, such as a Durable Power of Attorney for Health Care, a Natural Death Act Declaration or a living will.

II. The Home shall not condition the provision of care or otherwise discriminate against an individual based on whether or not the individual has executed an advance directive.

III. As the Home is a religious organization, the Home shall comply with the residents' wishes in accordance with the Home's written policies on feeding and hydration and cardiopulmonary resuscitation.

IV. The Home shall provide education to staff and the community on issues that concern advance directives. This education is to include:

A. annual inservices for staff
B. articles in Home newsletter for relatives and community
C. individual communication with applicants and residents
D. brochures distributed to applicants, residents, family, volunteers and community members.

V. For purposes of this policy, an admission is defined as the resident's initial move to the Home which is processed through the Admissions Department. In addition, an admission will include a resident in the Residential Care section who moves into the Nursing section either temporarily or permanently. This definition expressly excludes residents who leave the Home temporarily on leave of absence or hospital stay.

VI. If a resident is admitted to the Home and has no available family or designated representative, the Home will work with the resident to involve a representative from Jewish Family Services (JFS) to serve as the resident's surrogate decision maker. This representative shall meet with the resident to understand his or her wishes and will be provided information regarding the Home's policies and procedures related to advance directives and treatment decisions. The JFS representative will work with the Home's interdisciplinary team, including at least the resident's primary physician, social worker and licensed nurse, to make decisions on behalf of the resident who lacks capacity. If a resident does not have any representative and lacks capacity, the JHA interdisciplinary team will act on the resident's behalf.

Procedures

VII. New admissions

A. The Admissions staff shall provide to each new resident upon or prior to her or his admission:

1. brochure describing an individual's rights, based upon California statutes and court decisions, to accept or refuse medical or surgical treatment and to formulate advance directives; and
2. specific Home policies including Religious and Ethical Policy Statement, Feeding and Hydration Policy, and Cardiopulmonary Resuscitation Policy.

B. The Admissions staff will inquire as to the existence of an advance directive.

1. If the resident has a previously executed advance directive, the Admissions Department will request a copy and verify its validity. A copy will then be placed in the resident's medical record and social service file.
2. If the resident does not have an advance directive, the Admissions staff will encourage the resident and family to discuss issues related to medical treatment and will inform the new resident and family of the process by which these issues will be discussed with them after admission.

C. The Admissions staff shall document on the form "Documentation of Advance Directive:"

1. that the resident has received the information referred to in section VI. A 1 & 2
2. whether the resident has executed any kind of advance directive
3. whether a copy of the advance directive has been provided for the medical record.

This form shall be placed in the Advance Directives section of the resident's medical record.

D. As part of the initial medical assessment, the medical staff will:

1. determine existence of an advance directive
2. assess resident's decision-making capacity (see Section IX)
3. document decision-making capacity and any existing treatment decisions on treatment status sheet and medical face sheet (see Section X)
4. inform resident that Social Worker will be contacting them regarding further discussions.

E. During the second month of residency at the Home, the Social Worker shall meet with the new resident, whether or not the resident has an existing advance directive, to:

1. provide information about the Durable Power of Attorney for Health Care
2. review decisions the resident will be asked to make
3. explain Home policies related to advance directives
4. educate resident about CPR and artificial feeding and hydration through the use of vignettes
5. identify the resident's choice of a surrogate decision-maker.

F. Within two weeks of the above meeting, the Social Worker shall convene an appointment with the resident's primary medical doctor to include the resident, his/her surrogate decision-maker (if the resident so chooses) and the social worker. The social worker and primary medical doctor will again review the decisions the resident has been asked to make and answer any questions that the resident or surrogate decision-maker may have.

G. The resident will be encouraged to complete an advance directive and if she/he agrees, the Social Worker shall:

1. provide the Durable Power of Attorney for Health Care
2. arrange for the Long-Term Care Ombudsperson to be present during the execution of the advance directives (for nursing residents only)
3. ensure that copies are given to the resident and his or her surrogate decision-maker and copies are placed in the medical chart and social service file
4. update the form "Documentation of Advance Directive" and the MDS
5. advise physician of the completion of advance directive.

H. If no advance directive exists and the resident lacks decision-making capacity, the Social Worker shall:

1. send a letter to the family with vignettes related to CPR and tube feeding

2. offer to schedule a meeting with the primary physician to answer any questions they may have about treatment decisions
3. request that family indicate their understanding of the resident's wishes in writing
4. place the family statement in the Advance Directives section of the resident's medical record.

VIII. Transfers to nursing from residential care

A. The Medical Records Department shall initiate and Social Services Department shall provide to each resident who is admitted from the Home's Residential Care to Nursing Care the brochure described in section VII. A 1 within seven days of his or her transfer.
B. The medical staff, as part of the admission assessment, shall:

1. assess the resident's decision-making capacity (see Section IX)
2. determine existence of an advance directive and review with resident
3. document decision making capacity and treatment status on medical face sheet and treatment status sheet (see Section X).

If no advance directive exists, the medical staff will alert the social worker for further action as outlined in Section VII. E.

IX. Determination and documentation of decision-making capacity

A. The determination of decision-making capacity will be made by the medical staff based on historical and clinical information, as well as input from other members of the interdisciplinary team. There is no standard method for determining decision-making capacity; mental status test scores do not accurately reflect an individual's ability to make specific decisions. The determination is a clinical one that depends on the individual's ability to comprehend information, to weigh, in a rational manner at least some of the risks and benefits, and to understand the consequences of their decisions. The medical staff will clearly document this information on the medical face sheet according to the following categories:

- capable of making decisions
- capable of participating in decisions
- not capable of participating in decisions.

B. The interdisciplinary staff will review the decision-making capacity at the time of the care plan meetings. If the interdisciplinary team agrees that the documentation of decision-making capacity should be changed, the social worker will provide this input to the medical staff.

C. If, during the interim between care plan meetings, an interdisciplinary team member feels there has been a change in decision-making capacity, the following steps should be taken:

   1. The social worker (if not the person noting the change) should be notified.
   2. The social worker should discuss the change with the primary physician.
   3. If there is agreement on the change:

      a. The physician should update the medical face sheet.
      b. The social worker should:

         (1) update the MDS
         (2) contact the designated proxy to inform them of the change.

X. Documentation of treatment status

A. The medical staff shall be responsible for documenting the resident's treatment status based upon:

   1. The resident's/surrogate decision-maker's stated desires
   2. The resident's overall health condition
   3. The Home policies related to artificial feeding and hydration and cardiopulmonary resuscitation.

B. The medical staff shall document the resident's treatment status on:

   1. the treatment status sheet
   2. the medical face sheet
   3. physician's order sheet (as necessary).

C. If the resident's treatment status is Do Not Resuscitate, the medical staff will initiate the Do Not Resuscitate Form. The social worker will be responsible for obtaining the resident's or surrogate decision-maker's signature on this form.

XI. Review of advance directives and treatment status

A. For residents of nursing, the interdisciplinary team will review the resident's treatment status at the time of the quarterly care plan meeting. If the inter-disciplinary team feels that the treatment status should be re-assessed, the social worker will notify the physician.

B. For all residents, the advance directive and treatment decisions will be reviewed annually and at any significant change of condition by the medical staff. This review should include:

   1. Review of existing advance directives and treatment status desires
   2. Assessment of resident's overall health condition

3. Assessment of the resident's decision-making capacity
4. Discussion with the resident and/or designated representative regarding treatment desires
5. Review of findings with resident's social worker.

C. If changes in treatment status are indicated, the medical staff shall document and communicate this according to the procedure outlined in Section X.

1.2 Feeding and Hydration

Jewish Home for the Aging—Feeding and Hydration Policy

I. Purpose

A. The Feeding and Hydration Policy is designed to clarity, for residents, staff and family members, procedures for administration of artificial feeding and hydration for residents at the Jewish Home for the Aging.

Currently this policy relates only to those residents residing in the Home's nursing facilities, since state regulation does not currently allow a No Artificial Feeding or Hydration order in residential care facilities.

B. This policy is consistent with the Home's policy as it related to conformity with Jewish Law.

In recommending this statement of policy it relates only to the artificial feeding and hydration and is not to be considered as a precedent to be used in discussion of other treatments.

II. Basic policy

A. The general order of the Jewish Home for the Aging regarding treatment provided to all of its residents requires the administration of both nutrition and hydration at all times.

B. Every effort should be made to help residents obtain food and hydration orally.

C. If enteral feeding is necessary, and if, in the opinion of the attending physician, and after review of the Medical Director, Director of Nurses, and Director of Social Services, the resident meets the criteria outlined below, and if there is a written directive by the resident stating that he or she does not want artificial feeding and hydration, enteral feeding may be withheld or withdrawn.

1. coma or persistent vegetative state from which there is no reasonable medical probability of emerging, or
2. irreversible illness with the imminent death within a few months and when the anticipated burdens of enteral feeding exceed the benefits, and

3. the enteral feeding poses a greater threat to the resident's life than the probable benefit of such treatment, or
4. the enteral feeding causes tremendous persistent or recurrent pain.

D. Upon admission to the Jewish Home, all residents should be encouraged to sign a Durable Power of Attorney for Health Care (DPA).

As part of this process, the resident should be:

1. Informed about the medical care available at the Jewish Home, including procedures followed in emergency situations.
2. Informed about the policy on artificial feeding and hydration.
3. Encouraged to include in the Durable Power a statement that specifies what types of treatment they would or would not want, particularly artificial feeding and hydration.

Jewish Home for the Aging—Implementation of Feeding and Hydration Directive

I. New residents

A. Applicants to the Home will be requested to complete a DPA and the Artificial Feeding and Hydration Directive. A new, more concise form will be utilized by the Admissions Department.

B. After the resident is admitted, and should a DPA not have been completed, the Social Worker will meet with the resident and/or family in an attempt to obtain a completed DPA and Artificial Feeding form.

II. Current residents

In order to obtain a completed Artificial Feeding and Hydration Directive on current residents, the following procedures will be followed.

A. *Eisenberg Village*

1. Residential Care: The Social worker will meet with each resident at the time of his/her annual history and physical. The Clinic will furnish the Social Services Department with a list of residents due for annual H and Ps [histories and physical examinations] and for the following month. The Social Worker will schedule an appointment with the residents. The procedure will continue until all current residents have been contacted.
2. Nursing: Once a month, the social worker in each building will accompany the physician on his rounds in order for the social worker and physician to engage the resident in a conversation about the feeding and hydration. The conversation will be documented on the treatment status sheet and in the social service notes. The Feeding Directive will also be signed and placed in the chart.

B. *Grancell Village*

1. Residential Care: The social worker will meet with each resident at the time of his/her annual history and physical. The Clinic will furnish the Social Services Department with a list of residents due for annual H and Ps and for the following month. The Social Worker will schedule an appointment with the residents. The procedure will continue until all current residents have been contacted.
2. Nursing: The social worker will meet with each Nursing resident at the time of his/her quarterly review to engage the resident in a conversation about feeding and hydration. The conversation will be documented after consultation with the primary medical doctor on the treatment status form and signed by the primary medical doctor.

C. *Residents unable to sign the Feeding Directive*
Since there are currently residents who are unable to sign the Directive, the following procedures will be followed. Please note that the procedures listed below apply to residents who are unable to sign, who are living at the facility on or before August 1, 1991. After August 1, 1991, staff will look to the DPA/Feeding Directive for guidance in placement of a feeding tube. In the absence of a written note, artificial feeding will be implemented.

1. *Residents with a completed DPA*

   a. Does the resident meet the criteria outlined in the Feeding and Hydration policy which would preclude the insertion of a tube?
   b. Does the DPA address a desire not to be artificially fed and/or wishes and desires not to implement life-sustaining or prolonging treatments?

      - If both A and B are met, the feeding tube may be withheld.
      - If both A and B are not met, a feeding tube will be inserted.

2. *Residents without a completed DPA*
   If no DPA exists, a family conference will be convened to include at least the physician, social worker, and family members to ascertain the resident's desires regarding tube feeding. If family can clearly state that their relative would not want to be artificially fed, the physician and social worker should so document on the treatment status form and in the social services notes.

   Note: the intent of the Jewish Home Feeding and Hydration Policy is to feed and hydrate unless there is a directive and the resident's medical condition meets the policy criteria. In the event there is a disagreement between family members of the family and staff, the Administrator will call for a meeting with the family and representatives of the Ethics Committee.

Jewish Home for the Aging—Artificial Feeding and Hydration Directive

The Jewish Home has adopted a policy concerning feeding and hydration which is attached to this form.

In the event that I am in a nursing level of care and unable to give consent to receive food and liquids through tube—either inserted through my nose into my stomach or surgically inserted directly into my stomach—I wish to make my desires known in advance.

Should the Jewish Home staff feel that I am unable to take sufficient food and liquids by mouth, and I meet the criteria of the Jewish Home policy

_____ I would like to receive foods and liquids by tube for a trial period of several days and continued if it is found to be beneficial to me.

_____ I would like to receive food and liquids by tube.

_____ I do not want to receive food and liquids by tube.

____

Resident Signature

____

Resident Name

____

Date of Signature

____

Witness Signature

This form may be used an an attachment to the Durable Power of Attorney for Health Care.

1.3 Jewish Home for the Aging—Psychotropic Medication Policy (Revised and Approved by Clinical Practice Committee September 1992)

Purpose The objectives of this policy are to ensure that:

1. Residents with psychiatric and behavioral disorders are treated appropriately with psychotropic medications.

2. Psychotropic medications are prescribed for appropriate indications and in appropriate dosage regimens.
3. The response of target symptoms and behaviors to psychotropic medications are adequately monitored.
4. Side effects of psychotropic medications are minimized.

Policy This policy addresses the prescription of psychotropic medications for psychiatric and behavioral disorders. Commonly prescribed psychotropic medications are included on the list shown below. This list is not all inclusive, and some of the medications listed are prescribed for more than one indication.

1. Antidepressants, e.g.
   - Nortriptyline (Aventyl)
   - Desipramine (Norpramin)
   - Imipramine (Tofranil)
   - Protriptyline (Vivactil)
   - Doxepin (Sinequan)
   - Amitriptyline (Elavil)
   - Trazadone (Desyrel)
   - Fluoxetine (Prozac)
   - Lithium (Lithium)
   - Methylphenidate (Ritalin)
2. Anxiolytics, e.g.
   - Lorazepam (Ativan)
   - Oxazepam (Serax)
   - Alprazolam (Xanax)
   - Diazepam (Valium)
   - Clorazepate (Tranxene)
   - Buspirone (Buspar)
3. Hypnotics, e.g.
   - Chloral hydrate (Noctec)
   - Triazolam (Halcion)
   - Temazepam (Restoril)
   - Flurazepam (Dalmane)
4. Antipsychotics, e.g.
   - Haloperidol (Haldol)
   - Thiothixene (Navane)
   - Thioridazine (Mellaril)
   - Chlorpromazine (Thorazine)
   - Loxapine (Loxitane)
   - Molindone (Mobane)
   - Trifluoperazine (Stelazine)

General Guidelines

1. Psychotropic medications are to be prescribed for specific target symptoms and behaviors. The diagnosis underlying such symptoms and behaviors must be documented in the medical record.
2. Because many different medical conditions can cause psychological symptoms and behavioral changes, such medical conditions should be identified and treated before psychotropic medications are prescribed, unless a psychotropic is necessary to prevent the resident from harming himself or others.
3. Behavioral interventions should first be attempted before psychotropic medications are prescribed, unless the psychotropic is necessary to prevent immediate harm to himself or herself or others. These should include modifications of the resident's behavior or environment and include staff approaches to care to the largest degree possible to accommodate or change the resident's behavioral symptoms.
4. Residents who may require or who are prescribed an antidepressant, sedative, or antipsychotic, should have a psychiatric consultation.
5. New orders for psychotropic medications must be accompanied by:
   a. Specific indication(s) for the medication within the body of the order.
   b. A progress note specifying the diagnosis(es) and target symptom(s) and/or behavior(s) for which the psychotropic medication is being prescribed. The note should explain why these symptoms or behaviors are a problem for the resident or for the care of other residents.
6. Any changes in orders for psychotropic medications must be accompanied by a progress note describing the rationale for the change.
7. Psychotropic medication orders written by the psychiatry consultant do not need approval by the primary physician.

   Such orders may not be changed by the primary physician unless he or she has discussed the change with the consultant psychiatrist.

   If a difference of opinion between the primary physician and consultant psychiatrist cannot be resolved by discussion between the two parties, the medical director must be consulted.
8. After prescription of a pyschotropic medication, the response of target symptoms and behaviors must be monitored carefully.
   a. Licensed nursing staff, pharmacy, and social work will summarize their monitoring on a monthly "Psychotropic Medication Progress Note" form, which will then be reviewed and signed by the primary physician (see "Procedures" below).
   b. In addition to this form, progress notes written by the primary physician and consultant psychiatrist must contain a brief summary of the resident's response to the psychotropic medication.
9. Attempts must be made to reduce the dosage or discontinue psychotropic medications whenever clinically indicated based on the data from the monitoring of target symptoms and behaviors. (OBRA regulations require that

attempts at dose reduction be made twice in a one-year period for antipsychotics and anxiolytics and three times in a six-month period for sedative-hypnotics.)

Antidepressants Antidepressants should be considered for residents who meet DSM criteria for major depression or manic depressive illness, or who have depressive symptoms that are significantly interfering with their quality of life, physical function or general well-being. Pharmacologic treatment of depression must be accompanied by optimization of the management of coexistent medical conditions.

Several basic principles should be considered when prescribing antidepressants:

1. Antidepressants vary in their degree of sedation, anticholinergic properties, and cardiovascular side effects. The choice of an antidepressant should take into account these considerations as well as the resident's symptoms and comorbidities.
2. An adequate therapeutic trial should be given. For several antidepressants, blood levels are helpful in determining if therapeutic levels have been achieved and should be monitored periodically.
3. If a resident does not respond to an adequate therapeutic trial of one antidepressant, they may respond to a different type of antidepressant.

Anxiolytics Anxiolytics are useful in the short-term management of anxiety disorders. Medical conditions and depression that might underlie the anxiety should be excluded before an anxiolytic is prescribed.

Long-acting benzodiazepines should not be used in residents unless an attempt with a shorter-acting drug has failed, other possible reasons for resident's distress have been considered and ruled out, and its use in maintenance or improvement in the resident's functional status.

Barbiturates and other highly addictive agents should not be initiated for any reason. Newly admitted residents on these agents should receive gradual dose reductions as part of a plan to eliminate or modify the symptoms for which they are prescribed.

Daily use of any benzodiazepine for anxiety should not exceed four continuous months unless an attempt at a *gradual* dose reduction is unsuccessful. A *clinical contraindication* to dose reduction can be concluded if gradual dose reduction is attempted twice in one year without success.

Hypnotics Insomnia is a common complaint in the geriatric population. Age-related changes in sleep patterns, several medical conditions, depression, dietary and environmental factors (light, noise) can underlie this complaint and should be excluded. The use of a drug to induce sleep should result in the maintenance or improvement of the resident's functional status.

Residents should be encouraged to not become dependent on hypnotics. If a hypnotic is necessary, chloral hydrate is generally the best first choice at the present time. Short-acting benzodiazepines are effective, but have addictive properties and can cause rebound insomnia when they are discontinued. These agents should therefore be avoided whenever possible. Flurazepam and diazepam are long-acting and should be avoided.

Daily use of these medications should not exceed 10 days unless an attempt at gradual dose reduction is unsuccessful.

Antipsychotics Antipsychotic drugs should not be used unless the clinical record documents that the resident has one or more of the following specific conditions:

1. Schizophrenia
2. Schizo-affective disorder
3. Delusional disorder
4. Psychotic mood disorders (including mania depression with psychotic features)
5. Acute psychotic episodes
6. Brief reactive psychosis
7. Schizophreniform disorder
8. Atypical psychosis
9. Tourette's disorder
10. Huntington's disease
11. Organic mental syndromes (including dementia) with associated psychotic and/or agitated features as defined by:
    a. Specific behaviors as quantitatively documented by the facility which cause the resident to:
        (1) Present a danger to themselves,
        (2) Present a danger to others (including staff) or,
        (3) Actually interfere with staff's ability to provide care, or
        (4) Decrease the functional status of the resident.
    b. Psychotic symptoms (hallucinations, paranoia, delusions) not exhibited as specific behaviors listed in (a) above, but which cause the resident frightful distress.

Antipsychotics may *not* be used if (one or any more) of the following is/are the *only* indication:

1. Simple pacing
2. Wandering
3. Poor self-care
4. Restlessness
5. Crying out, yelling or screaming

6. Impaired memory
7. Anxiety
8. Depression
9. Insomnia
10. Unsociability
11. Indifference to surroundings
12. Fidgeting
13. Nervousness
14. Uncooperativeness

As needed or p.r.n. doses of antipsychotic drugs should be used to titrate the resident's total daily dose up to achieve symptom relief or down to avoid side effects to effect a gradual dose reduction.

Otherwise, antipsychotic medications prescribed on a p.r.n. basis can be given no more than 2 times in 7 days. If more doses are necessary, reassessment of the cause for the resident's behavioral symptoms and the development of a plan of care designed to attempt to reduce or eliminate the cause(s) for the harmful behavior is needed.

Residents who are prescribed antipsychotic medications should receive gradual dose reductions, and behavioral interventions, unless clinically contraindicated in an effort to discontinue the medication. **Behavioral interventions** means modification of the resident's behavior and/or the resident's environment, including staff approaches to care, to the largest degree possible to accommodate the resident's behavioral disturbances. **Gradual dose reductions** consist of tapering the resident's daily dose to determine if the resident's symptoms can be controlled by a lower dose or to determine if the dose can be eliminated altogether. **Clinically contraindicated** means that a resident has a diagnosis as described above, and has had gradual dose reductions attempted twice in one year and that attempt resulted in the return of symptoms for which the drug was prescribed to a degree that a cessation in the gradual dose reduction, or a return to previous dose levels was necessary.

Procedure

1. Psychiatric symptoms and behavioral disorders are reported to the primary physician and the social worker.
2. The primary physician will evaluate the resident for medical conditions or drug side-effects that may be contributing to the symptoms.
3. A care plan including behavioral interventions, environmental and staff interaction interventions, is attempted and monitored.
4. If significant symptoms persist or recur, a psychiatric consultation will be requested.
5. Psychiatric consultation may be requested by social work, psychologist and licensed nursing staff after discussion with the primary physician.
6. New orders for psychotropic medications must be accompanied by:

   a. Specific indication(s) for the medication within the body of the order.
   b. A progress note specifying the diagnosis(es) and target symptom(s) and behavior(s) for which the psychotropic medication is being prescribed.
7. When a psychotropic medication order is changed, a progress note must be written describing the rationale for the change.

   Primary physicians will not change psychotropic medication orders written by the consultant psychiatrist without discussing the change with the psychiatric consultant. When a disagreement occurs, the medical director will be consulted.
8. The response of target symptoms and behaviors to psychotropic medication and behavioral interventions will be documented quantitatively and qualitatively in a monthly "Psychotropic Medication Progress Note".
9. Attempts will periodically be made to reduce the dose or discontinue the psychotropic medication based on the documentation of response to target symptoms and behaviors at least twice per year. Residents with a chronic condition, such as an organic mood disorder or a primary dementia, may need ongoing maintenance therapy based on psychiatric assessments.

1.4 Jewish Home for the Aging—Physical Restraint Reduction/Elimination Policy (Revised July 1993)

Introduction Restraints in long-term care settings are commonly used when nursing or physician staff have concerns for safety of their residents, i.e., to assure adequate posture, to prevent injury due to falls and wandering, and for provision of medical treatment for life-threatening symptoms (e.g., feeding tubes, i.v. lines and catheters). While restraints have been used to prevent harm, studies have shown that in fact they may cause more harm than good. Use of restraints does not decrease the number of falls and may be responsible for more severe injuries. The goals of care in nursing homes emphasize achievement of the highest level of independent functioning for each resident. Restraints may interfere with achieving these goals.

OBRA 1987 regulations F203 states: "The resident has the right to be free from physical restraints imposed; or psychoactive drug administered for the purposes of discipline or convenience, and not required to treat the resident's medical symptoms." This policy is designed to adhere to these regulations with respect to physical restraints. A separate policy on psychotropic drugs has already been developed.

Definitions

Restraints (physical) are any manual method or physical or mechanical device, material, or equipment attached or adjacent to the resident's body that the individual cannot remove easily, which restricts freedom of movement or normal access to one's body. These physical restraints include: leg or arm restraints, hand mitts, soft ties or vest, safety bars, and geri-chairs. Seat belts are considered a restraint if the resident cannot demonstrate the ability to get out of them. Bed rails are also considered to be a restraint if both rails are up.

Discipline is any action taken by the facility for the express purpose of punishing or penalizing residents.

Convenience is any action taken by the facility to control resident behavior or maintain residents with the least amount of effort by the facility and not in the resident's best interest.

Psychoactive drugs are drugs prescribed to control mood, mental status, or behavior.

Purpose The objectives of this policy are to ensure that:

1. Physical restraints are used in a manner that will not preclude the resident from attaining or maintaining the highest level of mental, physical, and psychosocial well-being.
2. All possible less restrictive measures are evaluated and implemented before restraints are used.
3. Consultation with appropriate health professionals and implementation of recommendations are accomplished prior to use of restraints (e.g., gait evaluation by physical therapy).
4. The resident and/or resident's designated proxy has been fully informed of risks and benefits and has given consent for physical restraint use. Considerations should include the right to preserve dignity at the expense of possible risks to the resident's safety.
5. The restraint is evaluated at frequent regular intervals to assure no harm comes to the resident and to identify and implement less restrictive measures or alternatives to the restraints when possible.

General Guidelines

1. Physical restraints should be used sparingly in nonemergency situations after:
   a. Careful assessment of the resident and the environment including investigation and treatment aimed at understanding and eliminating the condition which precipitated a decision to restrain the resident.
   b. Documentation that provides substantial evidence that no safer, less restrictive alternative exists.
   c. Collaborative decision between resident, family, nursing staff, attending physician and other care providers including social worker, physical therapist, etc., is made.
2. Short-term use of restraints may be indicated emergently to manage a situation that poses substantial danger to the resident or others (e.g., delirium, psychosis).
3. Whenever restraints are used:

a. The least restrictive device should be used, e.g., a seat belt, pillow, or wedge which can easily be removed by the resident.
b. They must be padded to decrease the chance of pressure damage and abrasion to skin and underlying tissues.
c. The resident and restraint must be checked frequently and released periodically.
d. Attention to need for hydration, elimination, comfort and social interaction must be assured.
e. The need for the restraint and its effectiveness should be reassessed at reasonable intervals.
f. Frequent and regular assessment to identify a change in underlying behavior or to implement safer alternatives.

4. Education/quality/assurance
   a. Periodic staff education will be conducted regarding hazards of restraint use and alternative management strategies.
   b. Quality assurance audits will be conducted to assess the use of restraints and adherence to policy and procedures.

Procedures

1. There will be ongoing education about the use of physical restraints coordinated through Nursing Education. The education program will include:
   a. An overview including current literature review and epidemiologic studies.
   b. Incidents/behavior that lead to restraint use; alternatives/interventions; emergent use of restraints.
   c. Legal issues including: consent, use of restraints without approval, documentation.
   d. Policy implementation.
   e. Resident evaluation; continuous assessment.
2. Emergency use of physical restraints requires:
   a. Presence of a condition requiring emergent use of restraint to facilitate administration of life-saving treatment. Examples include: delirium, psychosis, dehydration, electrolyte imbalance, urinary blockage, drug overdoses or toxicities.
   b. Temporary restraint order renewed every 48 h.
3. If a resident is to be physically restrained in a nonemergent situation, the following criteria must be met:
   a. Written physician order.
   b. Physician and nurse documentation stating rationale for use of restraint.
   c. Documentation of informed consent. (See form: Documentation of Informed Consent for Restraints).
   d. Resident has been assessed for potentially treatable conditions that might underlie the need for restraints, e.g., pain, discomfort, infection,

constipation, dehydration, medication toxicity/side effects, emotional problems, delirium.

e. The resident's environment has been assessed for factors that might precipitate need for restraint, e.g., comfort, noise, lighting, etc.
f. Rehabilitation specialists (OT, PT) have been consulted whenever indicated to evaluate gait/balance problems or other dysfunctions relevant to restraint use.
g. Documentation of consideration of a less restrictive alternative.
h. The interdisciplinary care plan addresses the need for restraint. (See Form: Restraint Assessment for Nonemergent Use).

4. Restrained residents will be observed frequently for comfort, well-being and physical needs. Restraints will be released at least every 2 h and the resident will be repositioned.
5. Continuous assessment, evaluation and periodic trials of less restrictive interventions will be carried out.
   a. The need to continue use of restraints will be re-evaluated at least weekly. Trial periods without restraints will occur if the situation warrants.
   b. Residents at lowest risk for requiring restraints should be considered for alternatives before those at moderate or high risk.
6. Residents already restrained can be categorized into low, moderate or high risk groups as follows:
   - "Low"—one risk factor present.
   - "Moderate"—two risk factors present.
   - "High"—three or more risk factors present.

   Known risk factors for requiring restraints include:
   - Cognitive impairment
   - Poor body alignment
   - Physical frailty
   - Presence of monitoring or treatment devices (e.g., feeding tube, bladder catheter)
   - Safety awareness
   - Ability to transfer
   - History of previous falls.
7. If the resident has been determined to need restraint and refuses, the following procedure will be followed with documentation in the medical record:
   a. A team member will evaluate the understanding of the resident.
   b. The resident will be informed of health and safety consequences of refusal.
   c. Resident's or their proxy's signature on a release form will be obtained.

JEWISH HOME FOR THE AGING
Documentation of Informed Consent—Restraints

Resident Name ______________________________

1. **Type of Restraint**
   ☐ bed rail ☐ limb restraint ☐ seat belt
   ☐ trunk restraint ☐ chair prevents rising (if resident cannot release)

2. **Reason for Use of Restraint**
   ☐ history of falls/injuries ☐ poor safety judgment/awareness
   ☐ pulling out of treatment device ☐ appropriate body positioning
   ☐ resident/family request ☐ other ______________

3. **Less Restrictive Measures Attempted**
   ☐ frequent observation/monitoring ☐ periodic toileting
   ☐ lowering of bed ☐ softer surface around bed
   ☐ restorative care to enhance safe standing/walking
   ☐ visual and verbal reminders to use the call bell
   ☐ less restrictive devices (splint, support, brace, cushions)
   ☐ self-opening seat belt ☐ other ______________

4. **Resident Consent** (*if resident incapable of consenting; skip to 5*)
   Risks, benefits and alternatives discussed with resident:

   ____ Resident provided consent
   ____ Resident denied consent

5. **Family/Guardian consent** (*if resident incapable of consenting for him/herself*):
   Risks, benefits, and alternatives discussed with:

   ______________________ By ______________
   Name and Relationship Facility Representative

   On ____/____/____, ☐ By Telephone ☐ In Person

   ____ Family/guardian provided consent
   ____ Family/guardian denied consent

6. **Multidisciplinary Review**

____________	___/___/___	____________	___/___/___
Nurse	Date	Physician	Date
____________	___/___/___	____________	___/___/___
Social Worker	Date	Rehab Therapist	Date

1.5 Jewish Home for the Aging—Guidelines for Notification of Physicians and/or Nurse Practitioners of Changes in Resident Status

Policy

A. Specific signs, symptoms, and laboratory values suggestive of *acute* illness needing immediate medical assessment (as defined below) will be reported to the primary medical doctor (PMD) or nurse practitioner (NP) by the charge nurse or nursing supervisor as soon as possible after they are identified.

B. All acute changes in resident status reported to the medical staff on an immediate basis will be assessed and documented in the medical record by the nursing staff.

C. In the event of a witnessed cardiac or respiratory arrest (for residents who have full code status), "911" will be called, with later notification of PMD.

D. When contacting medical on-call coverage during night and weekend hours, nursing staff will have the following information available:

   1. Present problem with symptoms, signs, and results of physical assessment, including vital signs and mental status.
   2. Active medical diagnoses
   3. Relevant information about any recent hospitalization
   4. Current medications
   5. Allergies
   6. CPR status and/or hospitalization status
   7. Family contact/DPA
   8. Date of last PMD visit

E. Specific signs, symptoms, and laboratory values suggestive of *subacute* illness (as defined below) will be reported to the PMD or NP by the charge nurse or nursing supervisor, but not on an immediate basis (e.g., the next time the PMD makes rounds).

F. All subacute changes in resident status reported to the medical staff on a nonimmediate basis will be assessed and documented in the medical record by the nursing staff.

Procedure

I. *Immediate notification (acute) problems*

The following symptoms, signs, and laboratory values should prompt *immediate* notification of the PMD or NP.

Immediate implies that the PMD or NP should be notified as soon as possible either directly or by beeper (charge nurse must always inform the clinical supervisor prior to PMD or NP notification).

Situations requiring immediate *action* (i.e., transport of the resident to the emergency room) with later notification of the physician are rare.

These situations include:

1. Witnessed cardiac or respiratory arrest for residents who have full code status (*call 911*).
2. Rapid progression of signs or symptoms listed below before PMD or NP response is obtained. This applies only to residents with full code status (refer to transfer policy).

A. *Symptoms*

   1. Any complaint or apparent discomfort which is

      a. *Sudden* in onset
      b. *A marked change* (i.e., much more severe) in relation to usual complaints
      c. *Unrelieved* by measures which have already been prescribed (e.g., nitroglycerin for chest pain, antacid for abdominal pain, acetaminophen for other pain)

   2. Specific examples of symptoms (not meant to be all-inclusive)

      a. Shortness of breath
      b. Cough
      c. Chest pain, pressure, or tightness
      d. Nausea
      e. Diarrhea
      f. Musculosketal pain
      g. Severe headache
      h. Partial or complete loss of vision
      i. Dizziness or unsteadiness
      j. Weakness of an arm or leg
      k. Slurred speech
      l. New or worsening confusion
      m. Suicidal thoughts

B. *Signs*

   The following list of physical signs is not meant to be all inclusive. Any other sign about which you are uncertain should prompt PMD or NP notification.

   1. *Change* in vital signs
      General guidelines
      Temperature >101 degrees rectally
      Respiratory rate >28/min
      Pulse >110 or <55/min
      Blood pressure >200 systolic or <90 systolic
   2. Any loss of consciousness

3. Any seizure activity
4. Severe bleeding
   Examples
   Intractable nose bleed
   Hematemesis
   Melena
   Bright red blood in stool (not due to hemorrhoids)
   Profuse vaginal bleeding
   Gross hematuria
5. Laceration requiring sutures
6. Fall with any suspected serious injury (e.g., fracture)
7. New and/or severe gastrointestinal signs (not due to fecal impaction), including
   Nausea and vomiting
   Diarrhea
   Abdominal distention
8. Abnormal drainage, foul-smelling discharge, or wound complications
9. Sudden onset of new or severe worsening of confusion and/or agitation
10. New focal neurological sign, such as profound weakness of an extremity or slurring of speech

C. *Laboratory Results*

1. Any lab report, normal or abnormal, which the PMD or NP requests on a "stat" or "same day" basis.
2. In the event that "panic levels" are received from the laboratory, the PMD or NP will be notified *immediately* by phone or beeper.
3. Any of the following, *unless values are consistently at this level and PMD or NP is aware.*

   a. Hematocrit <30
   b. WBC $>12{,}000$
   c. Sodium (Na) <125
   d. Potassium (K) <3.0 or >5.5
   e. Glucose >250
      <90 in a diabetic on oral hypoglycemic or insulin
      <60 in anyone (diabetic or non-diabetic)
   f. BUN >40
   g. Positive urine culture ($>10^5$ col/ml of a pathogen) only if (1) the patient has symptoms and is not on treatment; *or* (2) the pathogen is *NOT sensitive to antibiotic which has been prescribed*
   h. X-ray report revealing an unsuspected finding which may require immediate intervention (e.g., pneumonia, new long bone fracture)

D. *Other*

1. Medication error (overdose or underdose)

   a. If it involves a cardiac or psychotropic drug
   b. If, in your judgment, the PMD or NP should be notified immediately because of the nature of the medication

II. *Nonimmediate notification (subacute) problems*
The following types of problems should be reported to the PMD or NP, *but not on an immediate basis* (*nonimmediate* implies that the PMD or NP should be informed of the problem or event, but not immediately):

A. *Symptoms*

1. **In general**
   Any *persistent* or *recurrent* complaint by a resident or family member that cannot be responded to satisfactorily with already existing understanding of the condition and/or orders for treatment.
2. Specific examples of symptoms (not meant to be all-inclusive):
   Constipation
   Weakness or fatigue
   Diminished appetite
   Sleep difficulty
   Itching
   Headache
   Change in vision
   Hearing loss
   Dyspnea or orthopnea
   Difficulty swallowing
   Abdominal discomfort (e.g., bloating, cramps, etc.)
   Urinary hesitancy or poor stream
   Urinary incontinence
   Vaginal discharge or spotting
   Musculoskeletal pain
   Dizziness
   Difficulty walking
   Recurrent falls
   Memory loss
   Depressive thoughts

B. *Signs*

1. Signs
   In general
   Any substantial *change* in physical condition, functional status, or *new* physical sign which does not require immediate notification should be discussed with the PMD or NP on rounds

2. Examples of signs and changes in condition (not meant to be all inclusive):
   Progressive weakness
   Diminished appetite
   Weight loss or weight gain (e.g., greater than 5 lb in a month or shorter time period)
   Sleep disturbance
   Difficulty swallowing
   Nocturia
   Incontinence of urine or stool
   Skin rash or pressure sore
   Edema
   Gait disturbances
   Forgetfulness or confusion
   Depressed affect
   Agitation or behavioral disturbance
   Personality change

C. *Other*

1. Consult reports requesting specific actions or changes in resident's management.
2. Observations in the course of routine nursing procedures that might require physician action. For example:
   a. Poorly controlled blood pressure in a patient on antihypertensive therapy
   b. Changes in urine or finger stick glucose values in diabetics (e.g., persistently high determinations in a patient who is normally well controlled)
   c. Symptoms unresponsive to recently prescribed treatment
   d. p.r.n. medications which are never used
3. Medication errors (that do not require immediate notification)
4. Special topics concerning a resident's family
5. Annual lab and diagnostic study results

1.6 Jewish Home for the Aging—Primary Care Physician Response to Calls from JHA Nursing Staff and Nurse Practitioners

Policy

Purpose of policy
To ensure that the timing and nature of the response of primary care physicians to calls from JHA staff are appropriate.

1. This policy is meant to complement the existing policies entitled "Guidelines for Notification of Physicians and/or Nurse Practitioners of Changes in Residential Status."
2. Nursing staff and nurse practitioners (NP) will call 911 for paramedics only when in their judgment a resident (who is not on "No CPR" status) will require cardiopulmonary resuscitation before Encino Hospital can be reached by ambulance.
3. Calls to primary care physicians should be limited to those situations requiring immediate notification, as outlined in "Guidelines for Notification of Physicians and/or Nurse Practitioners of Changes in Resident Status," unless otherwise requested in the physician's orders.
4. If there is any doubt about whether the primary care physician should be called, the nursing supervisor should make the decision and in doing so generally favor making the call if there is any question.
5. Primary care physicians will be notified of situations requiring non-immediate notification, as outlined in "Guidelines for Notification of Physicians and/or Nurse Practitioners of Changes in Resident Status," the next time they make rounds or are in clinic.
6. Primary care physicians must be available to respond to calls from JHA staff at all times during weekdays and nights.

   a. If they will not be available, they must arrange coverage by another member of the JHA primary care medical staff and inform the nursing staff of this change.

7. Weekend call schedules for each campus will be published monthly.
8. When a primary care physician is called, he or she should respond promptly, generally within 15 min.

   a. Response time should not exceed 30 min.
   b. Staff should call or page the physician again if he or she has not responded within 30 min.

9. If the primary care physician does not respond within 15 min of the second call, staff should contact, in the following order: (1) the medical director of their campus; (2) the medical director of the other campus; (3) the associate medical director.
10. Primary care physicians must be courteous and respectful when answering calls from JHA nursing staff and NPs. Verbal abuse of staff is a violation of the JHA Standards for Primary Physicians and will not be tolerated.

    a. If nursing staff or the NP feel that the primary care physician has been unnecesssarily discourteous or disrespectful when responding to a call, they will convey this to the medical director of their campus in writing.

b. If the nursing staff or NP is uncomfortable with the primary care physician's response and feel that the resident needs further attention, they will contact the medical director or associate medical director as outlined in item 9 above.
c. Situations in which a primary care physician has difficulty responding to a call or has been called inappropriately should be reported to the appropriate medical director.

1.7 Jewish Home for the Aging—Policy for Reporting Minor Skin Wounds, Medication Variances, Minor Occurrences and Incidents (Revised October 1994)

I. Purpose

The purpose of this policy is to provide a system which will ensure that all minor skin wounds, medication variances, minor occurrences and incidents are documented, reported, reviewed and monitoring in a manner that will enhance the quality of care provided at the Jewish Home.

II. Definitions

A. Minor skin wound
A minor skin wound is any small laceration, contusion or abrasion that in the nurse's opinion is not in need of immediate medical attention by a physician, does not meet criteria for significant injury (see below), and can be treated by a standard nursing protocol.
B. Medication variance
A situation in which a resident does not receive a prescribed medication properly. This may result from omission of a dose, the administration of the wrong medication, the administration of the correct medication in the wrong dose, the administration of the correct dose of the correct medication at the wrong time, or administration of a medication to the wrong resident.
C. Minor occurrence
An event which does not result in significant injury to the resident or need for medical staff assessment and treatment.
D. Incident
An event which results in significant injury to a resident, as defined below, either immediately or within 72 h.

The definition of significant injury is one or more of the following:

1. Change in mental status of level of consciousness
2. Complaints of new pain
3. Abnormal vital signs

4. New decrease in range of motion
5. Hematoma
6. Ecchymosis, abrasion, or contusion greater than 4 cm in its longest dimension
7. Skin laceration greater than 3 cm in length
8. Any fall with impact or injury to the head
9. Any injury not covered by the above, for which nursing staff feels medical input would be helpful.

III. Reporting Forms

Minor skin wounds, medication variances, and minor occurrences/incidents will be reported on different forms (one for each of these different events), in addition to documentation in the Medical Record.

IV. Procedures

A. The nursing supervisor and charge nurse are responsible for completing the reporting forms.

   (The nursing supervisor is responsible for determining, in questionable situations, whether a minor occurrence vs. an incident should be reported.)
B. All minor skin injuries, medication variances, minor occurrences and incidents will be documented in the Medical Record in addition to the reporting form.
C. Minor Skin Injury forms will be sent directly to the nursing office.
D. Medication Variance forms will be reviewed by the nursing supervisor immediately. The nursing supervisors then make a determination as to whether the physician needs to be notified immediately. They will then be forwarded to the office of the DON (Director of Nursing) and COO (Chief Operating Officer). In addition, a copy will be placed in the employee file.
E. For minor occurrences, forms will be kept in a folder at each nurse's station for 72 h. If injury becomes apparent during this time, then the Incident section on the back of the form will be completed and the form immediately sent to the DON for review. The nursing supervisor will be responsible for daily review of the folder to ensure that: (1) Appropriate follow up of residents suffering a minor occurrence takes place; (2) any correctible cause of the occurrence is identified and immediately addressed, if possible; (3) other concurrent minor occurrence reports on the same resident are not present; and (4) forms are forwarded to the DON after the 72 h has expired. Examples of correctible causes include faulty mechanical devices, environmental obstacles, and incorrect methods of transferring, If an incident occurs, or two or more minor occurrences develop in the same resident within 72 h, the attending

physician (or nurse practitioner/physician assistant) will be immediately notified.

F. For incidents, the completed form will be forwarded immediately to the DON, and the attending physician (or nurse practitioner/physician assistant) is immediately notified. The medical director will be notified on a regular basis of all incidents.

G. After completion, data from the forms will be entered daily onto a computer database. Incidents will be red-flagged and printed out immediately. On a weekly basis all minor occurrences and incidents will be printed out by both attending physician name and unit location, and distributed accordingly. Monthly and quarterly summary reports will be generated by computer and reviewed by the DONs, COO, the Medical Director, and the Quality Assurance Committee.

JEWISH HOME FOR THE AGING

Minor Occurrence/Incident Report (Nursing Care)

Resident ______________________ Date ___/___/___

Unit __________ Room __________ Time __:__ A.M. P.M.

PMD Name ______________________

1. **Type of Occurrence** (choose one)
   - ____ Fall while walking
   - ____ Fall while transferring
   - ____ Slipped from chair
   - ____ Fell from bed
   - ____ Found on floor
   - ____ Found Injured (not on floor)
   - ____ Other (______________)

2. **Location** (choose one)
   - ____ Bedroom
   - ____ Bathroom
   - ____ Hall
   - ____ Dining room
   - ____ Outside
   - ____ Other (______________)

3 **Cause of Occurrence** (mark all that apply)
   - ____ None
   - ____ Dizzy
   - ____ Lost Balance
   - ____ Tripped
   - ____ Slipped
   - ____ Other (______________)

4. **Protective Device in Use** (mark all that apply)
   - ____ None
   - ____ Postural Support
   - ____ Seat Belt
   - ____ Bed Rails (up)
   - ____ Other (______________)

5. **Significant change in mental status?** No/Yes*
6. **Did the resident lose consciousness?** No/Yes*
7. **Abnormal range of motion?** No/Yes*
8. **Any evidence of significant injury?** No/Yes*

   ** If yes to any of the above, complete opposite side of form*

9. **Vital Signs**

	BP	**P**
Supine	___/___	___
Stand (1 min)	___/___	___
Stand (3 min)	___/___	___
Stand (5 min)	___/___	___

Temp ____ Resp ____

10. **Family notification**

    Person Notified ______________________ Time __:__ A.M. P.M.

    ____ By Telephone (person) ____ By Telephone (machine) ____ In person

11. **Details of Occurrence**

____

Person Completing Form

THIS PAGE ONLY NEEDS TO BE COMPLETED IF THERE IS ABNORMAL RANGE OF MOTION OR EVIDENCE OF INJURY EITHER AT THE TIME OF THE OCCURRENCE <u>OR</u> WITHIN 72 HOURS OF THE OCCURRENCE.

12. **Description of Injury**

____ Significant hematoma/bruise (>4 cm)
____ Significant laceration (>3 cm)
____ Possible fracture
____ Head trauma/injury
____ Abnormal range of motion
____ Significant new pain

Comments:

13. **Physician Notification**

Physician ______________
Date ____/____/____
Time ___:___ A.M. P.M.*
____ In Person
____ Macine/voice mail
____ Office
____ Answering service
* *If physician does not respond within 20 minutes, notify the Medical Director*

14. **Orders**

____ X-ray
____ ER Evaluation
____ Hospitalize
____ Clinic Follow-up
____ Labs
____ Monitor (vital signs, neuro checks)
____ Other (specify):

15. **Outcomes**

X-ray
____ No fracture
____ Fracture

ER evaluation
____ Not hospitalized
____ Hospitalized

This side completed by ____________________________

Reviewed By: D.O.N./A.D.O.N. ____________________________

Administration ____________________________

JEWISH HOME FOR THE AGING
Minor Occurrence/Incident Report (Residential Care)

Resident ______________________________ Date ____/____/____
Unit __________ Room __________ Time ___:___ A.M. P.M.
PMD Name ______________________________

1. **Type of Occurrence** (choose one)
   ____ Fall while walking
   ____ Fall while transferring
   ____ Slipped from chair
   ____ Fell from bed
   ____ Found on floor
   ____ Found Injured (not on floor)
   ____ Other (______________)

2. **Location** (choose one)
   ____ Bedroom
   ____ Bathroom
   ____ Hall
   ____ Dining room
   ____ Outside
   ____ Other (______________)

3 **Cause of Occurrence**
   (mark all that apply)
   ____ None
   ____ Dizzy
   ____ Lost Balance
   ____ Tripped
   ____ Slipped
   ____ Other (______________)

4. **Protective Device in Use**
   (mark all that apply)
   ____ None
   ____ Postural Support
   ____ Seat Belt
   ____ Bed Rails (up)
   ____ Other (______________)

5. **Significant change in mental status?** No/Yes*
6. **Did the resident lose consciousness?** No/Yes*
7. **Abnormal range of motion?** No/Yes*
8. **Any evidence of significant injury?** No/Yes*

   ** If yes to any of the above, complete opposite side of form*

9. **Vital Signs**

	BP	**P**
Supine	____/____	____
Stand (1 min)	____/____	____
Stand (3 min)	____/____	____
Stand (5 min)	____/____	____

Temp ____ Resp ____

10. **Family notification**
    Does resident want facility to notify family?
    ____ No ____ Yes If yes, person notified ____________________

11. **Details of Occurrence**

____
Person Completing Form

THIS PAGE ONLY NEEDS TO BE COMPLETED IF THERE IS ABNORMAL RANGE OF MOTION OR EVIDENCE OF INJURY EITHER AT THE TIME OF THE OCCURRENCE OR WITHIN 72 HOURS OF THE OCCURRENCE.

12. **Description of Injury**

____ Significant hematoma/bruise (>4 cm)
____ Significant laceration (>3 cm)
____ Possible fracture
____ Head trauma/injury
____ Abnormal range of motion
____ Significant new pain

Comments:

13. **Physician Notification**

Physician ______________
Date ____/____/____
Time ___:___ A.M. P.M.*
____ In Person
____ Machine/voice mail
____ Office
____ Answering service
* *If physician does not respond within 20 minutes, notify the Medical Director*

14. **Orders**

____ X-ray
____ ER Evaluation
____ Hospitalize
____ Clinic Follow-up
____ Labs
____ Monitor (vital signs, neuro checks)
____ Other (specify):

15. **Outcomes**

X-ray
____ No fracture
____ Fracture

ER evaluation
____ Not hospitalized
____ Hospitalized

This side completed by ______________________________

Reviewed By: D.O.N./A.D.O.N. ______________________________

Administration ______________________________

JEWISH HOME FOR THE AGING
Minor Skin Wound Report

Resident ____________________________ Unit ________ Room ________

Date ____/____/____ Time ___:___ A.M. P.M.

1. **Type of skin wound**

____ Skin Tear
____ Abrasion
____ Laceration
____ Bruise

2. **Size:**

3. **Location:**

4. **Treatment Initiated:**

5. **Family Notification:**

____
Person Notified

____ By Telephone (reached person)
____ By Telephone (by message machine)
____ In Person

____
Person Completing Form

JEWISH HOME FOR THE AGING
Medication Variance Report

Resident ______________________________ Unit ________ Room ________

Date ____/____/____ Time ___:___ A.M. P.M.

1. **Medication(s) involved in variance:**

____

____

2. **Type of error:**

____ Wrong dose given
____ Wrong medication given
____ Other (Describe):

3. **Adverse effects:**

____ None
____ Adverse reaction (Describe):

4. **Physician notification:**

____ No ____ Yes* *If yes:

Physician ____

Date ____/____/____ Time ___:___ A.M. P.M.

____ In person ____ Machine/voice mail ____ Office ____ Answering service

____
Person Completing Form

Reviewed By: D.O.N./A.D.O.N. ________________________________

Administration ________________________________

1.8 Jewish Home for the Aging—Laboratory Monitoring Policy (July 11, 1996)

Policy

A. **Diuretics**

All residents on the following diuretics will have electrolytes, BUN, and creatinine measured at least three months. More frequent monitoring may be ordered by the prescribing physician as appropriate given the resident's clinical conditions. The specified diuretics are:

- furosemide (Lasix)
- metolazone (Zaroxolyn)
- bumetanide (Bumex)
- ethacrynic acid (Edecrin)
- torsemide (Demadex)
- amiloride (Midamor)
- spironolactone (Aldactone)
- triamterene (Dyrenium)
- chlorothiazide (Diuril)
- chlorthalidone (Hygroton)
- hydrochlorothiazide (HCTZ)
- indapamide (Lozol)

B. **Therapeutic drug monitoring**

All residents on the following medications will have drug levels measured at least every six months. The specified drugs are:

- phenytoin (Dilantin)
- carbamazepine (Tegretol)
- valproic acid (Depakene; Depakote)
- digoxin (Lanoxin)
- theophylline (Theodur)
- quinidine (Quinaglute)
- procainamide (do both procainamide and *N*-acetal procainamide (NAPA) levels) (Procan SR)

C. **Anticoagulation**

All persons on warfarin (Coumadin) will have a prothrombia time done at least monthly. More frequent monitoring is appropriate when therapy is initiated, dosage is changed, or drugs that can alter Coumadin's effects are stated or stopped.

Procedure

1. Unless otherwise specified in the physicians' orders, pharmacy will be responsible for adding monitoring orders consistent with the policy when the specified drugs are ordered.

2. Pharmacy will be responsible for monitoring adherence to the laboratory monitoring policy during the quarterly drug regimen review.

1.9 Policy and Procedures for Sending Resident Information to Consultants and Hospitals

I. Objectives

To transfer pertinent information to health care providers caring for a resident of the Jewish Homes for the Aging when the resident must be evaluated outside the facility.

This is necessary to improve understanding by consultants and emergency room personnel of the resident's overall health and medication history and to enhance the conveyance of their findings and new orders.

The overall goal is to help residents obtain maximum benefit from visits to caregivers when outside of the Jewish Homes for the Aging.

II. Transfer Forms

Two different checklist forms are to be used to assemble:

1. INFORMATION PACKET FOR CONSULTANTS
2. TRANSFER PACKET FOR HOSPITALS and EMERGENCY ROOMS

Each contains a list of necessary documents to be sent with the resident (Figs. A-1 and A-2).

III. Procedures

The nursing supervisor and charge nurse are responsible for completing the transfer forms.

A. The LVN charge nurse will oversee

   1. The timely photocopying of pertinent parts of the medical record
   2. Initial his/her name after each part is included

B. The RN nursing supervisor will

   1. Confirm that all necessary papers are in the information packet
   2. Sign his/her name certifying that the packet has been reviewed

C. Whenever possible, clerical personnel in the medical clinic will assist in the photocopying, collating, and completion of the above records.

D. The only occasion when the above information package would be waived is when

   1. The resident has a life-threatening condition
   2. Completion of the forms would delay immediate transfer by emergency medical services

Acute Hospitalization
Transfer Check List

		Initial
1.	Copy of Medical Face Sheet and Treatment Status Sheet (and Forms re: No CPR or No Artificial Feeding and Hydration, if applicable)	______
2.	Copy of last 2 progress note pages	______
3.	Copy of Medicare, Social Security, Medi-Cal cards	______
4.	Copy of latest computer-generated MD orders, plus any additional orders since printout	______
5.	Copy of latest complete H & P	______
6.	Copy of original admission H & P (if available)	______
7.	Copy of recent lab test results (CBC or hemoglobin, BUN, Creatinine, other lab done recently)	______
8.	Copy of last chest x-ray report	______
9.	Copy of last EKG	______
10.	Copy of DPA pages	______
11.	Check list of personal belongings (including dentures, hearing aid)	______
12.	Notify social worker and administration if resident is admitted	______
	(If DPA or conservatorship **not** available, let Social Worker know)	

The above papers were sent with ______________________________
Name of Resident

To:______________________________ On:_____/_____/_____
Name of Hospital Date

By:______________________________
Name of Person Preparing Packet

Figure A-1 Example of a checklist that is transferred to the acute care hospital with the resident.

Consultant Information
for Initial Consult

		Initial
1.	Copy of Consultation Request Form and a Progress Note page	______
2.	Blank Physician Order page	______
3.	Copy of Medical Face Sheet	______
4.	Copy of last 2 progress note pages	______
5.	Copy of Medicare, Social Security, Medi-Cal cards	______
6.	Copy of latest computer-generated MD orders, plus any additional orders since printout	______
7.	Copy of recent lab test results (CBC or hemoglobin, BUN, Creatinine, other lab tests done recently)	______
8.	Copy of last chest x-ray report	______
9.	Copy of last EKG	______
10.	Copy of latest complete H & P	______
11.	Copy of original admission H & P (if available)	______

The above papers were sent with ____
Name of Resident

To:____ On:_____/_____/_____
Name of Consultant Date

By:______________________________
Name of Person Preparing Packet

Figure A-2 Example of a checklist that is sent to consultants with the resident.

In such a situation, the information packet should still be assembled and its contents faxed or delivered to the receiving facility as soon as possible.

E. The original copy of the completed and signed transfer form should be sent with the documents and the resident to the receiving consultant or hospital. A photocopy of the transfer form is to be retained in the medical record.

2 EXAMPLES OF FORMS

2.1 Medical Face Sheet and Treatment Status Sheet

JHA JEWISH HOME FOR THE AGING

MEDICAL FACE SHEET

ACTIVE PROBLEMS

1. ______
2. ______
3. ______
4. ______
5. ______
6. ______
7. ______

PAST HISTORY

A. Acute hospitalizations since admission to JHA

	Diagnoses	Month/Year
1.	______	__/__
2.	______	__/__
3.	______	__/__

B. Major surgical procedures

	Procedure	Year
1.	______	____
2.	______	____
3.	______	____

C. Allergies

1. ______
2. ______

D. Antibiotic Prophylaxis required:
☐Yes ☐No

TREATMENT STATUS
(Document on Treatment Status Sheet)

A. Decision making capacity

☐ Capable of making own decisions
☐ Capable of participating in decisions, but proxy should be involved
☐ Not capable of participating in decisions, proxy should make decisions

B. Status
☐ Full code ☐ No CPR ☐No tube feeding
☐Do not hospitalize unless necessary for comfort

This form completed by: ______
Date: ___/___/___

______
Resident's Name

Bldg./Station	Room Number	JHA Record No.

NEUROPSYCHIATRIC STATUS

A. Cognitive impairment
☐ None
☐ Yes, but not criteria for dementia
☐ Dementia (by DSM criteria) present:
☐Alzheimer's ☐Mixed
☐Multi-infarct ☐Uncertain/other

B. Psychiatric/behavioral disorders
1. ______
2. ______

C. Usual mental status
☐ Alert, oriented, follows simple instructions
☐ Alert, disoriented, but *can* follow simple directions
☐ Alert, disoriented, *cannot* follow simple directions
☐ Not alert (lethargic, comatose)

D. Most recent mental status scores
1. MDS-COGS ___/10
2. MMS ___/30 (date ___/___/___)

FUNCTIONAL STATUS

A. Ambulation
☐ Unassisted ☐ With cane/walker
☐ Transfer: ☐ Ind ☐ Dep

B. Continence

	Cont	Inc
Urine	___	___
Stool	___	___

Indwelling bladder catheter: ☐ No ☐ Yes
If yes:
a. Date placed: ___/___/___
b. Placed in: ☐acute hospital ☐JHA ☐other
c. Reason: ☐urinary retention (PVR=); due to:
☐obstruction ☐poor bladder contraction
☐uncertain
☐skin condition ☐comfort/preference

C. Basic ADL

	Ind	Dep
Bathing	☐	☐
Dressing	☐	☐
Grooming	☐	☐
Feeding	☐	☐

Tube feeding: ☐No ☐Yes
If yes:
a. Date placed: ___/___/___
b. Reason: ☐swallowing dysfunction
☐severe dementia and poor nutrition
☐other: ______

D. Vision (w/glasses if used)
☐Adequate for regular print
☐Impaired - can read large print
☐Highly impaired - can get around
☐Severely impaired - has difficulty getting around

E. Hearing (w/aid if used)
☐Adequate ☐Minimal difficulty
☐Hears only when speaker adjusts
☐Highly impaired (no useful hearing)

JHA
JEWISH HOME FOR THE AGING

TREATMENT STATUS SHEET

Legibly document all conversations held about the resident's treatment status. Include the date, the participants, the resident's wishes if known, a concise summary of the discussion and the decisions made.

Resident's Name

Bldg./Station | Room Number | JHA Record No.

2.2 Monthly Progress Note

DATE	Note Progress of Case, Complications, Consultations, Change in Diagnoses, Condition on Discharge, Instructions to Patient			
	MONTHLY SKILLED NURSING VISIT			
	INTERIM HISTORY:			
	OTHER ACTIVE MEDICAL PROBLEMS:			
	MEDICATIONS:			
	NUTRITION:	Weight last month:	Weight this month:	
		Food intake: □ Adequate	□ Inadequate (Comment):	
	MOBILITY:	□ Ambulates unassisted	□ Cane	□ Walker
			□ Wheelchair	□ Bedbound
	PSYCHOSOCIAL: □ Stable	□ Unstable (Comment):		
	PHYSICAL EXAM:			
	Mental status/affect			
	V.S.: B/P:	Temp:	Pulse:	Resp:
	Skin:	CV:		
	Lungs:	Other:		
	Extremities:			
	LABS:			
	ASSESSMENT:			
	PLAN:			

Name_______________________________________ MRN #______________

Physician_____________________________________

PROGRESS RECORD

2.3 Fax Communication to Physician

FAX for nonimmediate communication

Nursing Section		
Patient Name	Station	Date/Time
Dr:		
Concern and Assessment		
Allergies	Pertinent Medications	
Signature:		
Physician Section		
Orders and relevant diagnoses		
Dr. Signature/Date:		

This form is faxed to the primary physician's office, who then completes the Physician Section and returns it to the Facility by FAX.

After: Keith Rapp, MD, CMD and Mary Pat Rapp, RN-C, MSN (with permission)

2.4 Summary of Interdisciplinary Team Meeting

Example of a Subacute Unit Weekly Interdisciplinary Team Conference Summary

Patient's Name: ____ Date: ______/______/______

Primary Physician: ____

Primary diagnosis(es) for subacute admission:
Other relevant diagnosis(es):
Major active medical/nursing problems ____Improving ____No change ____Regressing Comments:
Admitted to hospital from: ___Home ___Residential Care ___Nursing facility ___Other
Discharge plan: ___Home, no assistance ___Home/24h assistance ___Home/some assistance ___ Residential care ___ NH ___ Needs an order for Home Health ___Yes ___No
PT: ___Progressing ___No change ___Regressing ___N/A Safety Perception: ___ Good ___ Poor
OT: ___Progressing ___No change ___ Regressing ___N/A Equipment needed at discharge: ___Yes ___No
Speech: Dysphagia ___Yes ___No Communication: ___Improving ___No change ___Regressing
Nutrition: ___Weight loss ___Weight gain ___Stable
Pharmacy Issues:
Recommendations: Re-evaluate in ________days Purpose(s) for re-evaluation

2.5 Resident Transfer Form, Medical Transfer Summary, and Admission Orders

Resident Transfer Form—Nursing Home to Hospital

The form illustrated (Fig. A-3) contains information that should be transferred to the acute care hospital when a NH resident is hospitalized.

This form is modeled after Chutka DS, Freeman Pl, and Tangalos EG: Convenient form for transfer of patients from nursing home to hospital. *Mayo Clin Proc* 64:1324–1325, 1989.

(See also "Policy and Procedures for Sending Resident Information to Consultants and Hospitals," contained in this Appendix.)

Medical Transfer Summary—Acute Care Hospital to Nursing Home

The form illustrated (Fig. A-4) is used by primary care medical staff at the Jewish Homes for the Aging of Greater Los Angleles.

It is completed the day before or the morning of the resident's transfer back from the acute care hospital to the Jewish Home and is accompanied by a preprinted Physician's Readmission Order Form (Fig. A-5).

This summary form does *not* replace the hospital discharge summary, which is dictated, transcribed, and subsequently sent to the Jewish Home and placed in the resident's record.

This summary does meet all the documentation requirements for readmission. When the resident arrives back at the Jewish Home, a nurse practitioner reviews the form and orders, assesses the resident, and writes a medical readmission note.

Admission Orders

The illustrated format (Fig. A-5) is used by primary care physicians at the Jewish Homes for the Aging of Greater Los Angeles to write readmission orders for residents returning from the acute care hospital.

The physician order forms are preprinted and kept at the nursing stations in the acute care hospital. Each form has multiple copies so that no reproduction or transcribing of orders is necessary when the resident is readmitted.

Transfer Form - Nursing Home to Hospital

Name____
Last First

Code Status/Critical Care Plan____

Date of Birth_____/_____/_____ Age___ Physician________________________

Sex ___Male ___Female Nursing Home________________________

Religion______________________ Phone ( )________________

Relative/Guardian____________________ Family notified of transfer ___Yes ___No

Phone ( )________________

Social Security #__________ Medicare #__________ Medicaid #__________

Reason for Transfer____

____

____

____

Valuables accompanying patient________________________________

Medical Information

Diagnoses:

______________________ ______________________

______________________ ______________________

______________________ ______________________

______________________ ______________________

Medications - Dosages	Time Last Given	
______________________	__________	
______________________	__________	Diet______________
______________________	__________	Alergies______________
______________________	__________	
______________________	__________	

Usual Mental Status ___Alert ___Wanders ___Confused

___Oriented ___Combative ___Withdrawn

Vital signs HR_____ Resp_____ Temp_____ BP_____

Figure A-3 Example of a transfer form to go with residents when they are sent to the acute care hospital.

NURSING INFORMATION

ACTIVITIES OF DAILY LIVING

			COMMENTS
Ambulation	1. 2. 3. 4. 5.	Independence with two assistive device Walks with supervision Walks with continuous physical support Bed to chair (total help) Bedfast	
Transfer	1. 2. 3. 4. 5.	No assistance Equipment only Supervision only Requires transfer with two equipment Bedfast	
Bladder Control	1. 2. 3. 4. 5. 6.	Continent Rarely Occasional - once a week or less Frequent - up to once a day Total incontinence Catheter - indwelling	
Bowel Control	1. 2. 3. 4. 5.	Continent Rarely Frequent - once a week or more Total incontinence Ostomy	
Bathing	1. 2. 3. 4. 5.	No assistance Supervision only Assistance in shower/tub Is bathed in shower/tub Is bathed - bed bath procedure	
Dressing	1. 2. 3. 4.	Dresses self Minor assistance Partial help, completes 1/2 dressing Has to be dressed	
Feeding	1. 2. 3. 4.	No assistance Minor assistance - needs tray set up only Help in feeding/encouraging Is fed	

SENSORY/LANGUAGE IMPAIRMENTS

			AID/ PROSTHESIS
Sight	1. 2. 3. 4.	Good Vision adequate - unable to read fine print Vision limited - Gross object observation Blind	
Hearing	1. 2. 3. 4.	Good Hearing slightly impaired Limited hearing (e.g. must speak loudly) Virtually completely deaf	
Speech	1. 2. 3.	Speaks clearly with others of same language Some defect - usually gets message across Unable to speak clearly or not at all	

Figure A-3 *(Continued)*

MEDICAL TRANSFER SUMMARY

Encino Hospital to Jewish Homes for the Aging

Patient's name____

Primary physician____

Admission date_____/_____/_____ Discharge date_____/_____/_____

A. Discharge diagnoses:

1. ____

2. ____

3. ____

B. Surgical procedures and endoscopies during admission (include results and name of M.D. who performed the procedure):

1. ____Date_____/_____/_____

2. ____Date_____/_____/_____

3. ____Date_____/_____/_____

C. Laboratory values - please record the latest results:

HCT	______	BUN	______
NA	______	Creat	______
K	______	Glucose	______
Other:			

D. Results of other pertinent studies (radiology, CT, MRI, sonography, nuclear scans, etc.):

1. ____

2. ____

3. ____

- -**For JHA Use Only**

Resident	Bldg.	Room	JHA Record No.
______________________	__________	__________	______________

Figure A-4 Brief transfer summary completed at the time of discharge and sent to the nursing home. A complete dictated summary is sent subsequently.

Medical Transfer Summary
Page Two

E. Treatment decisions

Were No CPR and/or No Hospitalization orders discussed during admission?

______No ______Yes If yes,:

Orders decided: ______No CPR ______No Hospitalization

Reason for order(s):____

Discussed with:____

F. Comments on hospital course (complications, etc.):

____

____

G. Re-admission diagnoses for JHA: **(Please list all diagnoses for Medical Face Sheet)**

1. ____________________ 5. ____________________

2. ____________________ 6. ____________________

3. ____________________ 7. ____________________

4. ____________________ 8. ____________________

H. Is the patient aware of their diagnosis(es)? ______No ______Yes

If no, why not:

____

I. Is the patient a candidate for rehabilitation therapy? ______No ______Yes

1. State goals of rehabilitation:

____

2. Estimate rehabilitation potential:

______Good ______Fair ______Poor

Doctor's signature:______________________________Date______/______/______

- -**For JHA Use Only**

Resident	Bldg.	Room	JHA Record No.

Figure A-4 *(Continued)*

Re-Admission Orders to Jewish Homes for the Aging
PHYSICIAN'S ORDERS

Order Date	
	1. Readmit to __Board & Care __Nursing __Victory __Grancell
	2. Activity: __Up ad lib __Restricted; specify__________
	3. Diet:__________
	4. Vital signs: __ TPR q______ __Blood Pressure q______
	5. Weigh q______
	6. Other routine nursing orders: (Include catheter care, oxygen, turning, positioning, etc.)
	7. Standard orders: (Check the appropriate orders)
	____May participate in scheduled activities
	____May go out on day or overnight pass with family designee prn
	____Podiatry care prn for corns, calluses, fungus, nail debridement
	8. Therapies: (Check the appropriate orders)
	____Physical therapy for:__________
	____Occupational therapy for:__________
	____Respiratory therapy for:__________
	9. CPR Status: __Full Code __No CPR See note dated___/___/___
	10. Laboratory tests and frequency:
	11. Skin and wound care, if any:__________
	12. Medications (routine first, followed by prns; use additional page if necessary)

Date____/____/____ Time________

Physician's Name ______ Phone # ______ Alt Physician's Name ______ Phone # ______

Diagnosis ______ Allergies ______

Patient Name ______ Patient # ______ Station ______ Room Bed ______ Page ______

Figure A-5 Standard format for admission orders from the acute care hospital; these are completed by the primary care physician at the acute care hospital and transferred to the nursing home.

2.6 Infection Control Reporting Form (Revised December 21, 1994)

Name of Resident________________________ GV/EV Unit___________ Room___________
PMD________________ Date of Report________________ Reported by________________
I. Infection symptoms and signs (please complete or check off all that apply):
Temperature_________________PO/PR/Ax Chills?________________

1. Symptomatic urinary tract infection: (Complete if any present.) Foley Catheter ________
______ New burning pain on urinating, or urinary frequency or urgency
______ Flank or suprapubic pain/tenderness
______ New appearance of cloudy or foul smelling urine
______ Change in mental or functional status, or increased incontinence
2. Cellulitis/soft tissue/wound infection: (Complete if *pus*, *or* 3 or more other signs present.)
______ Pus present at site
______ Heat present at site Site_________________
______ Redness at site
______ Swelling at site
______ Pain/tenderness at site
______ Serious drainage from site
3. Upper respiratory tract infection: (Complete if 2 or more present.)
______ Nasal discharge or sneezing
______ Nasal congestion
______ Sore throat or hoarseness or difficulty swallowing
______ Dry cough
______ New swollen or tender/painful lymph nodes in neck
4. Lower respiratory tract infection: (Complete if 2 or more present.)
______ New or increased cough
______ New or increased sputum production
______ Pleuritic chest pain
______ New lung physical findings (rales, ronchi, wheezing, bronchial breathing)
______ New or worsened shortness of breath *or* increased respiratory rate (>25/min) *or* change in mental or functional status
5. Influenza-like illness: (Complete only if T > 100.4 *and* 2 or more present.)
______ Headache or eye pain
______ Myalgias (muscle aches)
______ Malaise or loss of appetite
______ Sore throat
______ Dry cough
6. Gastroenteritis: (Complete if any present.)
______ Three or more loose or watery stools (above what is normal for resident)/24 h period
______ Three or more episodes of vomiting/24 h period
7. Conjunctivitus: (Complete if any present, in one or both eyes.)
______ Pus or thick discharge from one or both eyes for >24 h
______ Conjunctival redness (with or without itching or pain) for >24 h
8. Dermatitis: (Complete if present.)
______ New itching/scratching *and* new rash Site_________________
9. Other site (Specify): ____

II. Lab data ordered: CBC____ RUA____ C & S (Specify site)______________ CXR____

III. Were antibiotics prescribed: ______ Yes ______ No Date ordered: ______________

Antibiotic #1 ____________________ Dose/Duration ____________________

Antibiotic #2 ____________________ Dose/Duration ____________________

2.7 Monthly Quality Assurance Data Collection Form

MONTHLY QUALITY ASSURANCE REPORT

	JAN	FEB	MAR	APR	MAY	JUNE	ETC.
Census							
Falls							
a. Found on floor after apparent fall							
b. Fall while ambulating							
c. Fall in or going to/from B.R.							
d. Fall during transfer							
e. Fall from or with chair or wheelchair							
f. Fall while getting in or out of bed							
g. Fall from bed							
TOTAL							
Injury from fall necessitating hospital visit							
Injury of other resident by resident							
Other injury							
Employee incident							
Physical restraints							
Residents with decubitus							
--Institution required							
--Admitted with							
TOTAL							
Residents started on antibiotics							
Total cultures							
Negative cultures							

MONTHLY QUALITY ASSURANCE REPORT (Page 2)

	JAN	FEB	MAR	APR	MAY	JUNE	ETC.
UTIs							
Number of catheters							
UTI in indwelling catheter							
Eye infections							
GI infections							
Incontinent urine							
Incontinent feces							
No toileting program							
5 lb weight loss in last 3 months							
10 lb weight loss in last 6 months							
Residents on special diets							
Residents with G-tubes							
Residents requiring assistance with feeding							
Hotline calls							
Admissions							
Discharge							
Deaths							
Residents on antipsychotic							
Residents taken off antipsychotic							
Residents put on antipsychotic							
Residents on antipsychotic dosage reduction							
Residents on anxiolytics							
Residents on antidepressants							

MONTHLY QUALITY ASSURANCE REPORT (Page 3)

	JAN	FEB	MAR	APR	MAY	JUNE	ETC.
Residents with <20 mm systolic drop in blood pressure							
Residents with <10 mm diastolic drop in blood pressure							
Residents with both							
No scheduled meds\resident							
PRN medications per resident							
RX orders per resident							
Average age							
Code 1							
Code 2							
Code 3							
No code status							
Consumer view							
Patient satisfaction index							
Contractures							
New contractures in facility							

3 OTHER MATERIALS

3.1 Nurse Practitioner Responsibilities, Clinical Privileges, and Standardized Procedures

Jewish Home for the Aging—Nurse Practitioner/Physician Assistant Responsibilities (September 1994)

All activities of the nurse practitioner/physician assistant will be assigned and supervised by the Medical Director or his or her designee. All such activities will also be approved by the Director of Nursing and the Chief Operating Officer. Notes and orders written by the nurse practitioner/physician assistant will be co-signed by a supervisory physician. Nurse practitioners will function within the scope of Nurse Practitioner Standardized Procedures as specified in the California Nursing Practice Act (see separate policy). Physician assistants function within specified protocols as specified in the California Code of Regulations Title 16 Article 4 (see separate policy).

Responsibilities of the nurse practitioner/physician assistant will include (but not necessarily limited to):

1. Complete history and physical examinations (post-admission, readmission, annual).
2. Monthly nursing facility evaluations.
3. Periodic screening/health maintenance/preventative medicine examinations.
4. Evaluation and treatment of acute problems and changes in status.
5. Evaluation and treatment of chronic medical conditions.
6. Evaluation of employee injuries.
7. Participation in the development and implementation of specialty clinics and services.
8. Participation in medical and nursing quality assurance activities, including medical care evaluation studies and appropriate committees.
9. Participation in all meetings of the medical staff, including interdisciplinary conferences and educational sessions.
10. Development of specific care protocols for use by nurse practitioners/physician assistants in the assessment and follow-up of Jewish Home for the Aging residents.
11. Provision on a periodic basis, educational sessions for various students, nursing staff, residents, family members, and others as requested.
12. Evaluation of own individual professional practice and identify needs for continuing education, independent study and/or networking with other professionals.
13. Facilitation of the development and implementation of clinical research projects.
14. Facilitation of and participation in teaching activities.
15. Maintaining current active licensure and providing copies to the Department of Medicine.

16. Maintaining theoretical and practical competencies for all clinical privileges granted.

Jewish Home for the Aging—Clinical Privileges for Nurse Practitioners/Physician Assistants (Revised September 1994)

Purpose

To establish a policy on clinical privileges for nurse practitioners and physician assistants.

Objectives

1. To define clinical privileges for nurse practitioners (NPs) and physician assistants (PAs) who are performing expanded role activities.
2. To delineate a systematic process for the requesting and recommendation of clinical privileges for individual NPs/PAs.

Definitions

1. Clinical privileges are defined as specific direct patient care processes, procedures, or activities that a NP or NA is qualified and authorized to perform, by reason of advanced preparation and training. Clinical privileges communicate clearly who is prepared and authorized to do what in direct patient care within the agency. They assure that specific health care services are provided by persons who have the prerequisite skills and knowledge to do so in a competent and professional manner.
2. Nurse practitioners are defined by the California Board of Registered Nursing as a Registered Nurse (RN) with additional preparation and skills in physical diagnosis, psychosocial assessment and management of health and illness in primary care. The NP functions within the scope of practice for all RNs as specified in the California Nursing Practice Act. Standardized procedures is the mechanism by which they are legally authorized to amplify their practice into areas overlapping the realm of medicine (Section 2725, Nursing Practice Act).
3. Physician assistants are trained to provide only medical care, under the supervision of a physician. The scope of their practice is governed under the California Code of Regulations Title 16, Article 4, Sections 1399.540, 1399.541, 1399.542, 1399.543, 1399.545, and 1399.546.

Policy

1. Clinical privileges may be granted to NPs and PAs who are qualified by education, training, and demonstrated competence to perform certain activities.
2. Clinical privileges reflect and are consistent with professionally recognized standards of practice, and are procedurally consistent with established criteria, and, for NPs, the ANA Standards of Gerontological Practice.
3. Clinical privileges are reviewed and granted by the Medical Director.

Procedure

1. The individual NP or PA completes an application for specific clinical privileges for which they are applying (see Attachment A).
2. The application will be reviewed by the Medical Director, who serves as the clinical privileging authority.
3. When the requirements for clinical skills and competencies are met they will be granted by the Medical Director. This will be kept on file in the Medical Department at all times. A copy of this will be sent to the Chief Operating Officer and the Director of Nursing.
4. Clinical privileges must be renewed at the time of the annual performance evaluation. If it has been less than 6 months since the initial granting of clinical privileges at the anniversary, they will not be reviewed again until the following anniversary. Thereafter, the clinical privileges and annual review will come due at the same time. Unless otherwise indicated, clinical privileges will be renewed at that time.

Duties

1. Individual NPs and PAs are responsible for initially applying for clinical privileges, and for maintaining both theoretical and practical competencies for all clinical privileges granted.
2. Both theoretical and practical performance aspects for the clinical privileges being applied for must be certified by the appropriate persons before consideration by the Medical Director for initial recommendation.
3. The Medical Director is responsible for assuring the competence of NPs and PAs performing clinical activities.

Jewish Home for the Aging—Application for Clinical Privileges (Revised September 1994)

I ________________________, am applying for the following privileges as a Nurse Practitioner/Physician Assistant (circle one):

1. Independent initiation of the orders listed below, which require a physician's co-signature:

    A. Verification and transcription of the following orders on Physician's Order Sheet:

        1. Admitting diagnosis
        2. Resident condition
        3. Activity level
        4. Diet order

    B. Renewing of prescribed medication
    C. Renewing of existing treatment intensity orders (e.g., no CPR, no enteral feeding, etc.)

2. Independent initiation of:

   A. Nursing care orders (i.e., weights, vital signs, fingersticks for blood glucose, catheter care, wound/skin care)
   B. Oral fluids
   C. Over the counter medications, non-narcotic antidiarrheals, antacids, antihistamines, decongestants, expectorants, non-narcotic analgesics, dermatologicals, vitamins
   D. Rehabilitation evaluations (OT/PT/ST)
   E. All diagnostic studies except: Radiocontrast studies, nuclear medicine studies, echocardiography, invasive studies, CT or MRI scans
   F. Oxygen therapy and respiratory therapy

3. Initiate treatment per standardized procedure and/or after MD consultation (see references)

   A. Consultants
   B. All other diagnostic studies and treatments

4. Administration of intravenous fluids and medications per institutional policy
5. Perform venipuncture for obtaining blood specimens
6. Perform ECGs
7. Interpretation of ECGs
8. Perform simple urodynamics, including post-void residual by ultrasound or catheterization, and simple cystometry
9. Remove sutures
10. Suturing of minor wounds
11. Debridement and packing of minor wounds and pressure sores
12. Irrigate ears and remove impacted cerumen
13. Pack anterior nares for epistaxis
14. Administration and interpretation of diagnostic skin testing according to established criteria
15. Insertion of intravenous lines and heparin locks
16. Drawing arterial blood gases
17. Performance of pulse oximetry

Jewish Home for the Aging—Nurse Practitioner Standardized Procedures (Revised September 1994)

I. Definitions

A. The nurse practitioner functions within the scope of practice for all registered nurses as specified in the California Nursing Practice Act. Standardized procedures are the mechanism by which they are legally authorized to amplify their practice into areas overlapping the realm of medicine (Section 2725, Nursing Practice Act).

B. There are two components of standardized procedures as described in the Nursing Practice Act: Policies and Protocols. Policies refer to the general intent to permit the nurse practitioner to perform specific clinical functions or services. Protocols refer to the rule and/or procedures to be authorized by policies.

II. Policy

A. Function

Overlapping medical functions performed by the nurse practitioner include:

1. Assessment and management of acute illnesses.
2. Assessment and management of chronic illnesses.
3. General evaluation of health status, disease prevention, health maintenance, and health promotion. This includes, but is not limited to, complete history and physical examinations and ordering of diagnostic procedures.

B. Requiremrents

The nurse practitioner has active licensure as a registered nurse and nurse practitioner in the State of California, is prepared at the Masters level in a program conforming to Board of Registered Nursing standards, or is certified by a national or state organization.

C. Setting

The nurse practitioner at the Los Angeles Jewish Home for the Aging works in a multi-level geriatric long-term care facility.

D. Physician consultation

During working hours, the nurse practitioner will have medical consultation available either in person or via telephone from the resident's attending physician, the Medical Director, the supervising physician, or other appropriate physician. Because the Jewish Home for the Aging is affiliated with the UCLA School of Medicine, geriatric fellows will often be the "appropriate designee" with whom the nurse practitioner confers.

E. Physician referral

Physician referral may include, but not be limited to, the following situations:

1. Acute decompensation of patient situation.
2. Problem not resolving as anticipated.
3. Emergent conditions requiring prompt medical intervention.
4. Unexplained historical, physical, or laboratory findings.
5. Indication of new medical illness requiring further medical attention.
6. Upon request of resident, family, or physician.

F. Evaluation

The Medical Director is responsible for assuring the competence of the nurse practitioner when hired and thereafter.

G. Record keeping

Documentation of care provided to residents will be made on Physician Progress Notes. New orders will be written on the Physician Order Sheet. The Medical Director, supervising physician, or other appropriate designee will co-sign all such documentation.

III. Process Protocols

Process-oriented protocols are utilized to outline the specific requirements for functions such as diagnosis and management. The parameter of action may be delineated without unnecessary restricting management options. Within these parameters, the nurse practitioner can evaluate and treat patients according to practice standards.

A. Management of acute illness:

1. Definition: the assessment, diagnosis, and treatment of acute illness.
2. Database:
    a. Subjective: Symptoms relevant to the presenting complaint and organ(s) systems involved.
    b. Objective: Physical examination appropriate to the presenting complaint. Laboratory/diagnostic tests appropriate to the database, as covered in the laboratory and test protocol (see item C below).
    c. Assessment: Interim/final diagnosis appropriate to the database.
    d. Plan:
        (1) With physician consultation initiate, alter, or discontinue medications as covered in the medication protocol (see item D below).
        (2) Consultation Referral: To the appropriate specialty consultant as needed.
        (3) Referral to other health care supportive services, i.e., PT, OT, ST relevant to the functional status and stability of the resident.
        (4) Prescription for diet, treatments, exercise and activity level as indicated by disease process and patient condition with physician consultation.
3. Physician referral: Physician referral may include, but not limited to the following situations:
    a. Acute decompensation of patient condition.
    b. Problem not resolving as anticipated.

c. Emergent conditions requiring prompt medical intervention.
d. Unexplained historical, physical, or laboratory findings.
e. Indication of new medical illness requiring further medical attention.
f. Upon request of resident, family, or physician.

B. Management of chronic illness

1. Definition: The assessment, diagnosis, and treatment of chronic illness.
2. Database:

   a. Subjective: Relevant historical information, symptoms relevant to the disease process, and organ system(s) involved.
   b. Objective: Physical examination appropriate to the disease process. Laboratory/diagnostic tests appropriate to the disease process as covered in the laboratory, and diagnostic testing protocol (see item C below). Present status of current symptoms.
   c. Assessment: Interim/final diagnosis appropriate to the database.
   d. Plan:

      (1) With physician consultation initiate, alter, or discontinue medications as covered in the medication protocol (see item D below).
      (2) Referral to other health care supportive services, e.g., PT, OT, ST.
      (3) Planning for level of care changes relevant to functional status and stability of the resident with physician collaboration.
      (4) Initiate or alter diet, treatments, exercise, and activity level as indicated by disease process and patient condition with physician consultation.

3. Physician referral: (see Section II, item E).

C. Ordering laboratory and diagnostic studies

1. Definition: the ordering and/or performing of laboratory studies, radiologic tests, and other relevant imaging studies that will aid in making or confirming possible diagnosis. Physician consultation and approval will be obtained for all invasive procedures.
2. Database:

   a. Subjective: Any physical complaints made by the resident that can be measured by laboratory/diagnostic testing.
   b. Objective: Physical signs/symptoms manifested by a patient that could be measured by laboratory/diagnostic testing.

c. Assessment: Successful diagnosis or the ruling out of potential disease process.
d. Plan: Order further laboratory/diagnostic tests with physician collaboration as necessary.

3. Physician referral (see Section II, item E).

D. Medications

1. With physician consultation initiate, alter, renew, or discontinue medication.
2. Database:

a. Subjective: any history or indication of allergic or adverse reactions.
b. Objective: Any indication of allergic or adverse reactions. Physical signs or symptoms manifested by a patient that could be treated by medication.
c. Assessment: Effectiveness of medication use or problems that result from its use.
d. Plan: With physician consultation initiate, alter, renew, or discontinue medication.

3. Physician referral (see Section II, item E).

IV. Approval and Periodic Review

1. These standardized procedures will be dated and signed by the nurse practitioner and by the Medical Director, Director of Nursing, and the Chief Operating Officer of the Jewish Home for the Aging (see Appendix A).
2. These standardized procedures will be reviewed by the nurse practitioner annually at the time of their annual performance evaluation.

Appendix A—Approval of Nurse Practitioner Standardized Procedures

The policies and protocols as contained in these standardized procedures have been accepted by the following persons:

Nurse Practitioner ______________________________ Date ____________

Medical Director ______________________________ Date ____________

Director of Nursing ______________________________ Date ____________

Chief Operating Officer ______________________________ Date ____________

3.2 Physician Assistant Agreements

Jewish Home for the Aging—Approved Supervising Physician's Responsibility for Supervision of Physician Assistant

SUPERVISORS:	*SUPERVISOR #1*	*SUPERVISOR #2*
NAME:	____________	____________
MEDICAL LICENSE #:	____________	____________
APPROVAL #:	____________	____________
EXPIRATION DATE:	____________	____________

The above named Supervisor(s) is(are) licensed to practice in California as a physician and surgeon. Hereinafter, the above named approved supervising physician(s) shall be referred to as the supervising physician(s).

SUPERVISION REQUIRED. The physician assistant (PA) named in the attached Delegation of Services Agreement will be supervised by the supervising physician in accordance with these guidelines, set forth as required by Section 1399.545 of the Physician Assistant Regulations, which have been read by the physician whose signature appears below.

The physician shall review, countersign, and date within seven (7) days the medical record of any patient cared for by the physician assistant for whom the physician's prescription was transmitted or carried out.

MEDICAL RECORD REVIEW. One or more of the following mechanisms, as indicated below, by a check mark (✓), shall be utilized by the supervising physician to **partially** fulfill his obligation to adequately supervise the actions of the physician assistant named:

____

(Give Name of Physician Assistant)

_____ Examination of the patient by a supervising physician the same day as care is given by the PA.

_____ The supervising physician shall review, audit, and countersign every medical record written by the PA within 30 days, except that every record of Medi-Cal patients shall be reviewed within 7 days of the encounter.

_____ The physician shall audit the medical records of at least 10 percent of patients managed by PA under any protocols which shall be adopted by the supervising physician and the physician assistant. The physician shall select for review those cases which by diagnosis, problem, treatment, or procedure represent, in his judgement, the most significant risk to the patient.

_____ Other mechanisms approved in advance by the Physician Assistant Examining Committee may be used. Written documentation of those mechanisms are located at ______________________________.

BACK UP PROCEDURES: In the event this approved supervising physician is not available when needed, the following physician(s) has(have) agreed to be a consultant(s) and/or to receive referrals:

______________________________ Phone: ______________.
______________________________ Phone: ______________.

The consultant and referral physicians are not authorized to act as a supervising physician for the PA unless they have received prior approval of the Medical Board of California to be a supervising physician.

PROTOCOLS. NOTE: This document does not meet the regulation requirement to serve as a protocol. Protocols, if adopted by the supervising physician, must fully comply with the requirements authorized in Section 1399.545(e)(3) of the Physician Assistant Regulations.

______________ ______________________________

DATE PHYSICIAN'S SIGNATURE

______________ ______________________________

DATE PHYSICIAN'S SIGNATURE

Jewish Home for the Aging—Delegation of Services Agreement between Supervising Physician and Physician Assistant (Title 16, CCR, Section 1399.540)

PHYSICIAN ASSISTANT ______________________________, P.A.

Physician assistant, graduated from the ______________________________

physician assistant training program, on _______/_______/_______.

He took (or is to take) the licensing examination for physician assistants recognized by the State of California (e.g., Physician Assistant National Certifying Examination or a specialty examination given by the State of California) on _____/_____/_____. He was first granted licensure by the Physician Assistant Examining Committee on _____/_____/_____, which expires on _____/_____/_____, unless renewed. (Or was granted interim approval by the Physician Assistant Examining Committee on _____/_____/_____, which expires on _____/_____/_____.

SUPERVISION REQUIRED. The physician assistant named above (hereinafter referred to as PA) will be supervised in accordance with the written supervisor guidelines required by Section 1399.545 of the Physician Assistant Regulations. The written supervisor guidelines are incorporated with the attached document entitled, "Approved Supervising Physician's Responsibility for Supervision of Physician Assistants."

AUTHORIZED SERVICES. The PA is authorized by the physician whose name and signature appear below to perform all the tasks set forth in subsections (a), (d), (e), (f), and (g) of Section 1399.541 of the Physician Assistant Regulations, when acting under the supervision of the herein named physician.

The PA is authorized to perform the following laboratory and screening procedures:

In Accordance with Section 1399.541 of the Physician Assistant Regulations, Subsection (b), (c): Kane RL, Ouslander JG, Abrass IB: *Essentials of Clinical Geriatrics*. McGraw-Hill, New York, NY 1994; Ouslander JG, Osterweil D, Morley J: *Medical Care in the Nursing Home*, 1st ed. McGraw-Hill, New York, NY, 1991, Hazzard WR, Bierman EL, Blass JP, Ettinger WH, Halter JB: *Principles of Geriatric Medicine and Gerontology*, 3d ed. McGraw-Hill, New York, NY, 1994.

The PA is authorized to assist in the performance of the following laboratory and screening procedures:

In Accordance with Section 1399.541 of the Physician Assistant Regulations.

The PA is authorized to perform the following therapeutic procedures:

In Accordance with Section 1399.541 of the Physician Assistant Regulations, Subsection (b), (c), (i): Kane RL, Ouslander JG, Abrass IB: *Essentials of Clinical Geriatrics*. McGraw-Hill, New York, NY 1994; Ouslander JG, Osterweil D, Morley J: *Medical Care in the Nursing Home*, 1st ed. McGraw-Hill, New York, NY, 1991; Hazzard WR, Bierman EL, Blass JP, Ettinger WH, Halter JB: *Principles of Geriatric Medicine and Gerontology*, 3d ed. McGraw-Hill, New York, NY, 1994.

The PA is authorized to assist in the performance of the following therapeutic procedures:

In Accordance with Section 1399.541 of the Physician Assistant Regulations.

CONSULTATION REQUIREMENTS. The PA is required to always and immediately seek consultation on the following types of patients and situations (e.g., patient's failure to respond to therapy; physician assistant's uncertainty of diagnosis; patient's desire to see physician; any conditions which the physician assistant feels exceeds his ability to manage, etc.):

The patients and situations that are not covered under the Physicians Assistant Regulations and Authorized Services under this protocol.

MEDICAL DEVICES AND PHYSICIAN'S PRESCRIPTIONS. The PA may transmit by telephone to a pharmacist, and orally or in writing on a patient's medical record to a nurse, the supervising physician's order for medication or medical device requiring a prescription in accordance with subsection (h) of Section 1399.541 of the Physician Assistant Regulations.

The PA may also enter an order on the medical record of a patient at Jewish Home for the Aging in accordance with the Physician Assistant Regulations and other applicable laws and regulations.

Any medication handed to a patient by the PA shall be authorized by the physician's prescription and be prepackaged and labeled in accordance with Sections 4047.5, 4048, and 4228 of the Business and Professions Code.

PRACTICE SITE. All approved tasks may be performed for care of patients in this office or clinic located at: Jewish Home for the Aging, 18855 Victory Boulevard, Reseda, California, 91335, and 7150 Tampa Avenue, Reseda, California, 19335.

EMERGENCY TRANSPORT AND BACKUP. In a medical emergency, telephone the 911 operator to summon an ambulance.

The Encino/Tarzana Regional Medical Center emergency room at (818) 995–5000 is to be notified that patient with emergency problem is being transported to them for immediate admission. Give name of admitting physician. Tell ambulance crew where to take patient and brief them on known and suspected health condition of patient.

Notify Physician on-call at Valley Geriatric Medical Group at (818) 343–9881 immediately (or within 5 minutes).

PHYSICIAN ASSISTANT DECLARATION

My signature below signifies that I fully understand the foregoing Delegation of Services Agreement, having received a copy of it for my possession and guidance, and agree to comply with its terms without reservations.

______/______/______ ______________________________
DATE PHYSICIAN SIGNATURE

____
PHYSICIAN'S PRINTED NAME

______/______/______ ______________________________
DATE PHYSICIAN SIGNATURE

____
PHYSICIAN'S PRINTED NAME

______/______/______ ______________________________
DATE PHYSICIAN SIGNATURE

____
PHYSICIAN'S PRINTED NAME

______/______/______ ______________________________
DATE PHYSICIAN ASSISTANT'S SIGNATURE

____
PHYSICIAN ASSISTANT'S PRINTED NAME

3.3 Format for Physician Evaluation at the Time of Nursing Home Admission

History

- Reason(s) for seeking admission
- Status of active medical problems
- Past medical history
  - Chronic medical conditions
  - Surgical procedures
  - Psychiatric history
- Preventive care
  - Vaccinations
  - Dental, optometric, podiatric care

- Medications
- Review of symptoms

Physical Examination
In addition to traditional system approach include:

- Orthostatic changes in blood pressure
- Nutritional status
- Screening for hearing problems
- Visual capabilities
- Mobility (i.e., direct observation of ability to ambulate or transfer)
- Cognitive function
- Affective status

Functional Status
Ability to perform:

- Instrumental activities of daily living
- Basic activities of daily living

Socioeconomic Status

- Nature of family relationships
- Relevant financial information (e.g., private pay, Medicaid, Medicare, other)

Advance Directives

- Designation of proxy decision maker
- Desired intensity of care

Recommendations

- Specific for medical, functional, psychosocial problems
- Level of care

3.4 Sample Format for Annual Physician Review of a Long-Staying Nursing Home Resident

1. Active problem list:
   a. Medical
   b. Functional
   c. Psychosocial
2. Medical history
   a. Description of acute medical conditions that have occurred in the past year
   b. Comment on results of laboratory tests done to monitor active medical problems

   c. Summarize symptoms relevant to active medical problems
   d. List current medications

3. Symptom review
   a. Review symptoms common in the nursing home population

4. Physical examination
   a. Note any new physical findings

5. Functional status*
   a. Briefly summarize current status, highlighting changes in:
      (1) Ability to perform basic activities of daily living
      (2) Mobility
      (3) Continence
      (4) Cognitive function
      (5) Affective status (including behavioral disturbances)
   b. Assess rehabilitation potential (if relevant)

6. Social status
   a. Review any family involvement, family concerns or problems

7. Health maintenance
   a. Review the results of screening evaluations including:
      (1) Audiologic
      (2) Ophthalmologic/optometric
      (3) Dental
      (4) Podiatric
      (5) Tuberculosis testing

8. Screening laboratory tests (not done for monitoring of active medical conditions)
   a. Brief summary of results

9. Advanced directive
   a. Existence of directive
   b. Identification of proxy
   c. Whether the resident is still capable of making or participating in decisions about their health care
   d. Intensity of care (e.g., no CPR, etc)

10. Plans
   a. Summarize overall goals for care
   b. List specific plans related to findings from the entire review

---

*Functional status is assessed in detail quarterly on the MDS

3.5 Examples of Centers for Disease Control (CDC) Definitions for Nosocomial Infections

The definitions included below are abstracted from Garner JS, Jarvis WR, Enori TG, et al: CDC definitions for nosocomial infections, 1988. *J Infect Control* 16:128–140, 1988.

Because of the nature of nursing home (NH) residents and the typical diagnostic evaluations that are done in NHs, these definitions may need to be modified for NH infection control programs.

Urinary tract infection

Urinary tract infection (UTI) includes symptomatic UTI, asymptomatic bacteriuria, and other infections of the urinary tract.

Symptomatic UTI must meet these criteria:

1. One of the following: fever (>38°C), urgency, frequency, dysuria, or suprapubic tenderness *and* a urine culture of $\geq 10^5$ colonies/ml urine with no more than two species of organisms.
2. Two of the following: fever (>38°C), urgency, frequency, dysuria, or suprapubic tenderness *and* any of the following:

   a. Dipstick test positive for leukocyte esterase and/or nitrite
   b. Pyuria [≥ 10 white blood cells (WBC)/ml^3 or ≥ 3 WBC/high-power field of unspun urine]
   c. Organisms seen on Gram stain of unspun urine
   d. Two urine cultures with repeated isolation of the same uropathogen with $\geq 10^2$ colonies/ml urine in nonvoided specimens
   e. Urine culture with $\leq 10^5$ colonies/ml urine of single uropathogen in patient being treated with appropriate antimicrobial therapy
   f. Physician's diagnosis
   g. Physician institutes appropriate antimicrobial therapy

Asymptomatic bacteriuria must meet either of the following criteria:

1. An indwelling catheter is present within 7 days before urine is cultured *and* patient has no fever (>38°C), urgency, frequency, dysuria, or suprapubic tenderness *and* has urine culture of $\leq 10^5$ organisms/ml urine with no more than two species of organisms
2. No indwelling urinary catheter is present within 7 days before the first two urine cultures with $> 10^5$ organisms/ml urine of the same organisms with no more than two species of organisms *and* patient has no fever (>38°C), urgency, frequency, dysuria, or suprapubic tenderness.

Eye, ear, nose, throat, and mouth infection

Eye infection includes conjunctivitis and other eye infections. Ear infections include otitis externa, otitis interna, and mastoiditis. Nose, throat, and mouth infections include oral cavity infections, upper respiratory infections, and sinusitis.

Conjunctivitis must meet either of the following criteria:

1. Pathogen isolated from culture of purulent exudate obtained from conjunctiva or contiguous tissues such as eyelid, cornea, meibomian glands, or lacrimal glands
2. Pain or redness of conjunctiva or around eye *and* any of the following:
   a. WCBs and organisms seen on Gram stain of exudate
   b. Purulent exudate
   c. Positive antigen test on exudate or conjunctival scraping
   d. Multinucleated giant cells seen on microscopic examination of conjunctival exudate or scrapings
   e. Positive viral culture on conjunctival exudate
   f. Diagnostic single antibody titer (IgM) or fourfold increase in paired serum samples (IgM) for pathogen

Otitis externa must meet either of the following criteria:

1. Pathogen isolated from culture of purulent drainage from ear canal
2. One of the following: fever (>38°C), pain, redness, or drainage from ear canal *and* organisms seen on Gram stain of purulent drainage

Sinusitis must meet either of the following criteria:

1. Organism isolated from culture of purulent material obtained from sinus cavity
2. One of the following: fever (>38°C), pain or tenderness over the involved sinus, headache, purulent exudate, or nasal obstruction *and* either of the following:
   a. Positive transillumination
   b. Radiographic evidence of infection

Upper respiratory tract infection (pharyngitis, laryngitis, epiglottis) must meet one of the following criteria:

1. Two of the following: fever (>38°C), erythema of pharynx, sore throat, cough, hoarseness, or purulent exudate in throat *and* any of the following:
   a. Organism isolated from culture of specific site
   b. Organism isolated from blood culture
   c. Positive antigen test on blood or respiratory secretions
   d. Diagnostic single antibody titer (IgM) or fourfold increase in paired serum samples (IgG) for pathogen
   e. Physician's diagnosis
2. Abscess seen on direct examination, during surgery, or by histopathologic examination

Pneumonia

Pneumonia is defined separately from other infections of the lower respiratory tract. The criteria for pneumonia involve various combinations of clinical, radiographic, and laboratory evidence of infection. In general, expectorated sputum cultures are not useful in diagnosing pneumonia but may help identify the etiologic agent and provide useful antimicrobial susceptibility data. Findings from serial chest X-ray studies may be more helpful than those from a single X-ray film.

Pneumonia must meet one of the following criteria:

1. Rales or dullness to percussion on physical examination of chest *and* any of the following:

    a. New onset of purulent sputum or change in character of sputum
    b. Organisms isolated from blood culture
    c. Isolation of pathogen from specimen obtained by transtracheal aspirate, bronchial brushing, or biopsy

2. Chest radiographic examination shows new or progressive infiltrate, consolidation, cavitation, or pleural effusion *and* any of the following:

    a. New onset of purulent sputum or change in character of sputum
    b. Organism isolated from blood culture
    c. Isolation of pathogen from specimen obtained by transtracheal aspirate, bronchial brushing, or biopsy
    d. Isolation of virus or detection of viral antigen in respiratory secretions
    e. Diagnostic single antibody titer (IgM) or fourfold increase in paired serum samples (IgG) for pathogen
    f. Histopathologic evidence of pneumonia

Lower respiratory tract infection (excluding pneumonia)

Lower respiratory tract infection (excluding pneumonia) includes infections such as bronchitis, tracheobronchitis, bronchiolitis, tracheitis, lung abscess, and empyema.

Bronchitis, tracheobronchitis, bronchiolitis, or tracheitis without evidence of pneumonia must meet either of the following criteria:

1. Patient has not clinical or radiographic evidence of pneumonia *and* has two of the following: fever ($>38°C$), cough, new or increased sputum production, rhonchi, wheezing, *and* either of the following:

    a. Organism isolated from culture obtained by deep tracheal aspirate or bronchoscopy
    b. Positive antigen test of respiratory secretions

Other infections of the lower respiratory tract must meet one of the following criteria:

1. Organisms seen on smear or isolated from culture of lung tissue or fluid, including pleural fluid
2. Lung abscess or empyema seen during surgery or by histopathologic examination
3. Abscess cavity seen on radiographic examination of lung

Skin and soft tissue infection

Skin infection must meet either of the following criteria:

1. Purulent drainage, pustules, vesicles, or boils
2. Two of the following at affected site: localized pain or tenderness, swelling, redness, or heat *and* any of the following:

   a. Organism isolated from culture of aspirate or drainage from affected site. If organism is normal skin flora, must be pure culture of single organism
   b. Organism isolated from blood culture
   c. Positive antigen test on infected tissue or blood
   d. Multinucleated giant cells seen on microscopic examination of affected tissue
   e. Diagnostic single antibody titer (IgM) or fourfold increase in paired serum samples (IgG) for pathogen

Decubitus ulcer infection, including both superficial and deep infection, must meet two of the following criteria: redness, tenderness, or swelling of wound edges *and* either of the following:

1. Organism isolated from culture of fluid obtained by needle aspiration or biopsy of tissue obtained from ulcer margin
2. Organism isolated from blood culture

Gastrointestinal system infection

Gastroenteritis must meet either of the following criteria:

1. Acute onset of diarrhea (liquid stools for more than 12 h) with or without vomiting or fever ($>38°C$) *and* no likely noninfectious cause (e.g., diagnostic tests, therapeutic regimen, acute exacerbation of a chronic condition, psychological stress)
2. Two of the following with no other recognized cause: nausea, vomiting, abdominal pain, or headache *and* any of the following:

   a. Enteric pathogen isolated from stool culture or rectal swab
   b. Enteric pathogen detected by routine or electron microscopy examination
   c. Enteric pathogen detected by antigen or antibody assay on feces or blood
   d. Evidence of enteric pathogen detected by cytopathic changes in tissue culture (toxin assay)
   e. Diagnostic single antibody titer (IgM) or fourfold increase in paired serum samples (IgG) for pathogen

3.6 Cardiopulmonary Resuscitation Vignette

The problem

Many health problems are so serious that they cause your heart to stop beating. This is called cardiac arrest. When that happens, you also stop breathing. The heart pumps blood to all organs in your body to give them oxygen.

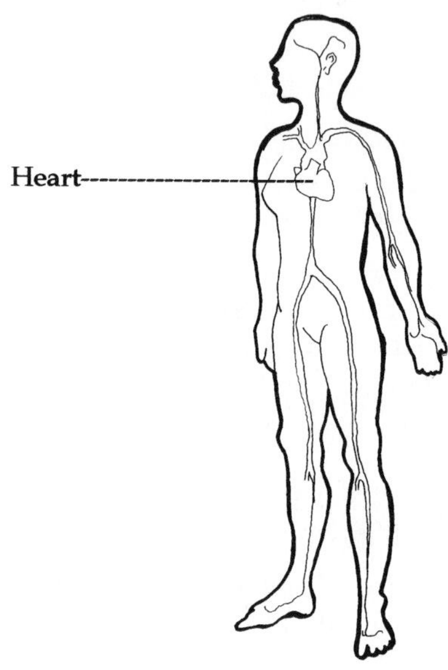

When your heart stops beating, your body and brain do not get enough oxygen for you to live.

Treatment option (choice)
There is only one treatment that is helpful when your heart stops beating. That treatment is cardiopulmonary resuscitation or **CPR**. CPR is done to try to restart the heartbeat and breathing. When your heart stops beating, CPR is the only treatment that will save your life.

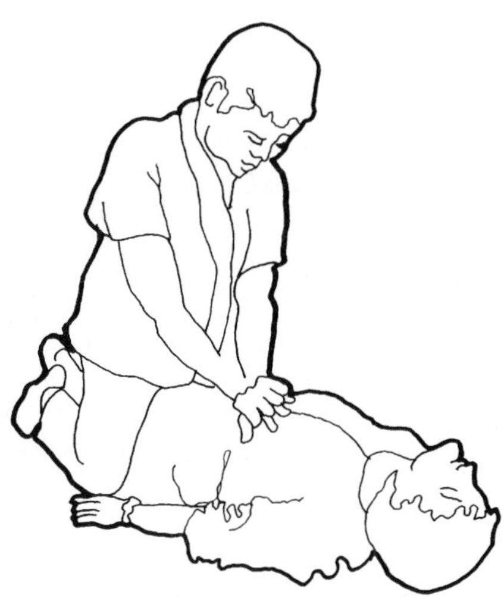

CPR includes rapidly pushing on the chest, medicines, electric shock, and placement of a tube through the mouth into the lungs to directly help you breathe.

CPR is a choice, and it is not done on everyone. Some people believe that when their time comes or their heart or breathing stops, nothing more should be done to keep them alive. Other people may want everything done to keep them alive. Neither of these choices is right or wrong. It is your decision.

What are my chances of surviving CPR?
Studies done in long-term care institutions show that about 1 in 20 (5 percent) persons given CPR survive. Of these survivors, some have permanent brain damage or other significant disabilities.

Some factors to consider
Although you are being asked to make a decision in your present circumstances, your health may change. Given what you know about CPR, would you choose to have CPR in your present state of health?

Here are some circumstances to think about as you make your decision about CPR:

1. If you enter a hospital with a severe illness or accident that requires intensive care and an uncertain life expectancy.

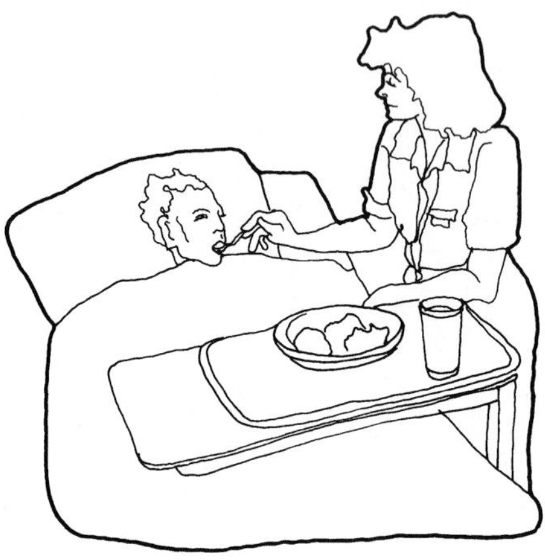

For example: if you are paralyzed from a stroke and unable to do anything for yourself, such as eating, dressing, or controlling your bladder and bowels, and then you have a cardiac arrest.

2. If you have a fatal disease and you are expected to live less than 6 months, no matter what type of treatment you receive.

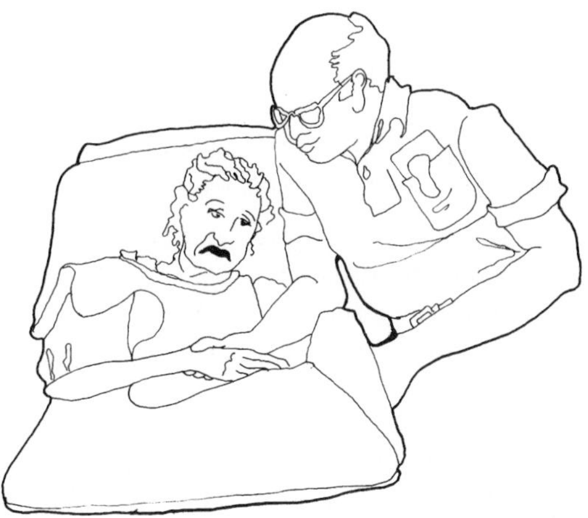

For example: you have advanced cancer and then have a cardiac arrest.

3. If your mind isn't what it used to be and you do not know your name or where you are and do not recognize anyone around you. Physically, however, you are in good condition.

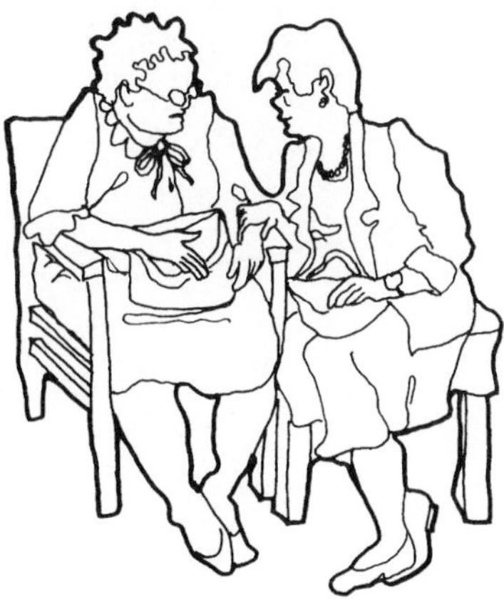

For example: you have severe dementia (such as Alzheimer's) and then you have a cardiac arrest.

These are just a few examples of circumstances in which CPR could be used. There are also many other situations that could result in illness or injury in which CPR would be an option to consider, but CPR alone does not cure your underlying illness.

What are the possible outcomes?

CPR may be successful by bringing you back from near death. It may bring you back to your original lifestyle. CPR efforts can also be the cause of complications and injuries. These complications may include:

1. Permanent brain damage may occur because of lack of oxygen to the brain.
2. Injuries such as broken ribs, collapsed lung, broken teeth, burned skin on the chest, and severe pain may result from CPR.
3. You may need a machine to breathe for the rest of your life.

Making the decision

The decision whether or not to have CPR may be a difficult one. You may want to discuss it with your doctor, social worker, nurse, rabbi, or family.

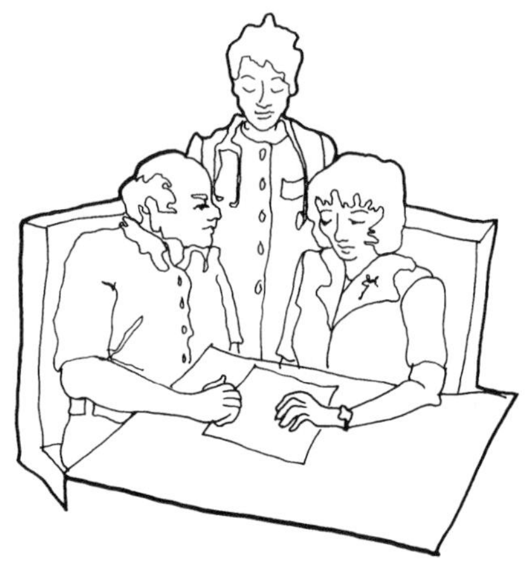

3.7 Feeding Tube Vignette

The problem

Many health problems may cause you to lose more and more of your mental and physical abilities. As a result, you may or may not be able to recognize people or be able to talk to them. The problems may become so serious that you can no longer eat all the food your body needs. If you do not get enough food, you will become very weak.

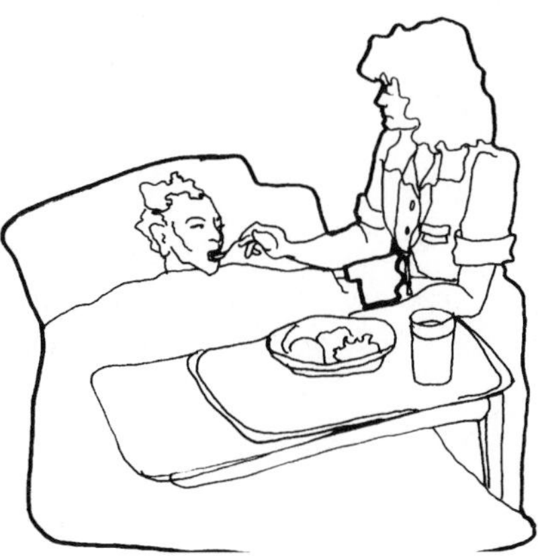

Nurses or others will feed you, but you may still continue to have trouble eating and may not be able to get all the food and fluids your body needs to maintain your health.

Treatment options (choices)

One treatment for eating problems is to have a feeding tube placed into your stomach. You would be fed liquids through the tube which provide all the nutrition you need.

Feeding tubes are not used for everyone. You have a choice about whether or not you want to have this treatment. Feeding tubes may be used for a short time or for the rest of your life.

Short term

This feeding tube can be used for a few days or weeks. The tube would be placed through your nose and down your throat into your stomach. You would receive liquid food several times per day. If you regain the ability to feed yourself, then the tube could be removed. This is used for acute medical illnesses when recovery is expected in a few days or weeks.

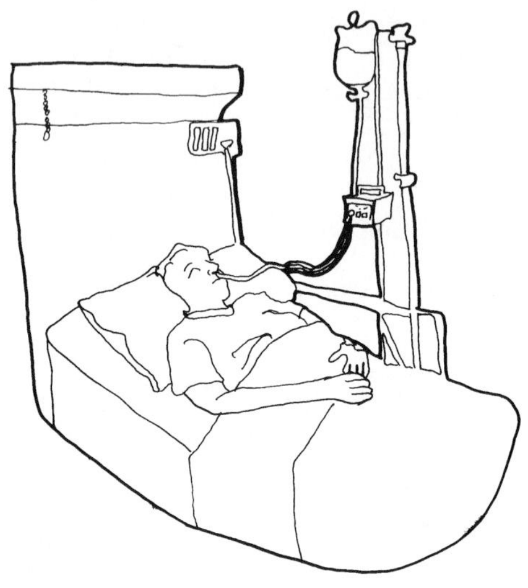

Long term

If a feeding tube is needed for longer than a few weeks, a tube could be placed into your stomach. This would require a small operation. If you regained the ability to eat on your own, this tube could be removed.

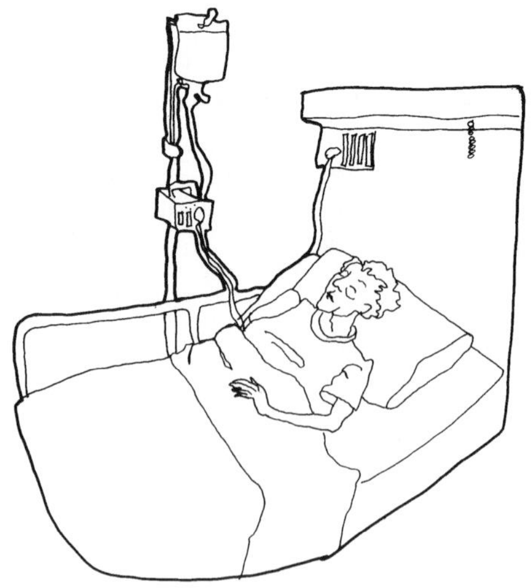

What is involved in the placing of the feeding tube?

In order to have the feeding tube inserted for longer than a few weeks, you would need a small operation. You would be given medication to make you comfortable. The doctor uses another tube through your mouth into the stomach to see inside. Then the doctor would make a small hole in your stomach so that the feeding tube can go through your skin into your stomach. You could be fed liquid food through the feeding tube that now goes directly into your stomach. This operation is usually safe and has been done often.

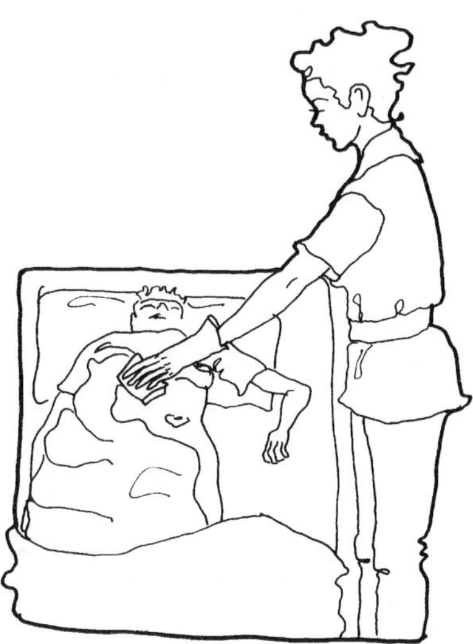

What are the possible results?

A feeding tube can supply you with the food and fluids your body needs. You may live longer than if you did not have the feeding tube. It will **not cure** the underlying disease that has made you unable to eat without the feeding tube. Without the tube you would probably die in a few weeks or months because your body would not be getting enough fluids or nourishment.

Possible complications

There are some complications that may occur whether or not you receive tube feedings.

1. You may develop sores on your skin.
2. You may get pneumonia.
3. You may get other infections that your body is too weak to fight.

Making the decision

The decision to have or refuse a feeding tube may be a difficult one. You may want to discuss it with your doctor, nurse, social worker, rabbi, or family. You may choose to have a tube feeding trial, which could then be stopped if the underlying illness shows no improvement after a specified period of time.

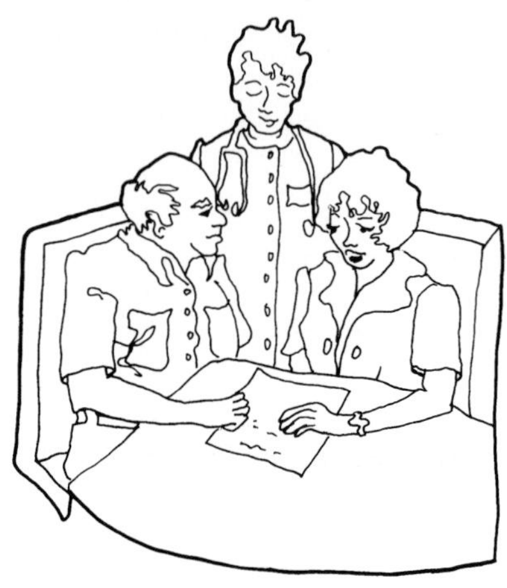

INDEX

Page references in *italic* indicate tables and illustrations

ISBN 0-07-048209-8